OSCE

and Clinical Skills Handbook

KATRINA F. HURLEY, MD

Emergency Medicine Resident
Dalhousie University
Royal College of Physicians and Surgeons
of Canada
Halifax, Nova Scotia, Canada

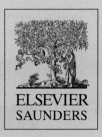

ELSEVIER
SAUNDERS

ELSEVIER
SAUNDERS

Notice

Medicine is an ever-changing field. Standard safety precautions must be followed, but as new research and clinical experience broaden our knowledge, changes in treatment and drug therapy may become necessary or appropriate. Every effort has been made to ensure that the drug dosage schedules are accurate and in accord with standards accepted at the time of printing. However, it is important to mention that the doses used in this publication do not necessarily conform to manufacturer's recommendations. Readers are advised to check the most current product information provided by the manufacturer of each drug to be administered to verify the recommended dose, the method and duration of administration, and contraindications. It is the responsibility of the licensed prescriber, relying on knowledge of the patient and experience, to determine the dosages and best treatment for each patient. Neither the publishers nor the editors assume any liability for any injury and/or damage to persons or property arising from this publication.

The Publisher

Library and Archives Canada Cataloguing in Publication

Hurley, Katrina F., 1976-
  OSCE and clinical skills handbook / Katrina F. Hurley.
Includes bibliographical references and index.
ISBN 0-7796-9902-5

  1. Internal medicine—Examinations, questions, etc.
2. Internal medicine—Outlines, syllabi, etc.   I. Title.
RC71.H87 2005   616'.0076   C2004-905182-2

Publisher: Ann Millar
Developmental Editor: Adrienne Shiffman
Projects Manager: Liz Radojkovic
Publishing Services Manager: Pat Joiner
Project Manager: David Stein
Cover, Interior Design: Julia Dummitt

Elsevier Canada
1 Goldthorne Ave., Toronto, ON, Canada M8Z 5S7
Phone: 1-866-896-3331
Fax: 1-888-359-9534

Printed in China.

1 2 3 4 5 09 08 07 06 05

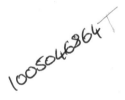

CONTRIBUTORS

Peter Green, MD, FRCPC
Program Director, Division of Dermatology
Associate Professor of Dermatology
Dalhousie University
Halifax, Nova Scotia, Canada
Chapter 7: Dermatology

Glen Jickling, MD
Neurology Resident
Dalhousie University
Halifax, Nova Scotia, Canada
Royal College of Physicians and Surgeons of Canada
Chapter 5: Nervous System

To my by'e and our sweet Noah.

"In spite of pain and injustice, life is good.
Under the badness, goodness lives;
and if good doesn't exist, we will make it exist; and we will save the world
although it might not want us to."

Rafael Barret
Great writer, journalist, and Spanish mathematician

PREFACE

STATEMENT OF PURPOSE

The *OSCE and Clinical Skills Handbook* was designed as a study aid for medical students preparing for Objective Structured Clinical Examinations (OSCEs). In my own experience as a student at Memorial University of Newfoundland, I found OSCE preparation difficult, because of the plethora of materials and the lack of a centralized study aid that suited the style of the examination. For this reason, I saw an opportunity to develop a book that not only summarized important history and physical examination skills in a centralized way, but also presented the information in a question-answer format. The format is designed to facilitate both individual and group study.

Your feedback and ideas are welcome; contact me at **kfhurley@dal.ca.**

DISCLAIMER

By no means is this book all-inclusive; while it contains a multitude of questions that may not be asked, it also fails to include every *possible* question. The *OSCE and Clinical Skills Handbook* has not been officially endorsed by medical schools, the Medical Council of Canada, or the United States Medical Licensing Examination (USMLE).

The scope of this book is primarily limited to basic clinical medicine and contains only a cursory review of anatomy that would be considered to be the minimum requirements needed to learn the core clinical competencies. Furthermore, physiology, therapy, and current management are beyond the scope of this book and students are encouraged to consult appropriate textbooks (such as those included in the **Resource List** and **References**) to review this information as the need arises.

Communication and interviewing skills are considered core clinical competencies in medicine and their importance cannot be overemphasized. The subtleties of interpersonal, cross-cultural, and interprofessional communication skills are not addressed in detail in this handbook. Students are assumed to have attained these core skills in their teaching curriculums early in their training. Consult appropriate references in the **Resource List** to review this information.

ACKNOWLEDGMENTS

Many thanks to the students who have contributed feedback and new ideas that have helped to improve this book during its development, namely those at Memorial University of Newfoundland who were the first to read the book, many editions ago. It was the positive response from these students that convinced me to carry on in this endeavor. Thanks to Dr. Jim Ducharme for support in reviving this project. Special thanks to the staff at Elsevier who made this publication possible, especially Ann Millar and Adrienne Shiffman. I am thankful for the substantial contributions of Drs. Peter Green and Glen Jickling who wrote the Dermatology and Nervous System chapters, respectively. Without these contributions, surely this project could not have been completed. I am also keenly grateful for the moral support and expert assistance provided by Dr. Graham Bullock in the redevelopment of MSK, which largely took place under some duress!

Thanks to Dr. Karen Mann who provided valuable mentorship and advice in the "final stretch" and through adversity. Thanks to Drs. Merril Pauls and John Campbell for their feedback and suggestions on Ethics, Dr. Jen McVey for her suggestions for Psychiatry, and Dr. Connie LeBlanc for her suggestions for MSK. Thanks to Dr. Susan

Campbell and Rose Chand who contributed their expertise on breast-feeding. Appreciation to medical students Monica Ott, Michelle Grinman, Jonathan Gaudet, and Genevieve MacDonell who provided some pointed feedback for this edition of the book and to the anonymous reviewers whose ideas also shaped the final product. Lastly, I am indebted to my family and friends who continue to support all my crazy ideas, especially my husband who has to live with me while I work on them!

RESOURCE LIST

ANATOMY AND PHYSIOLOGY

Blumenfeld H: *Neuroanatomy through clinical cases*, Sunderland, 2002, Sinauer Associates.

Guyton AC, Hall JE: *Textbook of medical physiology*, ed 10, Philadelphia, 2000, WB Saunders.

Moore KL, Dalley AF: *Clinically oriented anatomy*, ed 4, Philadelphia, 1999, Lippincott Williams & Wilkins.

Netter FH, Hansen JT: *Atlas of human anatomy*, ed 3, 2003, Novartis Medical Education.

COMMUNICATION

Buckman R: *How to break bad news: a guide for health care professionals*, Baltimore, 1992, Hopkins Fulfillment Service.

Feldman MD, Christensen JF, eds: *Behavioral medicine in primary care: a practical guide*, ed 2, New York, 2003, McGraw-Hill/Appleton & Lange.

Enelow AJ: *Interviewing and patient care*, ed 4, New York, 1996, Oxford University.

Gordon T, Edwards WS: *Making the patient your partner: communication skills for doctors and other caregivers*, Westport, 1995, Auburn House.

DEFINITIONS AND TERMINOLOGY

Dorland WAN: *Dorland's illustrated medical dictionary*, ed 30, Philadelphia, 2003, WB Saunders.

Stedman TL: *Stedman's medical dictionary*, ed 27, Philadelphia, 2000, Lippincott Williams & Wilkins.

OSCE

Dornan T, O'Neill P: *Core clinical skills: how to succeed in OSCEs in medicine*, Edinburgh, 2001, Churchill Livingstone.

Harden RM, Stevenson M, Downie WW, Wilson GM: Assessment of clinical competence using objective structured examination, *Br Med J* 1:447–451, 1975.

Hodges B, McNaughton N, Regehr G, Tiberius R, Hanson M: The challenge of creating new OSCE measures to capture the characteristics of expertise, *Med Ed* 36:742–748, 2002.

Jugovic PJ, Bitar R, McAdam LC: *Fundamental clinical situations: a practical OSCE study guide*, ed 4, Toronto, 2003, WB Saunders.

Mavis B. Self-efficacy and OSCE performance among second year medical students, *Adv Health Sci Educ Theory Pract* 6(2):93–102, 2001.

Rees J, Pattison JM, Williams G: *100 cases in clinical medicine*, London, 2000, Oxford University.

Singer P, Robb A: *Ethics OSCE Project*, Centre for Bioethics and Department of Medicine, University of Toronto; http://wings.buffalo.edu/faculty/research/bioethics

PHYSICAL EXAMINATION AND HISTORY TAKING

Bickley LS, Szilagyi PG: *Bates' guide to physical examination and history taking*, ed 8, Philadelphia, 2002, Lippincott Williams & Wilkins.

Fuller G: *Neurological examination made easy*, ed 2, New York, 1999, Churchill Livingstone.

Hoppenfeld S: *Physical examination of the spine and extremities*, East Norwalk, 1976, Prentice-Hall.

LeBlond RF, DeGowin RL, Brown DD: *DeGowin's diagnostic examination*, ed 8, New York, 2004, McGraw-Hill.

Munro JF, Campbell IW: *MacLeod's clinical examination*, ed 10, Edinburgh, 2000, Churchill Livingstone.

Seidel HM, Ball JW, Dains JE, Benedict GW, Kissane DW: *Mosby's guide to physical examination*, ed 5, St. Louis, 2002, Mosby.

Swartz M: *Textbook of physical diagnosis: history and examination*, ed 4, Philadelphia, 2001, WB Saunders.

INTRODUCTION

WHAT IS AN OSCE?

The Objective Structured Clinical Examination (OSCE) is a widely employed tool for measuring clinical competence. The OSCE was first described by Harden et al. at the University of Dundee in 1975. It was developed based on a need for improved evaluation of clinical performance in medical students. The first OSCE consisted of a number of timed stations through which students rotated and evaluators used itemized checklists with "controlled grading criteria." The authors found the results to be easily reproducible.

Since that time, OSCEs have been extensively studied in both undergraduate and postgraduate medical settings. The advantage of this tool has been its ability to test the many dimensions of clinical competence—physical examination, history taking, interpersonal skills, technical skills, problem solving, decision making, and patient treatment or management.

The OSCE has been adopted by most medical schools, residency programs, the Medical Council of Canada, and several Canadian specialty boards. The United States Medical Licensing Examination will be instituting an OSCE examination in addition to the traditional multiple choice examination.

The medical education literature is extensive on reliability or the reproducibility of a score amongst a set of observers. A wide range of reliabilities have been reported over the years for the OSCE, ranging from 0.19 to 0.91. The validity of the OSCE has been demonstrated using the construct of experience—more experienced residents perform at a higher level than junior residents who perform at a higher level than medical students.

OSCEs can be expected to vary from medical school to medical school across North America, in terms of specific scenarios, standardized patients, grading criteria, and time allowed for each scenario. Although I have attempted to eliminate my own biases, the evolution of this book reflects my own experiences with OSCEs at Memorial University of Newfoundland and Dalhousie University.

HOW IS AN OSCE GRADED?

Typically, a trainee's performance is evaluated using a standardized clinical scenario and structured binary checklist. The "observer" completing the checklist may be an examiner (who witnesses the examination), the standardized patient (on whom the student is performing the history or examination), or a combination of both.

Because of the difficulty in using a checklist to evaluate complex skills such as communication or professionalism, some OSCEs are evaluated using a Global Rating Scale. This type of scale takes into account not only whether particular questions were asked in the history, for example, but also the sequence in which they were asked and the organization of the interview.

For the specific objectives and format of the Medical Council of Canada Qualifying examination, checkout their webpage at *www.mcc.ca*. For specific information on the United States Medical Licensing Examination, see *www.usmle.org*.

HOW SHOULD I PREPARE FOR AN OSCE?

Prior academic performance is probably the best predictor of success in OSCEs. "Good performance" appears to be linked to learning styles as well. Well-organized study methods and learning styles characterized by desire to achieve and an orientation toward learning for meaning (rather than surface learning or rote learning) appear to be positively associated with better OSCE performance. Mavis (2001) found that OSCE performance was a "product of complex relationships between skills and knowledge, mediated by perceptions of anxiety, self-confidence and preparedness."

With these things in mind, remember that it may not be possible to prepare yourself for every question that *could* be asked on your OSCE. More important than "knowing" each question is to face each question with a method or strategy. When you come upon a question that you have not studied or begin to draw a blank, try to *relax*, take a deep breath, and:

- Read the "instructions to candidate" carefully.
- Suspend disbelief; treat the simulated patient the way you would treat a "real" patient.
- Ignore the presence of the examiner; don't be put off by what the examiner is doing with their checklist.
- Be sure to introduce yourself to the patient and find out the patient's name and/or confirm the patient's identity.
- Wash your hands.
- Develop a rapport with the patient.
- Be conscientious about patient comfort during physical examination.
- Ensure that you drape the patient properly.
- Explain aloud what you are doing in your examination of the patient. State what you are looking for and your findings (both for the patient and the examiner).

When in doubt of a history, rely on **CHLORIDE FPP** and be sure to ask about medications, past medical/surgical history, allergies, and family history. Use **VITAMINS C** to sort out the etiology of a symptom, and ask questions to narrow your differential diagnosis. When in doubt of a physical examination, use the **IPPA** format.

When in doubt . . . take a systematic approach:

Character	Vascular	Inspection
Location	Infectious	Palpation
Onset	Traumatic	Percussion
Radiation	Autoimmune/Allergic	Auscultation
Intensity	Metabolic	
Duration	Idiopathic/Iatrogenic	
Events associated	Neoplastic	
	Substance abuse and Psychiatric	
Frequency		
Palliative factors	Congenital	
Provocative factors		

HOW TO USE THIS BOOK

A list of abbreviations is provided at the end of the introduction. All abbreviations used in this book can be found in this alphabetized list.

This book is arranged in a question-answer format and contains questions suitable to a variety of learning levels, from the most basic physical examination skills, such as examining the liver, to questions that require a multisystem approach, such as assessing a patient with a complaint of "chest pain."

The material is divided into a systems-based approach. Chapters 1 to 6 and 8 to 13 reflect core competencies in clinical medicine. Chapter 7, *Dermatology*, provides a fundamental approach to the examination and description of some common skin problems. Dermatology is considered a subspecialty area and is thus not a core area of study in medical curricula. The problem-based scenarios in this chapter are examples of what you may commonly encounter in a primary care or emergency department setting and are not intended to be all inclusive; it is hoped that a background of some common problems will be helpful in guiding you to formulate a differential diagnosis and approach to other skin conditions not covered here.

Chapters 1 to 11 are divided into sections on *Objectives*, *Anatomy*, *Cardinal Signs and Symptoms*, *Essential Clinical Competencies*, *Sample OSCE Scenarios*, and *Sample Checklists*. In general, junior level students should focus on *Anatomy*, *Cardinal Signs and Symptoms*, and *Essential Clinical Competencies*. The *Sample OSCE Scenarios* are generally more advanced in structure and approach, appropriate for senior medical students. The *Sample Checklists* are worthy of review by learners at all levels.

Although the majority of the book is arranged in a systems-based fashion, Chapters 12 and 13 reflect specific populations, pediatrics and geriatrics, respectively. In general, the *Essential Clinical Competencies* presented in Chapters 1 to 11 can still be applied (at times, in a modified way).

Chapter 14, *Ethics*, differs from the other chapters with respect to format; an ethical scenario is presented, followed by a discussion of the principal learning points for the case and a performance summary of what "the student should" accomplish.

At the start of each chapter, a list of clinical objectives is provided outlining the essential history and physical examination skills that you should be able to accomplish prior to participating in an OSCE. Not all objectives are covered in this handbook. You are encouraged to use the list of objectives to identify your own weaknesses and use other references to supplement your learning as necessary.

Approach the material as a guide only. You need not perform the physical examination tasks or approach the history in the order presented in this handbook. However, you should take an organized approach, developing a consistent method that you can apply in each patient encounter.

Sample Checklists appear at the end of each chapter. These checklists are an example of the performance assessment sheets an OSCE examiner might use to grade your demonstrated skill-set at each timed station. These lists serve as a means of testing oneself or group members in preparation for the test. Consult Appendix B for a template to construct your own *sample checklists* using cases from this handbook.

PROFESSIONALISM

Medicine is often considered *the* paradigm of professionalism. A physician must fulfill the role of a healer and a professional simultaneously. The role of healer dates back to ancient times while the role as professional arose in the Middle Ages as a means of organizing health care delivery. The "profession" has the privilege of self-regulation and self-policing. Physicians were consequently granted prestige and status within the community under the assumption that altruism and moral behavior would be adopted by those undertaking medical practice. This still holds true today, leading to an obligation to maintain a code of professional conduct.

Cruess et al (2004) published a working definition of professionalism as follows: "Profession: An occupation whose core element is work based upon the mastery of a complex body of knowledge and skills. It is a vocation in which knowledge of some department of science or learning or the practice of an art founded upon it is used in the service of others. Its members are governed by codes of ethics and profess a commitment to competence, integrity and morality, altruism, and the promotion of the public good within their domain. These commitments form the basis of a social contract between a profession and society, which in return grants the profession a monopoly over the use of its knowledge base, the right to considerable autonomy in practice and the privilege of self-regulation. Professions and their members are accountable to those served and to society."

COMMUNICATION

Entire courses in medical curricula have been developed on the topic of communication. Below are a series of key pointers intended to refresh your memory.

- Setting up the interview: It is best to conduct patient interviews in a quiet, non-threatening setting. Avoid physical barriers such as sitting behind a desk. It is not always possible to arrange this type of setting (e.g., in the emergency department). In these situations, do your best to maintain patient privacy by drawing the curtains and speaking quietly (if the patient is not hard of hearing).
- Beginning the interview: Begin by establishing the identity of the patient. Make eye contact with the patient and introduce yourself. Determine how the patient would like to be addressed.
- Body language: Throughout the interview, it is important to avoid appearing rushed because this is likely to interfere with the patient's desire to disclose information. Maintain eye contact when possible. Remain nonjudgmental.
- Open-ended questions: It is optimal to start with an open-ended question such as, "What brought you in here today?" Do not interrupt the patient's account of his or her chief complaint. Physicians interrupt patients during their opening statement in 69% of encounters after a mean of only 18 to 23 seconds! It is helpful to prompt the patient for more information: "Tell me more about that."
- Directed questions may be used later to clarify specific points in the history.
- Be an active listener. Take the time to ensure that you have heard the patient's story correctly by summarizing from time to time: "So, what you are saying is . . . Is there anything else?"
- **FIFE:** Many find the FIFE mnemonic helpful. Use it to help you remember to elicit the patient's **F**eelings, **I**deas, **F**ears, and **E**xpectations about his or her complaint or illness. This can be very revealing.
- Closing remarks: Draw the encounter to a close by summarizing any findings. Outline the next steps in delineating and managing the patient's complaint and a broader action plan. Provide an opportunity for the patient to ask questions.

CROSS-CULTURAL COMMUNICATION

Lack of understanding of cultural issues can lead to impaired physician-patient communication and negative health outcomes. In our multicultural environment, it is important for physicians to take time to understand patients' religious and cultural beliefs and their impact on perceptions of health and illness. The **LEARN** tool provides a framework for physicians:

- **L**ook at the patient through the **LENS** of his or her cultural context.
- **A**cknowledge patient concerns.
- Make **R**ecommendations for next steps in investigation and management of a complaint.
- **N**egotiate with the patient in the context of cultural and religious beliefs to arrive at an acceptable action plan.

BREAKING BAD NEWS

The definition of "bad news" is in the eye of the beholder and varies somewhat from patient to patient. Death and dying are generally considered the main topics in this area, but patients getting a diagnosis of chronic pain or a psychiatric illness, for example, may experience a comparable degree of turmoil and difficulty. The encounter whereby such news is delivered may affect the patient's satisfaction with his or her care and any future coping mechanisms and level of hopefulness. Interestingly, whereas physician stress peaks during the clinical encounter, patient stress peaks afterward.

The main goals of this type of patient encounter are to gather information from the patient, deliver the "bad news," provide patient support, and collaborate with the patient in developing a plan. The **SPIKES** protocol, as outlined by Baile et al (2000), is presented as follows:

- **S**etting up the interview: Mentally rehearse the interview. Arrange for a private space for the encounter and involve significant others. Sit down because you do not wish to appear rushed. Maintain eye contact when possible.
- Assess the patient's **P**erceptions: Find out how the patient perceives his or her current situation: "What have you been told about your condition so far?"
- Obtain the patient's **I**nvitation: Find out at what level the patient wishes to have information disclosed (e.g., details versus the big picture). This is optimally done at the time particular tests are ordered.
- Pass along **K**nowledge to the patient: Precede the bad news with a "warning shot" so as not to take the patient off guard: "I have bad news to tell you." Avoid medical jargon and talk to the patient at a level he or she can understand. Check the patient's understanding of the information where possible.
- Address the patient's **E**motions: Offer support by identifying the patient's emotions and the reason for them. Be empathic.
- **S**trategy and **S**ummary: It is important to outline a plan of next steps for the patient, including another planned encounter. Having a plan provides some security for the patient and the patient's family. Written information and a planned second encounter to further discuss their concerns are vital, as patients are unlikely to retain most of the information disclosed after the "bad news."

Strategies for breaking bad news are elaborated on in Robert Buckman's book, *How to Break Bad News: A Guide for Health Care Professionals*, 1992, Hopkins Fulfillment Service.

MEDICAL HISTORY

"Hello my name is Joe/Jane Doe and I am a medical student." Wash your hands.

Identifying Data (ID): Name, age/date of birth, sex, race, place of birth, marital status, religion, etc. Ask yourself whether the historian is reliable. Inquire about the source of the referral (e.g., self, family doctor).

Chief Complaint (CC): One or more symptoms/concerns for which the patient is seeking care or advice. Use the patient's own words when possible.

History of Present Illness (HPI): Clarifies CC; chronological account of how each symptom developed and related events (**ChLORIDE FPP**). Ask when the patient last felt "well."

- **Ch**aracter: What is it like?
- **L**ocation: Where is it?
- **O**nset: When did it start?
- **R**adiation: Does it go anywhere else?
- **I**ntensity: How bad is it (scale of 1 to 10 with 1 being mild and 10 being the worst)?
- **D**uration: How long does it last? How has it changed/progressed since it started?
- **E**vents associated: What were you doing/where were you when the symptom began?
- **F**requency: Has this happened before? If so, how often does it happen?
- **P**alliative factors: What helps?
- **P**rovocative factors: What makes it worse?
- Remember to:
  1. Ascertain the patient's thoughts/feelings about his or her illness/symptom.
  2. Clarify the patient's concerns that led to seeking medical attention.
  3. Find out how the illness/symptom has affected the patient's life.
  4. Develop a rapport with the patient.

Past Medical History (PMH) and Past Surgical History (PSH): Chronologically explore past illnesses (including psychiatric illnesses and childhood illnesses), past hospitalizations, current medical illnesses, injuries, and medical/surgical interventions and anesthetics.

Medications (MEDS): Include all current medications (including prescription, over-the-counter, and alternative medicines), may include relevant past medications.

Allergies: Include drug allergies (prescription, over-the-counter, and alternative medicines) and environmental allergies, such as latex.

Social History (SH): Cigarette smoking, alcohol/street drugs, diet, sleep patterns, exercise/leisure activities, hazards/safety, employment, relationship with family/peers/partner, sexual history.

Immunizations: Especially important in children, persons with infectious diseases, and travelers.

Family history (FH): Age, health, and cause of death of each immediate family member (parents, siblings, and children).

Review of Systems (ROS): Ask about common symptoms in each major body system. Be sure to address the patient (as always) in language consistent with his or her level of understanding. ROS pertinent to the chief complaint should be included in the HPI.

- **General:** Current state of health (includes past medical problems relevant to the current state of health)
- **CVS:** Chest pain/pressure/tightness, palpitations, orthopnea, paroxysmal nocturnal dyspnea (PND), shortness of breath (SOB), pedal edema, claudication, varicose veins, history of rheumatic fever, heart murmur, hypertension (HTN), hyperlipidemia, mitral valve prolapse
- **Resp:** Cough, sputum, hemoptysis, dyspnea, pleuritic chest pain, wheezing, asthma, chronic obstructive pulmonary disease (COPD), recurrent respiratory infections, occupational exposures (e.g., asbestos, radiation), last chest x-ray (CXR), tuberculosis (TB), pulmonary embolism (PE), sleep patterns (snoring, sleep apnea)
- **GI:** Weight gain/loss, previous endoscopy and digital rectal examination (DRE), nausea/vomiting (N/V), diarrhea, constipation, hematemesis, hematochezia, melena, change in stool caliber, hemorrhoids, hepatitis, peptic ulcer disease (PUD), gastroesophageal reflux (GER) or "heartburn," dysphagia, difficulty chewing, belching/flatus, abdominal pain, appetite, diet
- **GU:** Dysuria, hematuria, nocturia, urinary frequency, polyuria, decreased force of urination, hesitancy, urgency, incontinence, nephrolithiasis, urinary tract infection (UTI), pyelonephritis
  1. **Female:** Menarche, menopause, menstrual cycle, premenstrual syndrome (PMS), date of last menstrual period (LMP), dysmenorrhea, postmenopausal bleeding, vaginal discharge, labial sores/lesions, sexually transmitted infections (STIs), sexual dysfunction, endometriosis, birth control method, breast lumps, nipple discharge, gravida/para/abortions, dyspareunia, date of last PAP, history of abnormal PAP, past mammography
  2. **Male:** Hernias, testicular masses/pain, penile discharge, penile sores/lesions, prostatitis, sexual dysfunction, STIs, prostate specific antigen (PSA) level, DRE
- **Neuro:** Headache, diplopia, blurred vision, eye pain/redness, cataracts, glaucoma, visual field losses, hearing loss, tinnitus, vertigo, dizziness, syncope, seizures, paresthesias, weakness/paralysis, tremor, pain, ataxia, falls, head injury
- **MSK:** Arthritis, joint stiffness/swelling, myalgias, gout, back pain
- **Skin:** Rashes, changing moles, birthmarks, dryness, pruritus, lumps, pigmentation change, hair loss, hirsutism, nail changes
- **Heme:** Blood type, anemia, easy bruising/bleeding, prior transfusions and reactions, lymph node enlargement, constitutional symptoms (pain, fatigue, fever, chills, night sweats), thromboembolic disease
- **Endo:** Polyuria, polydipsia, polyphagia, cold-heat intolerance, diabetes mellitus (DM), thyroid disease, goiter, tremors, osteoporosis, galactorrhea, hirsutism, purple striae, central obesity, amenorrhea
- **HEENT:** Sinusitis, postnasal drip, nasal polyps, epistaxis, teeth/gums, oral cavity ulcers/growths, sore throat, change in voice, hoarseness, glasses, contact lenses, dentures
- **Psych:** Depression, agitation, panic-anxiety, memory disturbance, confusion, personality disorders, hallucinations, delusions, mania, substance abuse

DOCUMENTATION

In general, documentation should be as complete as possible at all times. From the perspective of those reading and reviewing your documentation of the patient's history and physical examination, if it isn't documented, it didn't happen. Document not only positive findings but pertinent negative findings as well. It is important to be consistent in your approach to charting; you will be less likely to omit information if you approach it the same way every time. When time permits, document in the same format as the medical history outlined above, documenting the physical examination in a systems-based format.

Writing a **SOAP** note is a useful way to quickly summarize a patient encounter:

Subjective: Write the history in the patient's own words.

Objective: Write your physical examination findings and laboratory investigations.

Assessment: Write your provisional diagnosis and differential diagnosis.

Plan: Outline your plan to delineate or confirm the diagnosis and manage the patient's problems. It is useful to organize the plan using a *problem list*. Develop the problem list starting with the patient's chief complaint, positive symptoms identified in the ROS, and concurrent medical problems.

SUMMATIVE OBJECTIVES

The successful student should be able to:

- Perform a **complete history** and **physical examination** for a given patient.
  1. Elicit the presenting problems and relevant details.
  2. Elicit past medical/surgical history, family history, social history, medications, and allergies.
  3. Perform an appropriate review of systems to detect other health problems.
  4. Show sensitivity and respect during the physical examination, explaining the procedures to the patient in understandable language.
  5. Demonstrate proper use of medical instruments (e.g., stethoscope, otoscope, ophthalmoscope, sphygmomanometer).
  6. Perform the examination in logical sequence, focusing on particular systems when appropriate.
  7. Demonstrate proper use of draping to position the patient for optimal exposure, while maintaining patient dignity and privacy.
- Establish a comfortable rapport with the patient.
- Exhibit empathy, tact, and compassion, maintaining a professional and ethical code of conduct.
- Concisely communicate the history and physical examination.
- Present significant positive and negative findings in a systematic fashion.
- Formulate a problem list and differential diagnoses **(VITAMINS C).**

ABBREVIATIONS

a: artery

A$_2$: aortic component of 2nd heart sound

AAA: abdominal aortic aneurysm

AAL: anterior axillary line

ABG: arterial blood gas

AC: acromioclavicular

ACA: anterior cerebral artery

ACE: angiotensin-converting enzyme

ACS: acute coronary syndrome

ACTH: adrenocorticotropic hormone

AD: autosomal dominant

ADH: antidiuretic hormone

AFB: acid-fast bacilli

AGA: appropriate for gestational age

AIDS: acquired immunodeficiency syndrome

AMI: acute myocardial infarction

AN: anorexia nervosa

AP: anterior-posterior

APGAR: appearance, pulse, grimace, activity, respiratory

AR: aortic regurgitation

AS: aortic stenosis

ASA: acetylsalicylic acid

ASD: atrial septal defect

ASIS: anterior superior iliac spine

AV: arteriovenous/atrioventricular

AVM: arteriovenous malformation

BCC: basal cell carcinoma

BCG: Bacille bilié de Calmette-Guérin (TB vaccine)

BM: bowel movement

BMZ: basement membrane zone

BN: bulimia nervosa

BP: blood pressure

BPH: benign prostatic hypertrophy

BPPV: benign paroxysmal positional vertigo

BRCA-1 and 2: mutant tumor suppressor genes (breast cancer)

ca: carcinoma

CABG: coronary artery bypass graft

CAD: coronary artery disease

CAH: congenital adrenal hyperplasia

CC: chief complaint

CF: cystic fibrosis

CHF: congestive heart failure

CHOL: cholesterol

CI: contraindications

CMC: carpometacarpal

CMV: cytomegalovirus

CN: cranial nerve

CNS: central nervous system

CO: cardiac output

COPD: chronic obstructive pulmonary disease

CP: chest pain

CPA: cerebellopontine angle

CPR: cardiopulmonary resuscitation

C-section: cesarean section

CSF: cerebrospinal fluid

CTS: carpal tunnel syndrome

CVA: cerebral vascular accident/costovertebral angle

CVP: central venous pressure

CVS: cardiovascular system

CXR: chest x-ray

D & C: dilatation and curettage

DBP: diastolic blood pressure

DDH: developmental dysplasia of the hip

DDST: Denver Developmental Screening Test

DD$_X$: differential diagnosis

DEJ: dermoepidermal junction

DHEAS: dehydroepiandrosterone sulfate

DIPJ: distal interphalangeal joint

DM: diabetes mellitus

DNR: do not resuscitate

D/O: disorder

DRE: digital rectal examination

DTaP: diphtheria, tetanus, and acellular pertussis

DTR: deep tendon reflexes

DVT: deep vein thrombosis

D$_X$: diagnosis

Dz: disease
EBV: Epstein-Barr virus
ECF: extracellular fluid
ECG: electrocardiogram
ED: emergency department
EDC: estimated date of confinement
Ej: early systolic ejection sound
ENT: ear, nose, throat
EOM: extraocular eye movements
EtOH: alcohol
FB: foreign body
FEV_1: forced expiratory volume in 1st second
FH: family history
FOB: fecal occult blood
FRC: functional residual capacity
FSH: follicle stimulating hormone
FVC: forced vital capacity
GBS: Group B *streptococcus*
GER: gastroesophageal reflux
GH: growth hormone
GI: gastrointestinal
GN: glomerulonephritis
GU: genitourinary
HBV: hepatitis B virus
HCG: human chorionic gonadotropin
HDL: high-density lipoprotein
HEENT: head, eyes, ears, nose, and throat
Hep B: hepatitis B vaccine
Hgb: hemoglobin
Hib: *Haemophilus influenzae* type b conjugate vaccine
HIV: human immunodeficiency virus
HPF: high power field
HPI: history of present illness
HPV: human papillomavirus
HR: heart rate
HRT: hormone replacement therapy
HSP: Henoch-Schönlein purpura
HSV: herpes simplex virus
HTN: hypertension
Hz: hertz
H_X: history
IBD: inflammatory bowel disease

IBS: irritable bowel syndrome
ICH: intracranial hemorrhage
ICP: intracranial pressure
ICS: intercostal space
ID: identifying data
IHD: ischemic heart disease
IPJ: interphalangeal joint
IPV: inactivated polio vaccine
IUGR: intrauterine growth restriction
IV: intravenous
IVC: inferior vena cava
JVP: jugular venous pressure
LAP: left atrial pressure
LDH: lactate dehydrogenase
LDL: low-density lipoprotein
LEEP: loop electrocautery excision procedure
LGA: large for gestational age
LGI: lower gastrointestinal
LH: luteinizing hormone
LLL: left lower lobe (lung)
LLQ: left lower quadrant (abdomen)
LMNL: lower motor neuron lesion
LMP: last menstrual period
LOC: loss of consciousness
LP: lumbar puncture/lichen planus
L/S: lecithin to sphingomyelin ratio
LSCS: lower segment cesarean section
LUL: left upper lobe (lung)
LUQ: left upper quadrant (abdomen)
LV: left ventricle
LVF: left ventricular failure
LVH: left ventricular hypertrophy
MAL: midaxillary line
MAOI: monoamine oxidase inhibitor
MCA: middle cerebral artery
MCL: midclavicular line
MCPJ: metacarpophalangeal joint
MEDS: medication
MEN: multiple endocrine neoplasia
Mets: metastasis
MI: myocardial infarction
MLF: medial longitudinal fasciculus
mm: millimeter

mm Hg: millimeters of mercury

MMR: measles, mumps, and rubella vaccine

MR: mitral regurgitation/mental retardation

MS: mitral stenosis/multiple sclerosis

MSK: musculoskeletal

MTPJ: metatarsophalangeal joint

MVP: mitral valve prolapse

n: nerve

NARES: nonallergic rhinitis with eosinophilia syndrome

Neuro: neurologic

NHL: non–Hodgkin's lymphoma

NO_2: nitrous oxide

NSAID: nonsteroidal antiinflammatory drug

NSVD: normal spontaneous vaginal delivery

NTG: nitroglycerin

N/V: nausea/vomiting

OCD: obsessive-compulsive disorder

OCP: oral contraceptive pill

O/E: on examination

OM: otitis media

OR: operating room

OS: opening snap (of stenotic mitral valve)

OSCE: objective structured clinical examination

OTC: over-the-counter (medications)

P_2: pulmonary component of 2nd heart sound

PAP smear: Papanicolaou test

PAT: paroxysmal atrial tachycardia

PCOS: polycystic ovarian syndrome

PCR: polymerase chain reaction

PDA: patent ductus arteriosus

PE: pulmonary embolism

PFT: pulmonary function test

PG: phosphatidylglycerol

PI: pulmonary infarction

PID: pelvic inflammatory disease

PIH: pregnancy induced hypertension

PIPJ: proximal interphalangeal joint

PMH: past medical history

PMR: polymyalgia rheumatica

PMS: premenstrual syndrome

PND: paroxysmal nocturnal dyspnea

POF: premature ovarian failure

PPD: purified protein derivative

PPH: postpartum hemorrhage

PPROM: prolonged premature rupture of membranes

PR: *per rectum*

PRL: prolactin

PRO: protein

PROM: premature rupture of membranes

PSA: prostate specific antigen

PSH: past surgical history

PSIS: posterior superior iliac spine

Pt: patient

PTH: parathyroid hormone

PTHrp: parathyroid hormone-related protein

PTSD: posttraumatic stress disorder

PTU: propylthiouracil

PUD: peptic ulcer disease

PUVA: psoralen plus ultraviolet A

PV: *per vaginam*

PVC: premature ventricular contraction

PVD: peripheral vascular disease

RA: rheumatoid arthritis

RAM: rapid alternating movements

RBC: red blood cell

RDS: respiratory distress syndrome

Resp: respiratory

RIND: reversible ischemic neurologic deficit

RLL: right lower lobe (lung)

RLQ: right lower quadrant (abdomen)

RML: right middle lobe (lung)

ROM: range of motion/rupture of membranes

ROS: review of systems

RR: respiratory rate

RUL: right upper lobe (lung)

RUQ: right upper quadrant (abdomen)

RVF: right ventricular failure

RVH: right ventricular hypertrophy

S_1: 1st heart sound
S_2: 2nd heart sound
S_3: 3rd heart sound
S_4: 4th heart sound
SAH: subarachnoid hemorrhage
SBP: systolic blood pressure
SCC: squamous cell carcinoma
SCM: sternocleidomastoid muscle
SES: socioeconomic status
SGA: small for gestational age
SH: social history
SI: sacroiliac
SIADH: syndrome of inappropriate ADH
SLE: systemic lupus erythematosus
SOB: shortness of breath
SOBOE: shortness of breath on exertion
SOL: space occupying lesion
SSSS: staphylococcal scalded skin
    syndrome
STI: sexually transmitted infection
SVC: superior vena cava
TA: therapeutic abortion
TB: tuberculosis
TCA: tricyclic antidepressant

Td: tetanus and diphtheria vaccine
TG: triglycerides
TIA: transient ischemic attack
TIBC: total iron binding capacity
TM: tympanic membrane
TMJ: temporomandibular joint
TORCH: toxoplasmosis, other, rubella,
    CMV, herpes simplex virus
t-PA: tissue plasminogen activator
TSH: thyroid stimulating hormone
U & E: urea and electrolytes
UGI: upper gastrointestinal
UMNL: upper motor neuron lesion
URTI: upper respiratory tract infection
U/S: ultrasound
UTI: urinary tract infection
UVB: ultraviolet B
VDRL: Venereal Disease Research
    Laboratories (test for syphilis)
VPL: ventral posterolateral nucleus
VSD: ventricular septal defect
WHO: World Health Organization
WPW: Wolff-Parkinson-White syndrome

CONTENTS

CHAPTER 1

Cardiovascular System

OBJECTIVES

ANATOMY
　　REVIEW OF HEART SOUNDS

CARDINAL SIGNS AND SYMPTOMS

ESSENTIAL CLINICAL COMPETENCIES
　　PALPATION: THE APICAL IMPULSE
　　AUSCULTATION: THE HEART
　　APPROACH TO EVALUATING A HEART MURMUR
　　APPROACH TO EVALUATING EXTRA HEART SOUNDS
　　PERFORM A FOCUSED PHYSICAL EXAMINATION FOR AORTIC STENOSIS
　　PERFORM A FOCUSED PHYSICAL EXAMINATION FOR AORTIC REGURGITATION
　　PERFORM A FOCUSED PHYSICAL EXAMINATION FOR MITRAL STENOSIS
　　PERFORM A FOCUSED PHYSICAL EXAMINATION FOR MITRAL REGURGITATION
　　PERFORM A FOCUSED PHYSICAL EXAMINATION FOR MITRAL VALVE PROLAPSE
　　PERFORM A FOCUSED PHYSICAL EXAMINATION OF THE JUGULAR VENOUS PRESSURE (JVP) AND
　　　　DESCRIBE HOW TO DIFFERENTIATE THE JVP FROM THE CAROTID PULSE
　　PERFORM AN ACCURATE MEASUREMENT OF BLOOD PRESSURE

SAMPLE OSCE SCENARIOS
- A 60-year-old patient with diabetes presents with a 6-month history of calf pain when walking. The pain resolves with rest. Perform a focused physical examination.
- A 58-year-old male with a history of hypertension presents for a "check-up." Perform a focused history and physical examination.
- A 22-year-old female presents to her family doctor after checking her blood pressure at a local pharmacy. She is worried that she has "high blood pressure." Take a detailed history, exploring possible etiologies, and perform a focused physical examination.
- A 55-year-old male presents to his family physician for the results of routine blood work he had drawn last month. His total cholesterol is 7.0 mmol/L and low-density lipoprotein is 4.5 mmol/L. Take a detailed history, and perform a focused physical examination.
- A 35-year-old female presents to the emergency department complaining that her "heart is beating out of her chest." This happened to her once before but resolved spontaneously. Take a detailed history, exploring possible etiologies, and perform a focused physical examination.
- A 79-year-old male with a history of "heart failure" presents to the emergency department with worsening shortness of breath and swelling in his legs. Take a detailed history, exploring possible etiologies, and perform an appropriate physical examination.
- A 39-year-old male presents to the emergency department with sharp chest pain that is most severe when lying down. He feels unwell and is having "trouble breathing." Take a detailed history, exploring possible etiologies, and perform a focused physical examination.
- A 56-year-old female presents to the emergency department with 3 hours of severe left-sided chest pain. The nurse hands you an electrocardiogram (ECG). Take a detailed history, exploring possible etiologies, and perform an appropriate physical examination. Interpret the ECG.

Continued

SAMPLE CHECKLISTS

❑ Demonstrate how you would measure blood pressure in a patient referred to you for evaluation of hypertension. Explain what you are doing, and document the patient's blood pressure measurement.

❑ Examine this patient's lower extremities for evidence of peripheral arterial insufficiency. Describe your findings.

❑ A 40-year-old male with ankylosing spondylitis has been referred to the cardiology clinic for evaluation of possible aortic regurgitation. Perform a focused physical examination, and describe your findings.

OBJECTIVES

*The successful student should be able to take a **focused history** of the cardiovascular system, including:*

- Chest pain
- Shortness of breath (SOB)
- Exercise tolerance
- Orthopnea
- Paroxysmal nocturnal dyspnea (PND)
- Palpitations
- Dizziness, syncope
- Peripheral edema
- Claudication
- History of known heart murmur, rheumatic fever
- Risk factors for cardiovascular disease:
  - Age (men, >55 years; women, >65 years)
  - Cigarette smoking
  - Hypertension (HTN)
  - Diabetes mellitus (DM)
  - Hyperlipidemia
  - Obesity (body mass index [BMI], >30)
  - Physical inactivity
  - Family history of premature cardiovascular disease (men, <55 years; women, <65 years)

*The cardiovascular **examination** will include:*

Inspection

- Color (e.g., cyanosis, plethora, pallor)
  - Differentiate peripheral cyanosis from central cyanosis.
- Clubbing
- Inspection of lower extremities for signs of arterial and venous insufficiency
- Measurement of the jugular venous pressure (JVP), including:
  - Patient positioning
  - Location of JVP in relation to surface anatomy
  - Determination of height and waveforms
  - Differentiation from the carotid pulse
- Thoracic deformity
  - Pectus excavatum/carinatum
  - Scoliosis, kyphosis
  - Barrel chest

Palpation

- Palpate the dorsalis pedis, posterior tibial, popliteal, femoral, radial, ulnar, brachial, and carotid pulses.

■ Describe rate, rhythm, contour, and volume of pulse.

■ Examine for symmetry of pulses.

- Pitting edema: Lower limbs, presacral area
- Hepatojugular reflux
- Palpate the precordium, noting the apical impulse and any thrills or heaves.

Auscultation

- Appropriate use of the stethoscope (diaphragm and bell)
- Technique for taking accurate blood pressure (BP)
- Use positional and respiratory maneuvers to optimize auscultation and localize murmurs and extra heart sounds.
- Identify the heart sounds.
- Note the presence of any murmurs, and describe salient features.
- Note the presence of pericardial rubs.
- Bruits: Carotid, femoral, aortic, and renal

ANATOMY

- The heart is enclosed in a thin sac of parietal pericardium. A small amount of pericardial fluid lubricates the space between the heart and the pericardium.
- The heart comprises four chambers (Figure 1-1). Blood enters the right atrium from the superior and inferior venae cavae, passing through the **tricuspid valve** and into

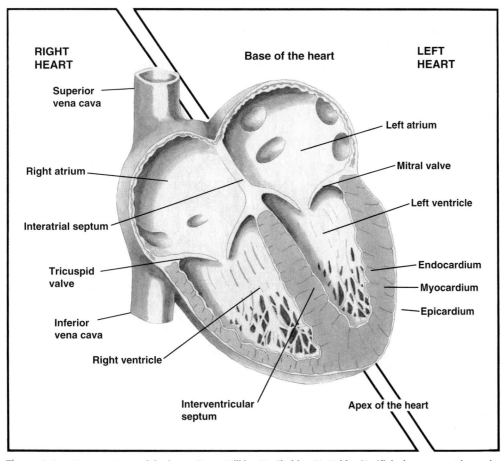

Figure 1-1   Gross anatomy of the heart. (From Wilkins RL, Sheldon RL, Krider SJ: *Clinical assessment in respiratory care*, ed 4, St. Louis, 2000, Mosby, Figure 9-1.)

the right ventricle. The deoxygenated blood then leaves the heart through the **pulmonic valve** into the pulmonary artery—the only artery in the body that carries deoxygenated blood. Once oxygenated in the pulmonary vascular bed, blood enters the left atrium through the pulmonary vein—the only vein in the body that carries well-oxygenated blood. Blood passes through the **mitral valve** into the left ventricle and exits the heart, passing through the **aortic valve** into the aorta.

Surface Anatomy (Figure 1-2)

- The **right atrium** forms the right border of the heart and is usually not identifiable on physical examination.
- The **right ventricle** occupies most of the anterior cardiac surface, narrowing superiorly to meet the pulmonary artery at the level of the third left costal cartilage.
- The **left atrium** lies mostly posterior and cannot be examined directly.
- The **left ventricle** lies to the left of and behind the right ventricle, forming the left border of the heart. The tip of the left ventricle produces the **apical impulse**—a systolic beat usually found in the fifth intercostal space (ICS).

Landmarks for Palpable Pulses (Figure 1-3)

- **Dorsalis pedis pulse:** Between the tendons of extensor hallucis longus and extensor digitorum longus
- **Posterior tibial pulse:** Two to 3 cm posterior to the medial malleolus
- **Popliteal pulse:** Deep within the popliteal fossa (hold the knee in 15 degrees flexion)
- **Femoral pulse:** Inferior to the inguinal ligament, midway between the pubic symphysis and anterior superior iliac spine (ASIS)—lateral corners of the pubic hair triangle
- **Radial pulse:** Anterolateral aspect of wrist (Remember the forearm is supinated in the anatomic position.)
- **Ulnar pulse:** Anteromedial aspect of the wrist
- **Brachial pulse:** Medial to the biceps tendon in the cubital fossa
- **Carotid pulse:** Between the trachea and the sternocleidomastoid (SCM) muscle at the

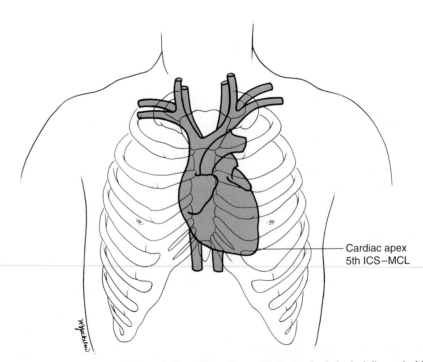

Cardiac apex
5th ICS–MCL

Figure 1-2   Surface anatomy of the heart. (Adapted from Swartz M: *Textbook of physical diagnosis: history and examination,* ed 4, Philadelphia, 2002, WB Saunders, Figure 13-4.)

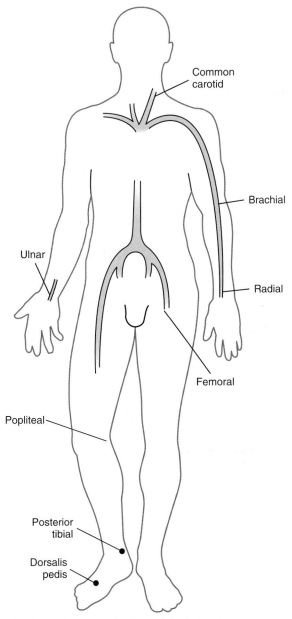

Figure 1-3 Areas for palpating peripheral pulses. (Adapted from Tilkian AG, Conover MB: *Understanding heart sounds: with an introduction to lung sounds,* ed 4, Philadelphia, 2001, WB Saunders, p 51, Figure 6-2.)

level of the thyroid cartilage. (Ensure there are no carotid bruits before palpating the carotid pulse, and never palpate both carotids simultaneously.)

REVIEW OF HEART SOUNDS

- Heart sounds are produced by the sudden deceleration of blood flow when the heart valves close and their timing relates to events within the cardiac cycle (Figure 1-4).
- The cardiac cycle is initiated by the conduction of an impulse generated by the **sinoatrial node** in the right atrium. This impulse propagates through the atria to the **atrioventricular node**. The impulse then continues to be propagated through the bundle of His, the right and left bundle branches, and the Purkinje fibers (Figure 1-5).

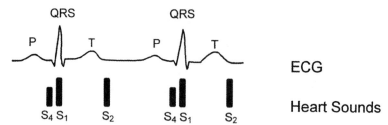

Figure 1-4   Timing of the heart sounds with the electrocardiogram (ECG).

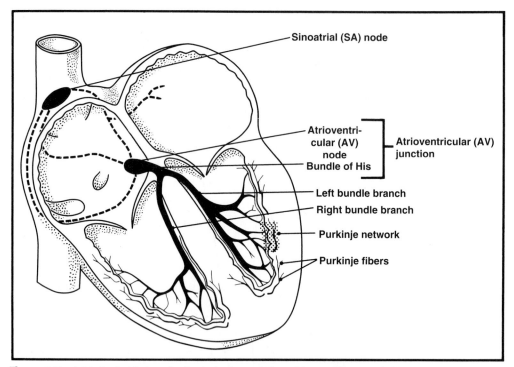

Figure 1-5   Intrinsic electrical conduction in the heart. (Adapted from Wilkins RL, Sheldon RL, Krider SJ: *Clinical assessment in respiratory care*, ed 4, St. Louis, 2000, Mosby, Figure 9-2.)

- At the onset of systole, contraction of the ventricles increases interventricular pressure, causing closure of the mitral and tricuspid valves and opening of the aortic and pulmonic valves. The closure of the mitral and tricuspid valves is heard as the **first heart sound (S_1).**
- As diastole begins the ventricles relax and interventricular pressure decreases, allowing the aortic and pulmonic valves to close, producing the **second heart sound (S_2).**
- A period of rapid ventricular filling follows and may be marked by a **third heart sound (S_3).**
- Although not often heard in normal adults, a **fourth heart sound (S_4)** marks atrial contraction and immediately precedes S_1 of the next beat.
- Pressures in the right side of the heart are significantly lower than pressures in the left side of the heart. As such, right-sided events usually occur slightly later than those on the left, a phenomenon that contributes to the splitting of heart sounds.
  - Normal inspiratory splitting of S_2 refers to the separation of S_2 into A_2 and P_2, which corresponds to the closure of the aortic and pulmonic valves, respectively. Splitting of S_2 on expiration or persistent splitting suggests an abnormality.
  - S_1 also has two components: an earlier mitral and a later tricuspid sound. Splitting of S_1 does not vary with respiration, and it is best heard at the lower left sternal border.

CARDINAL SIGNS AND SYMPTOMS

Shortness of Breath
- **Paroxysmal nocturnal dyspnea** is acute SOB that appears suddenly at night, often waking the patient from sleep. It results from left-sided heart failure with mobilization of fluid from dependent areas after lying down, leading to pulmonary congestion.
- **Orthopnea** is SOB, which is brought on or exacerbated by lying flat.

Swelling
- **Edema** is the accumulation of excessive fluid in cells or tissues. Edema may result from cardiac failure. **Pitting edema** is edema that retains the indentation of your fingers when pressure is applied. Look for edema in dependent areas such as the lower extremities in mobile persons and the presacral region in persons who are bedridden.

Loss of Consciousness
- **Syncope** is loss of consciousness and postural tone caused by decreased cerebral blood flow. This may be the presenting feature of dysrhythmia or severe aortic stenosis (AS).

Pulses
- **Pulsus tardus** describes a pulse contour with slow upstroke and prolonged downstroke; the peak is blunted and forms a plateau (Figure 1-6).
- **Water-hammer pulse** describes a pulse contour with rapid and forcible upstroke, followed by precipitous collapse, characteristic of aortic regurgitation (AR; see Figure 1-6).
- **Pulsus bisferiens** is effectively a double beat that may be perceived by light palpation of the carotid or auscultation of the compressed brachial artery (see Figure 1-6). It may occur in moderate AS with severe AR.
- **Pulsus alternans** is a regular pulse whose waves alternate between those of greater and lesser volume, varying beat to beat. It is indicative of serious left ventricular (LV) dysfunction (see Figure 1-6).
- **Pulsus paradoxus** refers to an inspiratory decrease in systolic blood pressure (SBP) that is >10 mm Hg (see Figure 1-6). The exaggerated waxing and waning in pulse volume may be detected by a palpable decrease in pulse amplitude on quiet expiration, or it may be **measured by a sphygmomanometer.** As the patient quietly breathes, lower the cuff pressure to the level of the first Korotkoff sound, which identifies the *highest systolic pressure* during the respiratory cycle. Then lower the pressure slowly until sounds can be heard throughout the respiratory cycle; note the pressure level as that of the *lowest systolic pressure.*
  - The difference between the highest and lowest systolic pressures is *normally* no greater than 3 to 4 mm Hg.
  - A difference of >10 mm Hg indicates a paradoxical pulse and may suggest severe asthma/chronic obstructive pulmonary disease (COPD), tension pneumothorax, pulmonary embolism (PE), pericardial tamponade, or constrictive pericarditis.
  - Evaluate the JVP, and check for **Kussmaul's sign**—a high JVP that paradoxically increases with inspiration.
- **Pulse pressure** is the difference between the systolic and diastolic values in mm Hg. Pulse pressures <30 mm Hg are considered **narrow** and may occur in severe AS. Pulse pressures >30 to 40 mm Hg are considered **wide.**

Types of Pain
- **Visceral pain** originating in the thoracic organs is carried by afferent fibers that enter the same thoracic dorsal ganglia. The pain from these organs (heart, lungs, and esophagus) is poorly localized (gnawing, burning, stabbing, or achy) and indistinct.

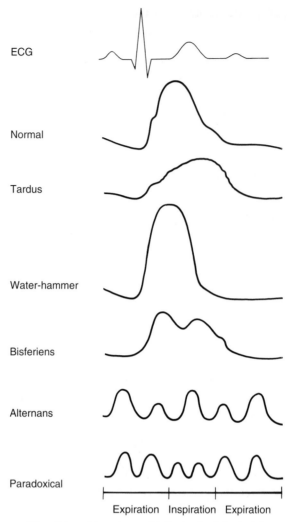

ECG

Normal

Tardus

Water-hammer

Bisferiens

Alternans

Paradoxical

Expiration   Inspiration   Expiration

Figure 1-6   Pulse abnormalities. (Adapted from Swartz M: *Textbook of physical diagnosis: history and examination,* ed 4, Philadelphia, 2002, WB Saunders, Figure 13-36.)

- **Parietal pain** originating in the parietal pericardium and parietal pleura tends to be sharp and well localized over the involved structure. It is somatically innervated.
- **Referred pain** is pain that is felt at the level of somatic innervation (dermatome) to which the sympathetic pain carrying nerves innervate. Pain from thoracic viscera may be felt anywhere from the epigastrium to the mandible.
- **Claudication** is pain classically caused by ischemia of the muscles. It is most commonly characterized as calf pain brought on by walking; the condition may occur in other muscle groups.

ESSENTIAL CLINICAL COMPETENCIES

PALPATION: THE APICAL IMPULSE

Patient Positioning
- Supine, with head of the bed elevated at 30 degrees.

Inspection
- Inspect the precordium for the apical impulse. Tangential lighting may improve the visibility of impulses.

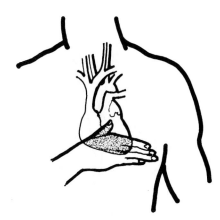

Figure 1-7   Palpation of the apical impulse. (From Tilkian AG, Conover MB: *Understanding heart sounds: with an introduction to lung sounds,* ed 4, Philadelphia, 2001, WB Saunders, p 50, Figure 6-1.)

Palpation
- Palpate the apical impulse using the pads of your fingers (Figure 1-7). Describe the location, amplitude, diameter, and duration of the apical impulse.
  - The apical impulse is usually found in the fifth ICS, at or just medial to the mid-clavicular line (MCL).
  - Normal **amplitude** is a gentle tap. Increases in amplitude may be caused by exercise, hyperthyroidism, severe anemia, and pressure or volume overload of the LV.
  - The **diameter** is usually <2.5 cm, or the size of a nickel or quarter.
  - Estimate the proportion of systole occupied by the apical impulse. A normal apical impulse lasts through the first two-thirds of systole.

Positional Maneuvers
- The following maneuvers may accentuate the apical impulse and are useful to identify left ventricular hypertrophy.
  - Ask the patient to exhale and hold his or her breath at the end of expiration; **OR**
  - Ask the patient to turn onto his or her left side. Once the apex is located, ask the patient to return to a supine position.

AUSCULTATION: THE HEART

Patient Positioning
- Supine and upright with the chest exposed

Auscultation
- The **diaphragm** is better for auscultating relatively high-pitched sounds such as S_1, S_2, the murmurs of aortic and mitral regurgitation, and pericardial friction rubs. The bell is more sensitive to low-pitched sound such as S_3, S_4, and the murmur of mitral stenosis (MS). Apply the **bell** lightly with just enough pressure to produce an air seal with its full rim. Applying too much pressure to the bell effectively converts it to a diaphragm.
- Auscultate for high-pitched sounds by placing the diaphragm of the stethoscope firmly against the patient's chest in the right second ICS close to the sternum. Listen for a few cycles to become accustomed to the rate and rhythm of the heart sounds. Make note of the following:
  - S_1 and S_2. If you cannot tell which sound is S_1, continue to auscultate while palpating the carotid pulse; S_1 just barely precedes the carotid pulsation.
  - Extra sounds in systole and diastole

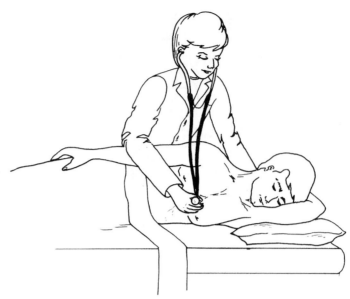

Figure 1-8   Auscultation in the left lateral decubitus position to accentuate left-sided S_3 and S_4 and the murmur of mitral stenosis. (From Tilkian AG, Conover MB: *Understanding heart sounds: with an introduction to lung sounds,* ed 4, Philadelphia, 2001, WB Saunders, p 211, Figure 16-12.)

  - Murmurs
  - Rubs
- Place the diaphragm along the left sternal border in the left second ICS. Listen for each heart sound. Continue listening in the left third, fourth, and fifth ICSs and at the site of the apical impulse. Finally listen in the axillae (where mitral murmurs may radiate) and over the carotids (where aortic murmurs may radiate).
- Repeat this sequence for low-pitched sounds using the bell of the stethoscope.

Positional Maneuvers
- Ask the patient to roll partly onto the left side into the left lateral decubitus position (Figure 1-8). Listen with the bell over the apical impulse. This position accentuates left-sided S_3 and S_4 and the murmur of MS.
- Ask the patient to sit up, lean forward, exhale completely, and hold this position (Figure 1-9). Listen with the diaphragm along the left sternal border and in the left second ICS. This position accentuates the murmur of AR.
- To help identify murmurs associated with mitral valve prolapse (MVP) and hypertrophic cardiomyopathy, ask the patient to do one of the following while you auscultate:
  - **Valsalva maneuver** (Figure 1-10): When a person takes a deep breath and bears down on a closed glottis (hold no longer than 8 to 10 seconds), venous return to the heart decreases, resulting in dynamic narrowing of the LV outflow tract. A murmur that gets louder with performance of the Valsalva maneuver is almost diagnostic of hypertrophic cardiomyopathy.
  - **Standing and squatting:** Squatting improves venous return, causing increased stroke volume and LV size. Standing then causes a relative decrease in venous return. This may accentuate the murmur of MVP.

APPROACH TO EVALUATING A HEART MURMUR

Inspection
- Inspect for the apical impulse and the ventricular movements of a left-sided S_3 or S_4. Tangential lighting may improve the visibility of impulses.

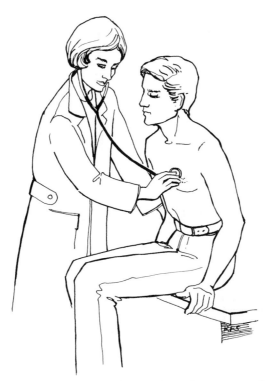

Figure 1-9   Auscultation with the patient seated and leaning forward to accentuate the murmur of aortic regurgitation. (From Tilkian AG, Conover MB: *Understanding heart sounds: with an introduction to lung sounds,* ed 4, Philadelphia, 2001, WB Saunders, p 202, Figure 16-6.)

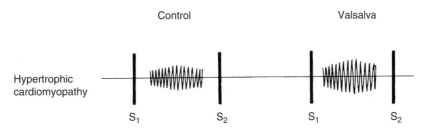

Figure 1-10   Effect of the performance of the Valsalva maneuver on the murmur of hypertrophic cardiomyopathy. (Adapted from Tilkian AG, Conover MB: *Understanding heart sounds: with an introduction to lung sounds,* ed 4, Philadelphia, 2001, WB Saunders, p 258, Figure 20-3.)

Palpation
- Palpate the impulses using the pads of your fingers, exerting light pressure for an S_3 or S_4 and firmer pressure for S_1 or S_2. Thrills often accompany loud, harsh, or rumbling murmurs such as those of AS and MS. Thrills are best felt using the ball of your hand pressed firmly on the chest.

Auscultation
- See pp 9 and 10 for auscultatory techniques.
- Describe the following features of an identified murmur:
  - **Timing** (Figure 1-11): Relationship to systole and diastole (e.g., holosystolic versus mid or late systolic). If you cannot tell which sound is S_1, continue to auscultate while palpating the carotid pulse. S_1 just barely precedes the carotid pulsation.
  - **Shape** (Figure 1-12): Crescendo, decrescendo, crescendo-decrescendo, or plateau
  - **Location** (Figure 1-13) of maximal intensity in relation to sternum, ICSs, and MCL
  - **Radiation** to carotids or axillae; represents direction of blood flow and intensity
  - **Pitch:** High, medium, or low
  - **Quality:** Blowing, harsh, rumbling, or musical

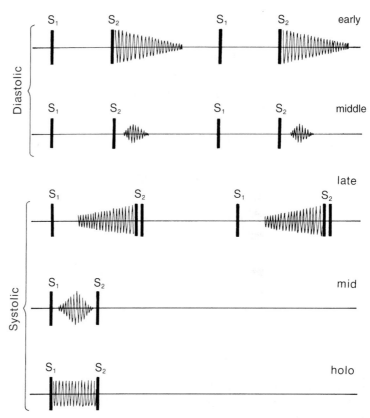

Figure 1-11   Description of the timing of murmurs in the cardiac cycle. (Adapted from Tilkian AG, Conover MB: *Understanding heart sounds: with an introduction to lung sounds*, ed 4, Philadelphia, 2001, WB Saunders, p 135, Figure 12-3.)

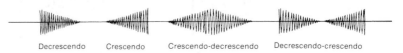

Decrescendo   Crescendo   Crescendo-decrescendo   Decrescendo-crescendo

Figure 1-12   Description of the "shape" of a murmur. (From Tilkian AG, Conover MB: *Understanding heart sounds: with an introduction to lung sounds*, ed 4, Philadelphia, 2001, WB Saunders, p 135, Figure 12-4.)

- **Intensity:** Grades I through VI, ranging from faint to audible with the stethoscope entirely off the chest. The intensity of the murmur is not related to the severity of disease (e.g., AR).
- Effect of patient positioning and respiratory maneuvers.

Positional Maneuvers
- Listen at the apex with the patient in the left lateral decubitus position to accentuate the murmur of MS.
- To accentuate AR, auscultate with the patient sitting up and leaning forward after exhaling completely.
- Maneuvers such as squatting and bearing down on a closed glottis help identify the murmurs of MVP, hypertrophic cardiomyopathy, and AS.

Respiratory Maneuvers
- Inspiration may augment right-sided murmurs. Expiration accentuates the murmur of AR.

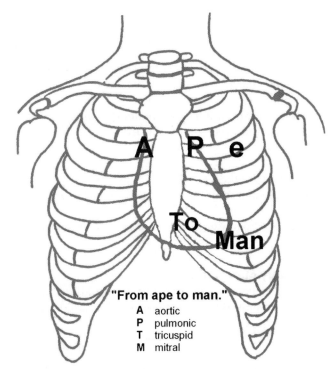

Figure 1-13   Auscultatory anatomy: Identifying the source of the murmur.

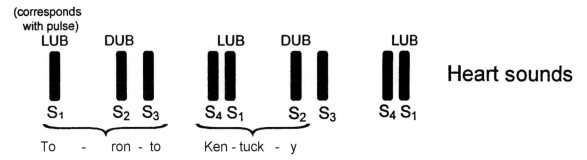

Figure 1-14   Timing of extra heart sounds in the cardiac cycle.

APPROACH TO EVALUATING EXTRA HEART SOUNDS

Definition (Figure 1-14)
- S_3 is the sound produced by the period of ventricular filling in diastole after S_2 **(To-ron-to)**. It may be normal in children and young adults but is usually pathologic in those >40 years old. It is often found in patients with heart failure (e.g., poor myocardial contractility).
- S_4 is the sound that occurs after atrial contraction, immediately before S_1 **(Kentuck-y)**. It is often known as the "atrial gallop." It is a marker for decreased ventricular compliance (i.e., "atrial kick" into a stiff ventricle). S_4 is **absent** in patients with atrial fibrillation because coordinated atrial contraction is absent.

Inspection
- Inspect for the apical impulse and the ventricular movements of a left-sided S_3 or S_4. Tangential lighting may improve the visibility of impulses.

Palpation

- Palpate using light pressure to identify an S_3 or S_4.
  - **Left-sided S_3 and S_4:** Best felt at the apex with the patient in the left lateral decubitus position, may be accentuated by having the patient exhale and briefly stop breathing. A brief mid-diastolic impulse indicates an S_3. A presystolic movement that is maximal at the apex represents an S_4.
  - **Right-sided S_3 and S_4:** Best felt when the patient is supine. Place your index finger in the subxiphoid area and push gently toward left shoulder.

Auscultation

- The bell is more sensitive for the low-pitched S_3 and S_4.
  - **Left-sided S_3 and S_4:** Listen with the patient in the left lateral decubitus position at the apex.
  - **Right-sided S_3 and S_4:** Listen with the patient supine over the lower left sternal border or subxiphoid.

Positional and Respiratory Maneuvers

- Maneuvers that increase venous return, such as squatting, accentuate S_3 and S_4. S_3 and S_4 can also be accentuated by expiration (left sided) and inspiration (right sided).

PERFORM A FOCUSED PHYSICAL EXAMINATION FOR AORTIC STENOSIS

Definition

- Aortic stenosis is pathologic narrowing of the aortic valve.

DD$_X$ VITAMINS C

- **Autoimmune/Allergic:** Rheumatic valvular disease
- **Idiopathic/Iatrogenic:** Degenerative valve calcification, hypertrophic cardio-myopathy
- **Congenital/genetic:** Congenital bicuspid valve

Patient Positioning

- Sit up and lean forward with breath held in exhalation to accentuate the murmur of AS.

Inspection

- Inspect for the apical impulse and the ventricular movements of a left-sided S_3 or S_4. Tangential lighting may improve the visibility of impulses.

Palpation

- Palpate the impulses using the pads of your fingers, exerting light pressure for an S_3 or S_4 and firmer pressure for S_1 and S_2. The apical impulse may be enlarged, sustained, and displaced because of left ventricular hypertrophy (LVH). Palpate for systolic thrills over the base of the heart and at the carotids. Thrills are best felt using the ball of your hand pressed firmly on the chest. Palpate the carotid pulse, noting its contour and volume.

Auscultation

- Listen for the high-pitched murmur with the diaphragm held firmly against the chest wall. Also listen at the apex with the bell with the patient in the left lateral decubitus position.
  - Expect a loud systolic crescendo-decrescendo murmur of medium pitch (higher pitch at the apex). It is often described as harsh and is best heard in the second right ICS. It is also often heard along the left sternal border and radiates to the neck.

- In significant valvular calcification A_2 is diminished or absent. During expiration S_2 may be split, a phenomenon known as **paradoxical splitting.** An S_4 is frequently audible.

Other Signs of AS
- Pulsus tardus
- Narrowed pulse pressure

PERFORM A FOCUSED PHYSICAL EXAMINATION FOR AORTIC REGURGITATION

Definition
- **Aortic regurgitation** refers to the reflux of blood through an incompetent aortic valve back into the left ventricle. It is also known as aortic insufficiency.

DD$_X$ VITAMINS C
- **V**ascular: Acute aortic dissection, dilatation of the aortic root (Marfan's syndrome)
- **I**nfectious: Bacterial endocarditis, syphilis of the aorta
- **T**raumatic
- **A**utoimmune/**A**llergic: Rheumatic valvular disease, ankylosing spondylitis, collagen vascular disease
- **I**diopathic/**I**atrogenic: Idiopathic valvular degeneration
- **C**ongenital/genetic: Congenital bicuspid valve

Patient Positioning
- Sit up and lean forward with breath held in exhalation to accentuate the murmur of AR.

Inspection
- Inspect for the apical impulse and the ventricular movements of a left-sided S_3 or S_4. Tangential lighting may improve the visibility of impulses.

Palpation
- Palpate the impulses using the pads of your fingers, exerting light pressure for an S_3 or S_4 and firmer pressure for S_1 and S_2. The apical impulse may be enlarged, sustained, and displaced because of LVH. Palpate for systolic thrills over the base of the heart and the carotids. Thrills are best felt using the ball of your hand pressed firmly on the chest. Palpate the carotid pulse, noting its contour and volume.

Auscultation
- Listen for the high-pitched murmur with the diaphragm held firmly against the chest wall. Also listen at the apex with the bell with the patient in the left lateral decubitus position.
  - Expect an early, blowing, decrescendo diastolic murmur that is high pitched. It is heard with maximal intensity in the second to fourth left ICSs. If the murmur is loud it may radiate to the apex or right sternal border.
  - A_2 is often accentuated, and the presence of an S_3 or S_4 suggests severe disease.

Other signs of AR
- **Musset's sign** is head nodding accompanying carotid pulsations.
- **Quincke's sign** describes the presence of pulsations in the nail beds.
- **Widened pulse pressure**
- **Hills' sign** is an increased BP in the legs compared with the arms.
- **Water-hammer pulse**

- **Corrigan's sign** is a prominent carotid pulsation characterized by *bounding* and *increased volume*; similar to the *water-hammer pulse*.
- **Pulsus bisferiens**
- **Duroziez's sign** is a femoral diastolic murmur with slight compression. It reflects flow backward up the aorta and indicates severe disease. It is related to *pulsus bisferiens*.
- A **pistol shot sound** over the femorals is produced by the front of a high-pressure arterial pulse wave striking the femoral arterial wall.

PERFORM A FOCUSED PHYSICAL EXAMINATION FOR MITRAL STENOSIS

Definition
- **Mitral stenosis** is pathologic narrowing of the mitral valve. It is the only major valvular disease that does not cause LVH (AR, AS, and mitral regurgitation [MR] all result in LVH).

DD$_X$ VITAMINS C
- Autoimmune/Allergic: Rheumatic valvular disease
- Idiopathic/Iatrogenic: Idiopathic valvular degeneration
- Neoplastic: Atrial myxoma
- Congenital/genetic: Congenital valvular lesion

Patient Positioning
- Use the left lateral decubitus position to accentuate the murmur of MS.

Inspection
- Inspect for the apical impulse and the ventricular movements of a left-sided S_3 or S_4. Tangential lighting may improve the visibility of impulses.

Palpation
- Palpate the impulses using the pads of your fingers, exerting light pressure for an S_3 or S_4 and firmer pressure for S_1 and S_2. If right ventricular hypertrophy (RVH) develops because of pulmonary HTN, a right ventricular heave may be palpable. Palpate the carotid pulse, noting its contour and volume.

Auscultation
- This murmur is low pitched and heard best with the bell at the apex.
  - An opening snap (OS) often follows S_2 and initiates the murmur of MS. The OS is best heard along the left sternal border, second to fourth ICSs with the diaphragm.
  - Expect a **rumbling** murmur, resembling the roll of a drum. The murmur may have two components: mid-diastolic (during rapid ventricular filling) and a presystolic crescendo that disappears in the presence of atrial fibrillation. S_1 is usually accentuated, and P_2 is also accentuated if pulmonary HTN is present.
  - Mild exercise may accentuate the murmur, and it is often better heard in exhalation.
  - An associated murmur termed the Graham Steell's murmur indicates pulmonic regurgitation. It is virtually indistinguishable from the murmur of AR, but it is usually less loud and transmitted less widely with the absence of peripheral signs of AR. It is caused by dilatation of the pulmonic valve in pulmonary HTN.

Other Signs of MS
- Malar flush
- Irregularly irregular pulse (in presence of atrial fibrillation)
- Increased JVP (in presence of right ventricular failure [RVF])

- Ortner's syndrome: Hoarseness caused by left vocal cord paralysis due to compression of left recurrent laryngeal nerve by a dilated left atrium

PERFORM A FOCUSED PHYSICAL EXAMINATION FOR MITRAL REGURGITATION

Definition
- Mitral regurgitation refers to the reflux of blood through an incompetent mitral valve back into the left atrium.

DD$_X$ VITAMINS C
- **V**ascular: Ruptured chordae tendineae or papillary muscles (secondary to ischemia)
- **I**nfectious: Bacterial endocarditis
- **A**utoimmune/**A**llergic: Rheumatic valvular disease, rheumatoid arthritis
- **I**diopathic/**I**atrogenic: MVP
- **C**ongenital/genetic: Dilatation of the mitral ring

Patient Positioning
- Use the left lateral decubitus position to accentuate the murmur of MR.

Inspection
- Inspect for the apical impulse and the ventricular movements of a left-sided S_3 or S_4. Tangential lighting may improve the visibility of impulses.

Palpation
- Palpate the impulses using the pads of your fingers, exerting light pressure for an S_3 or S_4 and firmer pressure for S_1 and S_2. The apical impulse may be enlarged, sustained, and displaced because of LVH. Palpate the carotid pulse, noting its contour and volume.

Auscultation
- Auscultate the precordium, and listen for the medium- to high-pitched murmur of MR with the diaphragm held firmly against the apex. Unlike the murmur of tricuspid regurgitation, the intensity of the murmur of MR does not change with respiration.
  - A loud, blowing, pansystolic (holosystolic) murmur with maximal intensity at the apex, radiating to the axilla is expected. S_1 is often decreased; the presence of an apical S_3 indicates LVH.
  - In extreme cases there may be a widened splitting of S_2 caused by premature emptying of the LV causing an early A_2. Rarely an apical diastolic rumble is present.

Other Signs of MR
- Irregularly irregular pulse (in presence of atrial fibrillation)

PERFORM A FOCUSED PHYSICAL EXAMINATION FOR MITRAL VALVE PROLAPSE

Definition
- **Mitral valve prolapse** is an echocardiographic diagnosis rather than a clinical one; therefore, although you may be asked to examine a patient with MVP, you would not be asked to diagnose MVP using only physical examination. MVP occurs when the valve undergoes a degenerative process creating redundant valve tissue, leading to enlargement of the valve annulus and elongation of the chordae tendineae. During

systole the valve leaflets are propelled backward into the atrium and billow out, accounting for the association with MR.

Patient Positioning
- Standing erect accentuates the murmur of MVP. Auscultation after exercise may elicit a murmur not audible at rest.

Inspection
- Inspect for the apical impulse and the ventricular movements of a left-sided S_3 or S_4. Tangential lighting may improve the visibility of impulses.

Palpation
- Palpate the impulses using the pads of your fingers, exerting light pressure for an S_3 or S_4 and firmer pressure for S_1 and S_2. Thrills are best felt using the ball of your hand pressed firmly on the chest. Palpate the carotid pulse, noting its contour and volume.

Auscultation
- Auscultate the precordium. Listen for the high-pitched murmur with the diaphragm held firmly against the chest wall.
  - This murmur is heard best at the apex and is a short, high-pitched murmur occurring late in systole, giving an impression of a crescendo sound and described as a "cooing" or a "whooping." Heard best at the apex, it may radiate to the back to the left of the spine. The intensity is variable.
  - Wide splitting of S_2 may occur with an audible S_3. A snapping or clicking sound is sometimes heard in mid-systole, corresponding to an observable retraction in the apical region.

Positional Maneuvers
- The murmur is softer and shorter when squatting and becomes more pronounced after standing again (Figure 1-15).

Other Signs of MVP
- The patient may have signs and symptoms associated with dysrhythmia. Associated dysrhythmias include premature ventricular contractions (PVCs), paroxysmal atrial

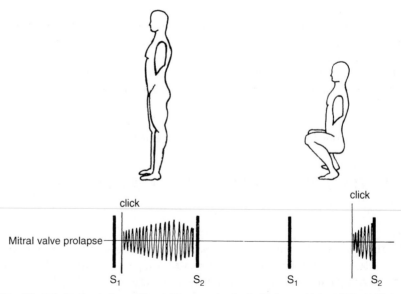

Figure 1-15   Effect of standing and squatting on the murmur of mitral valve proplapse. (Adapted from Tilkian AG, Conover MB: *Understanding heart sounds: with an introduction to lung sounds*, ed 4, Philadelphia, 2001, WB Saunders, p 255, Figure 20-2.)

tachycardia (PAT), atrial fibrillation/flutter, sinus bradycardia, and sick sinus syndrome.

- MVP is sometimes associated with connective tissue diseases such as *Marfan's syndrome*. Stigmata of Marfan's syndrome include arachnodactylism, hyperextensible joints, ectomorph build, and dislocated lenses.

PERFORM A FOCUSED PHYSICAL EXAMINATION OF THE JUGULAR VENOUS PRESSURE (JVP) AND DESCRIBE HOW TO DIFFERENTIATE THE JVP FROM THE CAROTID PULSE

Definition

- Pressure in the jugular veins reflects **right atrial pressure**. Jugular venous pressure is defined as the highest point of oscillation of the internal jugular vein measured as vertical distance from the sternal angle **(angle of Louis)**. The sternal angle is approximately 5 cm above the right atrium. A JVP of >3 to 4 cm is considered elevated and may be noted in RVF, pericardial tamponade, tension pneumothorax, or superior vena cava obstruction; it is decreased in hypovolemia. The JVP cannot reliably be used as an indication of hydration status; however, in the setting of other physical findings and an appropriate history, it is a useful physical sign.

Patient Positioning

- Position the patient supine with head on a pillow and SCM muscle relaxed (mouth open and head slightly away from inspecting side). Begin with the head of the bed elevated to 30 degrees, and adjust the position to maximize visibility of pulsations.

Inspection

- Use tangential lighting, and examine both sides of the neck. The right internal jugular vein is straighter than the left internal jugular vein. The JVP should be evaluated using the right internal jugular vein whenever possible.
- The internal jugular vein is located deep to the SCM muscle; look for pulsations between the heads of the SCM muscle as they are transmitted through surrounding soft tissues (Table 1-1). Identify the highest point of oscillation, and measure the vertical distance from the sternal angle (manubriosternal joint or angle of Louis). Place the ruler vertically on the sternal angle, and place a long rectangular object perpendicularly and adjust such that it rests at the highest point of oscillation; read the vertical distance from the ruler. Round off to the nearest centimeter (Figure 1-16).

Palpation

- **Hepatojugular reflux:** Place your hand in the right upper quadrant (RUQ) of the patient's abdomen, and press firmly upward under the costal margin. A sustained increase in JVP (elevation >10 seconds or three respiratory cycles) indicates venous congestion. Carotid pulsation is unaffected by hepatojugular reflux.

PERFORM AN ACCURATE MEASUREMENT OF BLOOD PRESSURE

- The width of the bladder should be approximately 40% of the circumference of the arm; the length should be 80% of the circumference. Cuffs that are too short or too narrow give falsely high readings. A loose cuff may also lead to falsely high readings.
- The patient should avoid smoking or ingesting caffeine for at least 30 minutes and should rest for at least 5 minutes.
- Position the patient comfortably sitting with both feet on the floor. The brachial artery should be at heart level (roughly the fourth ICS). If the brachial artery is below heart level, BP measurements may be falsely high.

Table 1-1 Differentiating Internal Jugular Pulsations from Carotid Pulsations

Mnemonic – "POLICE"	Internal Jugular Pulsations	Carotid Pulsations
Palpability	Rarely palpable (e.g., severe tricuspid regurgitation)	Palpable
Occludability	Pulsations eliminated by light pressure on the veins just above the sternal end of the clavicle	Not occludable
Location	Pulsations seen between heads of SCM muscle	Pulsations may be seen just medial to SCM muscle
Inspiration (effect of)	Level of pulsation descends with inspiration	Level of pulsation unaffected by inspiration
Contour	Rapid, undulating quality; two waveforms (two elevations, a wave and v wave)	Visible thrust with single elevation
Erect position (effect of)	Level of pulsation changes with position, decreasing as patient becomes more erect	Level of pulsation is unaffected by position

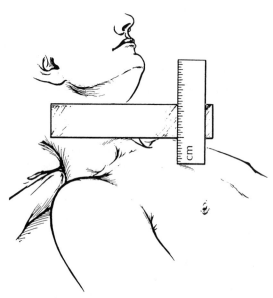

Figure 1-16 Measurement of the jugular venous pressure. (From Wilkins RL, Sheldon RL, Krider SJ: *Clinical assessment in respiratory care*, ed 4, St. Louis, 2000, Mosby, Figure 4-2.)

- The patient's own effort to support the arm may increase BP; therefore, the arm should be supported to ensure accuracy in BP measurement.
- Anxiety is a frequent cause of high BP (otherwise known as "white coat syndrome"). Try to get the patient relaxed, and repeat measurements later in the encounter.
- Apply an appropriately selected BP cuff to the arm, ensuring proper positioning with respect to the brachial artery.
- First estimate the SBP by palpation to avoid error caused by an auscultatory gap. Palpate the radial artery. Inflate the BP cuff beyond the point where the pulse is no longer palpable. Deflate the cuff at 2 to 3 mm Hg/sec. The estimated SBP is the point at which the pulse becomes palpable again.
- Wait 2 to 5 minutes before rechecking the BP *(this is not possible in an examination situation)*. Position the stethoscope over the brachial artery. Inflate the cuff 20 to 30 mm Hg beyond the estimated SBP. Deflate the cuff at 2 to 3 mm Hg/sec. Note the point at

which the first Korotkoff sound is heard (SBP). Continue to auscultate until the Korotkoff sounds disappear (diastolic BP [DBP]).

- Measure BP in both arms. If there is a pressure difference, subsequent readings should be made on the arm with the higher pressure.
- BP may be measured with the patient sitting, standing, or supine. To detect orthostatic changes, first measure the BP with the patient supine. Then ask the patient to sit or stand up as you reassess the BP in this upright position.

SAMPLE OSCE SCENARIOS

> INSTRUCTIONS TO CANDIDATE: A 60-year-old patient with diabetes presents with a 6-month history of calf pain when walking. The pain resolves with rest. Perform a focused physical examination.

Definition
- Intermittent **claudication** is characterized by attacks of pain, weakness, fatigue, or numbness in the calf brought on by exercise and relieved by rest. It may also occur in the foot, thigh, hip, or buttocks. In advanced disease claudication may be present at rest.

DD$_X$ VITAMINS C
- **V**ascular: Peripheral vascular disease (PVD; occlusive arterial disease), deep venous thrombosis (DVT)
- **I**diopathic/**I**atrogenic: Thromboangiitis obliterans, spinal stenosis (lumbar)

6 Ps of arterial insufficiency
- **Pain**
- **Pulselessness**
- **Pallor**
- **Polar** (cool temperature)
- **Paresthesia**
- **Paralysis**

Inspection (Table 1-2)
- Inspect both legs from the groin and buttocks to the feet, comparing both legs. Note the following:
    - Size and symmetry
    - Venous pattern and enlargement (varicose veins)
    - Integrity of skin and nails, including scars, ulcers, and atrophy (shiny)
    - Color of skin and nail beds
    - Distribution of hair growth

Palpation (see Table 1-2)
- Pulses: Dorsalis pedis, posterior tibial, popliteal, and femoral
- Capillary refill (normal <3 seconds)
- Temperature of feet and legs using back of your fingers, comparing one side with the other
- Pitting edema over dorsum of feet, behind medial malleoli, and over shins
- Note any tenderness of calves
    - **Homans's sign:** Flex the patient's knee. Forcefully and abruptly dorsiflex the ankle. This produces pain in some patients with DVT but may also be positive with intervertebral disk herniation and other conditions.
- Ischemic peripheral neuropathy: Check **vibration sense** using a tuning fork (128 Hz) placed over a bony prominence such as the medial malleolus. Check sensation of **light touch** using a cotton swab.
- Test muscle power, tone, and reflexes in the lower extremities to clinically rule out spinal stenosis.
- **Buerger's test:** Ask the recumbent patient to elevate his or her legs to 60 degrees. Maintenance of color or slight pallor is normal, whereas marked pallor is a positive sign of arterial insufficiency. Ask the patient to sit up and dangle legs over the side of the bed. Pink color normally returns in 10 seconds. Venous filling of the feet and

Table 1-2	Differentiating Arterial from Venous Insufficiency	
	Advanced Arterial Insufficiency	**Advanced Venous Insufficiency**
Pulses	Decreased or absent	Normal or difficult to palpate because of edema
Color	Marked pallor on elevation; dusky red on dependency	Brown pigmentation in chronic disease
Temperature	Cool	Normal
Edema	Absent to mild	May be marked
Skin	Thin and shiny with loss of hair; thick rigid nails	Brown pigmentation; stasis dermatitis
Ulceration	At points of trauma (e.g., toes, plantar aspect of feet)	Medial aspect of ankles, anterior tibia
Capillary refill	Slow	Normal
Bruits	May be present	Absent
Buerger's test	Positive	Negative
Trendelenburg's test	Negative	Positive

ankle normally takes approximately 15 seconds. Persisting rubor and plethora on dependency suggest arterial insufficiency. Normal findings with decreased arterial pulses suggest good collateral circulation around an arterial occlusion.

- **Trendelenburg's test:** Elevate one leg to 90 degrees, and stroke the veins toward the heart until they are empty. Manually occlude the great saphenous vein in the upper thigh with a tourniquet. Ask the patient to quickly stand and watch for venous filling. Normally arterial blood flow from below fills the venous system over 30 to 35 seconds. Rapid filling indicates incompetent valves in the communicating system (perforators). Release the tourniquet, and observe any further sudden venous filling, indicating incompetent valves in the great saphenous vein.

Auscultation
- Listen for femoral and iliac bruits.

INSTRUCTIONS TO CANDIDATE: A 58-year-old male with a history of hypertension presents for a "check-up." Perform a focused history and physical examination.

Definition
- **Hypertension** (HTN) refers to elevated BP (Table 1-3). It cannot be diagnosed clinically without accurate measurement of BP with a sphygmomanometer. HTN should only be diagnosed based on the mean of two or more seated measurements on each of two or more examinations. The most common type of HTN is primary idiopathic or essential. Secondary HTN is rare, although often correctable.

History
- Patients are usually **asymptomatic**.
  - How are you feeling? Any changes in your health lately?
  - Headaches? Suboccipital, pulsating headaches are common.
  - Visual disturbance? Nausea/vomiting (N/V)?
  - Chest pain? SOB on exertion (SOBOE)? Exercise tolerance?
- **Risk factors** for cardiovascular disease:
  - Age (men, >55 years; women, >65 years)
  - Cigarette smoking

Table 1-3 2003 Classification of Hypertension			
BP Classification	**Systolic BP (mm Hg)**		**Diastolic BP (mm Hg)**
Normal	<120	and	<80
Prehypertension	120-139	or	80-89
Stage 1 hypertension	140-159	or	90-99
Stage 2 hypertension	≥160	or	≥100

Adapted from Chobanian AV, Bakris GL, Black HR, et al. The Seventh Report of the Joint National Committee on Prevention, Detection, Evaluation, and Treatment of High Blood Pressure: The JNC 7 report. *JAMA* 289:2561, 2003 (Table 1).

- HTN
- DM
- Hyperlipidemia
- Obesity (BMI, >30)
- Physical inactivity
- Family history of premature cardiovascular disease (men, <55 years; women, <65 years)
- **Past medical history (PMH)/past surgical history (PSH):** Other medical/surgical problems
- **Medications (MEDS):** Nonsteroidal antiinflammatory drugs (NSAIDS), cyclooxygenase-2 (COX-2) inhibitors, steroids, or sympathomimetics
  - Consider compliance with antihypertensive medications.
- **Social history (SH):** Diet (including sodium intake), exercise, smoking, EtOH, street drugs, and psychosocial stressors
- **Family history (FH):** Lipid disorders, obesity, HTN, endocrine disease, or polycystic kidney disease

Physical Examination
- **Vitals:** Heart rate (HR), BP, respiratory rate (RR), and temperature
- To assess the effects of HTN one must assess its effect on end organs (e.g., eyes, heart, vasculature, brain, and kidneys).
  - **Vitals:** HR, BP, RR, and temperature
  - Ascertain the **height** and **weight** of the patient. BMI = weight (kg)/height^2 (m)
  - **Head, eyes, ears, nose, and throat (HEENT):** Perform a careful funduscopic examination for signs of retinopathy (e.g., narrowed arterioles, copper/silver wire appearance, exudates, hemorrhages, and papilledema).
  - **Cardiovascular system (CVS):** Measure the JVP (increased venous pressure in congestive heart failure [CHF]). Palpate peripheral pulses, and auscultate for bruits (e.g., carotid, aortic, renal, iliac, and femoral). Inspect and palpate the apical impulse (enlarged, sustained, and displaced with LVH). Palpate for thrills and heaves. Auscultate the heart looking for an S_3 or murmurs. Examine for signs of arterial insufficiency in the lower limbs.
  - **Abdomen:** Palpate the abdomen, and note any pulsatile masses.
  - **Neurologic (Neuro):** Mental status (encephalopathy)

INSTRUCTIONS TO CANDIDATE: A 22-year-old female presents to her family doctor after checking her blood pressure at a local pharmacy. She is worried that she has "high blood pressure." Take a detailed history, exploring possible etiologies, and perform a focused physical examination.

Definition

- Secondary HTN is uncommon but often amenable to treatment. *Clues* that HTN may be secondary to other disease:
  - Age of onset <25 years or >55 years
  - HTN that is severe, sudden, and difficult to manage medically

DD$_X$ VITAMINS C

- **V**ascular: Renal vascular disease (e.g., fibromuscular dysplasia), coarctation of the aorta
- **M**etabolic: Drugs, endocrine disease (Conn's syndrome, Cushing's syndrome, hyperthyroidism, acromegaly, or congenital adrenal hyperplasia [CAH])
- **I**diopathic/**I**atrogenic: Sleep apnea, renal parenchymal disease
- **N**eoplastic: Pheochromocytoma

History

- Patients are usually **asymptomatic**.
  - How are you feeling? Any changes in your health lately?
  - Headaches? Suboccipital, pulsating headaches are common.
  - Visual disturbance? N/V? Weakness?
  - Chest pain? SOBOE? Exercise tolerance?
  - Last menstrual period (LMP)? Are you pregnant?
  - Cushing's syndrome: Weight gain? Stretch marks? Easy bruising?
  - CAH: Hirsutism?
  - Pheochromocytoma: Palpitations? Sweating? Flushing?
  - Hyperthyroidism: Weight loss? Heat intolerance? Diarrhea?
  - Acromegaly: Enlarged hands/feet? Hyperpigmentation? Carpal tunnel syndrome?
- **Risk factors** for cardiovascular disease:
  - Age (men, >55 years; women, >65 years)
  - Cigarette smoking
  - HTN
  - DM
  - Hyperlipidemia
  - Obesity (BMI, >30)
  - Physical inactivity
  - Family history of premature cardiovascular disease (men, <55 years; women, <65 years)
- **PMH/PSH:** Systemic lupus erythematosus (SLE), hyperthyroidism, acromegaly, congenital heart disease, or coarctation of the aorta
- **MEDS:** NSAIDS, COX-2 inhibitors, sympathomimetics, oral contraceptive pill (OCP), or steroids
- **SH:** Diet (including sodium intake), exercise, smoking, EtOH, and street drugs
- **FH:** Multiple endocrine neoplasia (MEN), obesity, HTN, DM, polycystic kidney disease, or collagen vascular diseases

Physical Examination

- **Vitals:** HR, BP (use accurate technique via sphygmomanometer in at least one arm and leg), RR, and temperature
- Ascertain the **height** and **weight** of the patient. BMI = weight (kg)/height^2 (m)
- **Inspect** for signs associated with the following secondary causes of HTN:
  - Cushing's syndrome: Moon-facies, buffalo hump, supraclavicular fat pad, central obesity, purplish striae on abdomen and in axillae, acne, and proximal muscle wasting
  - CAH: Hirsutism, ambiguous genitalia
  - Pheochromocytoma: Paroxysmal tachycardia, diaphoresis, and flushing
  - Coarctation of the aorta: Decreased femoral pulses, radial-femoral delay, aortic bruits, and arm BP > leg BP

- ■ Acromegaly: Enlarged hands, feet, mandible, nose, lips, and tongue; increased space between the teeth; coarse facial features; oily skin; bitemporal hemianopsia; hyperpigmentation; and carpal tunnel syndrome
  - ■ Hyperthyroidism: Goiter, hyperreflexia, atrial fibrillation, widened pulse pressure, exophthalmos, lid lag, and periorbital edema
- **HEENT:** Perform a careful funduscopic examination for signs of retinopathy (narrowed arterioles, copper/silver wire appearance, exudates, hemorrhages, and papilledema). Inspect the neck for any masses, and palpate the thyroid gland.
- **CVS:** Measure the JVP. Palpate peripheral pulses, and auscultate for bruits (carotid, aortic, renal, iliac, and femoral). Note any radial-radial delay or radial-femoral delay. Note pulse volume, contour, and rhythm. Inspect and palpate the apical impulse (enlarged, sustained, and displaced with LVH). Palpate for thrills and heaves. Auscultate the heart, looking for extra heart sounds or murmurs. Coarctation is associated with a soft bruit heard in the second left or right ICS radiating to the thoracic spine.
- **Abdomen:** Palpate the abdomen for masses. Palpate the kidneys (polycystic kidney, aldosterone/renin-secreting neoplasms)
- **Neuro:** Mental status

INSTRUCTIONS TO CANDIDATE: A 55-year-old male presents to his family physician for the results of routine blood work he had drawn last month. His total cholesterol is 7.0 mmol/L and low-density lipoprotein (LDL) is 4.5 mmol/L. Take a detailed history, and perform a focused physical examination.

Definition

- **Hyperlipidemia** is an abnormally high amount of circulating lipids in the blood. The desirable total cholesterol and LDL levels vary according to cardiovascular risk.

DD$_x$ Secondary Hypercholesterolemia (VITAMINS C)

- It is important to rule out treatable causes of hypercholesterolemia.
- **Metabolic:** Hypothyroidism, DM, cholestasis
- **Idiopathic/Iatrogenic:** Nephrotic syndrome, obesity (nonalcoholic steatohepatitis)

History

- Patients are usually **asymptomatic.**
  - ■ Have you ever been told you had high cholesterol?
  - ■ How long have you had this problem?
  - ■ Is it being treated (medications, lifestyle modifications)?
  - ■ Is it improving, getting worse, or staying the same?
  - ■ Any other problems (angina, stroke, abdominal pain, pancreatitis, liver disease, ischemic bowel, or claudication)?
  - ■ Hypothyroidism: Weight gain? Cold intolerance? Constipation? Lethargy? Facial swelling?
  - ■ DM: Polyuria? Polydipsia?
  - ■ Nephrotic syndrome: Frothy urine? Edema? Increased abdominal girth (ascites)?
  - ■ Cholestasis: Jaundice? Pruritus? Anorexia? Steatorrhea?
- **Risk factors** for cardiovascular disease:
  - ■ Age (men, >55 years; women, >65 years)
  - ■ Cigarette smoking
  - ■ HTN
  - ■ DM
  - ■ Hyperlipidemia
  - ■ Obesity (BMI, >30)

- Physical inactivity
- Family history of premature cardiovascular disease (men, <55 years; women, <65 years)
- **PMH/PSH:** Pancreatitis
- **MEDS:** β-Blockers, glucocorticoids, thiazides, or in femates, OCP, estrogens, or progestin
- **SH:** Diet, exercise, smoking, and EtOH
- **FH:** Lipid disorders, obesity, HTN, DM, or liver disease

Physical Examination
- **Vitals:** HR, BP, RR, and temperature
- Ascertain the **height** and **weight** of the patient. BMI = weight (kg)/height^2 (m)
- **Inspect** for signs associated with the following secondary causes of hypercholesterolemia:
  - Hypothyroidism: Narrowed pulse pressure, bradycardia; dry, coarse, sallow skin; nonpitting edema in face, hands, and feet; coarse, brittle hair; slow return phase of deep tendon reflexes (DTRs), and carpal tunnel syndrome
  - Nephrotic syndrome: Anasarca, ascites, and muscle wasting
  - Cholestasis: Jaundice, excoriations
- **Skin:** Inspect for **tendon xanthoma** on ankles, extensor surface of elbows, and tendons of palms.
- **HEENT:** Inspect for **xanthelasma palpebrarum** (yellow deposits on the eyelids) and **corneal arcus** (granular fatty deposits on cornea). Examine the thyroid gland.
- **CVS:** Measure the JVP. Palpate peripheral pulses, and auscultate for bruits (carotid, aortic, renal, iliac, and femoral). Note pulse volume, contour, and rhythm. Inspect and palpate the apical impulse (enlarged, sustained, and displaced with LVH). Palpate for thrills and heaves. Auscultate the heart, looking for extra heart sounds or murmurs.
- **Abdomen:** Examine the liver, spleen, and kidneys.

INSTRUCTIONS TO CANDIDATE: A 35-year-old female presents to the emergency department complaining that her "heart is beating out of her chest." This happened to her once before but resolved spontaneously. Take a detailed history, exploring possible etiologies, and perform a focused physical examination.

Definition
- **Palpitations** are an unpleasant awareness of one's own heartbeat.

DD$_X$ VITAMINS C
- **V**ascular: Supraventricular tachycardia (SVT), rapid atrial fibrillation, and ventricular tachycardia
- **M**etabolic: Fever, anemia, hyperthyroidism, and acromegaly
- **N**eoplastic: Pheochromocytoma
- **S**ubstance abuse and **P**sychiatric: Drug ingestion (e.g., sympathomimetics) or drug withdrawal, anxiety
- **C**ongenital/genetic: Wolff-Parkinson-White syndrome (WPW)

History
- **C**haracter: What are the palpitations like? What were you doing when the palpitations began?
- **O**nset: When did the palpitations begin? Did it start suddenly or gradually?
- **I**ntensity: How severe are the palpitations on a scale of 1 to 10? How does it affect your activities of daily living?

- Duration: How long does it last? How long has this been happening to you (acute versus chronic)?
- Events associated:
  - How was your health before the palpitations began?
  - Chest pain, SOB, edema, diaphoresis, N/V, or dizziness/syncope?
  - Hyperthyroidism: Goiter, weight loss, heat intolerance, diarrhea, or exophthalmos
  - Pheochromocytoma: Diaphoresis, flushing
  - Anxiety (diagnosis of exclusion): Lightheadedness, diaphoresis, trembling, choking sensation, palpitations, numbness or tingling in hands and feet, chest pain, nausea or abdominal pain, depersonalization/derealization, flushes or chills, fear of dying, fear of going crazy or doing something uncontrolled
- Frequency: How often does it occur? When was the last time this happened?
- Palliative factors: Is there anything that makes it better? If so, what?
- Provocative factors: Is there anything that makes it worse? If so, what?
- **PMH/PSH:** Arrhythmias, valvular disease, rheumatic fever, ischemic heart disease (IHD), MEN (pheochromocytoma), hyperthyroidism, or psychiatric disorders
- **MEDS:** Thyroid replacement, antiarrhythmics, salbutamol, or medication withdrawal (antidepressants, EtOH, opiates)
- **SH:** Caffeine, smoking, EtOH, and street drugs
- **FH:** MVP, cardiomyopathy, MEN, or psychiatric disorders

Physical Examination

- **Vitals:** BP and HR lying and sitting or standing, RR, and temperature
- **General:** Diaphoresis, flushing, cyanosis, peripheral edema
- **HEENT:** Examine the thyroid gland.
- **Respiratory (Resp):** Chest expansion (symmetry), auscultation (breath sounds, adventitious sounds)
- **CVS:** Measure the JVP. Palpate peripheral pulses. Note pulse volume, contour, and rhythm. Inspect and palpate the apical impulse (enlarged, sustained, and displaced with LVH). Palpate for thrills and heaves. Auscultate the heart, looking for extra heart sounds or murmurs.
- **Abdomen:** Examine for ascites and organomegaly.
- **Neuro:** Mental status (adequate brain oxygenation)

INSTRUCTIONS TO CANDIDATE: A 79-year-old male with a history of "heart failure" presents to the emergency department with worsening shortness of breath and swelling in his legs. Take a detailed history, exploring possible etiologies, and perform an appropriate physical examination.

Definition

- **Heart failure** is a syndrome resulting in inadequate cardiac output to meet the body's metabolic demands. Congestive symptoms may be noted in the systemic or pulmonary circulation or both (Table 1-4). Patients with heart failure are at risk for complications such as thromboembolic disease, pneumonia, and renal failure. **Etiologies** include:
  - Intrinsic heart muscle disease (cardiomyopathy, ischemia), valvular heart disease, cardiodepressive toxidrome (e.g., calcium channel blockers, β-blockers, digitalis), restrictive filling (constrictive pericarditis, sarcoidosis), and inadequate HR
  - High output states leading to myocardial failure: Anemia, thyrotoxicosis, Paget's disease, and pregnancy
  - The commonest cause of RVF is LVF.

Table 1-4 Symptoms of Heart Failure

Symptoms of RV Failure	Symptoms of LV Failure
Exertional dyspnea	Dyspnea
Peripheral edema	Orthopnea
Abdominal distension (ascites)	Paroxysmal nocturnal dyspnea
Fullness in neck (jugular venous distension)	Cough and wheeze (cardiac asthma)
Nocturia (increased venous return when supine increases venous return to kidneys)	Hemoptysis/pink froth (pulmonary congestion)
Wasting (cardiac cachexia), fatigue	Wasting (cardiac cachexia), fatigue
RUQ pain (hepatic congestion)	

DD$_X$ VITAMINS C
- **V**ascular: CHF, acute coronary syndrome (ACS), and pulmonary embolism (PE)
- **I**nfectious: Pneumonia
- **T**raumatic: Pneumothorax
- **M**etabolic: Diabetic ketoacidosis (DKA)
- **I**diopathic/**I**atrogenic: COPD/asthma, massive atelectasis
- **N**eoplastic: Large pleural effusion

- **First evaluate A**irway, **B**reathing, and **C**irculation. It may be necessary to perform an immediate intervention, such as supplemental O$_2$, IV access, or intubation.
  - Is the patient able to talk? Swallow? Cough?
  - Are both lungs ventilated? Is the patient oxygenating (mentation, pulse oximetry)?
  - Abnormal vitals? Peripheral circulation (pulses, capillary refill)?
  - If no immediate interventions are required, proceed to take the history, and perform the physical examination.

History
- **Ch**aracter: Describe the nature of your breathing difficulty.
- **L**ocation: Where is the swelling in your legs? Both sides? Any other swelling?
- **O**nset: How did the SOB start (sudden versus gradual)? What were you doing when you became SOB? Exertion? Lying down?
- **I**ntensity: How severe is your SOB right now on a scale of 1 to 10 with 1 being mild and 10 being the worst? Has it gotten worse? Have your legs ever been this swollen?
- **D**uration: How long have you been SOB? How long have you had leg swelling?
- **E**vents associated:
  - Decreased appetite (liver and gastrointestinal [GI] congestion)? Abdominal distension (ascites)?
  - Weight gain (fluid retention), weakness, and fatigue (decreased CO)?
  - Orthopnea, PND, and pink frothy sputum (pulmonary edema)?
  - Chest pain? Diaphoresis?
  - PE: Hemoptysis, pleuritic chest pain, DVT
  - Pneumonia, other infections: Fever/chills, rigors, increased sputum production, cough
- **F**requency: Has this ever happened to you before? If so, how often does it happen? When was the last time you became SOB?
- **P**alliative factors: Is there anything that makes your SOB better? If so, what?
- **P**rovocative factors: Is there anything that makes your SOB worse? If so, what?
  - Exertion?
  - Position (sitting up versus lying down)?
  - Exposure to cold air?

- ■ Infection?
- ■ Allergies?
- **Risk factors** for cardiovascular disease:
  - ■ Age (men, >55 years; women, >65 years)
  - ■ Cigarette smoking
  - ■ HTN
  - ■ DM
  - ■ Hyperlipidemia
  - ■ Obesity (BMI, >30)
  - ■ Physical inactivity
  - ■ Family history of premature cardiovascular disease (men, <55 years; women, <65 years)
- **PMH/PSH:** IHD, valvular disease, PVD, COPD, stroke, or malignancy
- **MEDS:** Calcium channel blockers, β-blockers, digitalis, diuretics, angiotensin-converting enzyme (ACE) inhibitors, or bronchodilators
  - ■ Consider noncompliance with medications.
- **SH:** Smoking, EtOH, and street drugs
- **FH:** Cardiomyopathy, IHD, HTN, increased cholesterol, obesity, or stroke
- **Immunizations:** Pneumococcal vaccine, influenza vaccine, childhood vaccinations, and Bacille bilié de Calmette-Guérin (BCG) vaccine

Physical Examination (Table 1-5)

- **Vitals:** HR and rhythm, RR (depth, effort, and pattern), BP, and temperature
  - ■ In end-stage failure, the patient may be hypothermic.
- **General:** Respiratory distress, diaphoresis, cachexia
- **Skin:** Check capillary refill in distal extremities. Palpate for pitting edema over tibia, behind medial malleolus, dorsum of the foot, and presacral area. Note any peripheral cyanosis or pallor.
- **HEENT:** Look in the mouth for central cyanosis. Assess tracheal position.
- **Resp:** Inspect for thoracic deformity and chest expansion (symmetry). Perform tactile fremitus and percussion. Decreased tactile fremitus and flat percussion may indicate pleural effusion. Auscultate the lungs, and describe the breath sounds and adventitious sounds. You may note inspiratory crackles in pulmonary edema or expiratory wheezes (cardiac asthma).

Table 1-5   Physical Findings in Heart Failure

Signs of RHF	Signs of LHF
Increased venous pressure: • Elevated JVP, jugular venous distension (JVD) • Positive hepatojugular reflux may be demonstrated even before elevated JVP	Apical impulse: • Enlarged • Sustained • Displaced
Peripheral pitting edema: • Feet and ankles, extending proximally • Vulva/scrotum • Presacral area	Pulmonary edema: • Inspiratory crackles • Frothy, blood-tinged sputum
Hepatomegaly: • Congested, tender liver • Splenomegaly may be a late finding	Pulsus alternans
Ascites	Pleural effusion (commonly right sided)
Right-sided S_3	Left-sided S_3 or S_4

- **CVS:** Measure the JVP and hepatojugular reflux (increased venous pressure in CHF). Palpate peripheral pulses. Note pulse volume, contour, and rhythm. Pulses may be decreased, or pulsus alternans may be present. Inspect and palpate the apical impulse (enlarged, sustained, and displaced with LVH). Palpate for thrills and heaves. Auscultate the heart, looking for an S_3 or murmur.
- **Abdomen:** Inspect for ascites (bulging flanks, protuberant abdomen, umbilical herniation). Percuss the abdomen, noting any shifting dullness. Assess liver span. Palpate the liver and spleen.
- **Neuro:** Mental status (adequate brain oxygenation)

PEARL
- Manifestations of pulmonary edema on chest radiography (Figure 1-17):
  - Alveolar infiltrates, usually symmetric bilaterally
  - Kerley B lines (engorged lymphatics)
  - Pleural effusion (blunting of costophrenic angles)
  - Enlarged cardiac silhouette (chronic CHF)
  - Pulmonary vascular redistribution (enlarged vasculature in the apices)

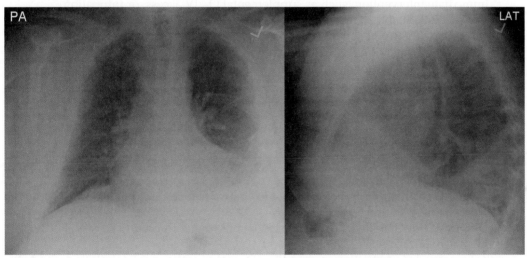

Figure 1-17 Posteroanterior and lateral views of the chest. The heart is moderately enlarged. There is a left-sided pleural effusion, and the lungs demonstrate vascular redistribution with increased interstitial and air-space disease at the lung bases, consistent with congestive heart failure.

> INSTRUCTIONS TO CANDIDATE: A 39-year-old male presents to the emergency department with sharp chest pain that is most severe when lying down. He feels unwell and is having "trouble breathing." Take a detailed history, exploring possible etiologies, and perform a focused physical examination.

Definition
- **Pericarditis** is inflammation of the pericardium surrounding the heart. Although the etiologies of pericarditis are numerous, most are idiopathic. Etiologies include Dressler's syndrome (post–myocardial infarction [MI] inflammation), infections (bacterial/viral/fungal), collagen vascular disease, trauma, uremia, medications (e.g., procainamide, hydralazine), radiotherapy, and malignancy.
- Symptoms of pericarditis:
  - Knifelike pain
  - Retrosternal; may radiate to shoulders
  - Prodrome of fever and myalgias

■ Relieved by sitting forward
■ Worsened by lying down or swallowing

DD$_X$ Chest Pain (VITAMINS C)

- **V**ascular: Aortic dissection, MI, PE, and pulmonary infarction
- **I**nfectious: Pericarditis, pneumonia, bronchiectasis, tuberculosis (TB), empyema, sub-phrenic abscess, and herpes zoster
- **T**raumatic: Pneumothorax, fractured rib, and chest wall injury
- **A**utoimmune/**A**llergic: SLE (serositis)
- **M**etabolic: DKA
- **I**diopathic/**I**atrogenic: Dressler's syndrome, esophageal spasm, peptic ulcer disease (PUD), and gastroesophageal reflux (GER)
- **N**eoplastic: Malignant pericarditis
- **S**ubstance abuse and **P**sychiatric: Cocaine (coronary vasospasm), other sympatho-mimetic ingestion, and anxiety
- **C**ongenital/genetic: Hiatal hernia

- **First evaluate A**irway, **B**reathing, and **C**irculation. It may be necessary to perform an immediate intervention, such as supplemental O$_2$, IV access, or intubation.
    - Is the patient able to talk? Swallow? Cough?
    - Are both lungs ventilated? Is the patient oxygenating (mentation, pulse oximetry)?
    - Abnormal vitals? Peripheral circulation (pulses, capillary refill)?
    - If no immediate interventions are required, proceed to take the history, and perform the physical examination.

History

- **Character:** Describe the pain.
- **Location:** Where exactly is the pain?
- **Onset:** When did the pain begin (sudden versus insidious)?
- **Radiation:** Does the pain go anywhere else?
- **Intensity:** How bad is it on a scale of 1 to 10, with 1 being mild pain and 10 being the worst pain?
- **Duration:** How long has the pain lasted (acute versus chronic)?
- **Events associated:**
    - Tamponade/constrictive pericarditis: Dyspnea, orthopnea, palpitations, and distension of neck veins
    - MI: N/V, diaphoresis
    - Pneumonia: Fever/chills, rigors, increased sputum production, cough
    - Trauma
- **Frequency:** How often does this pain occur? When was the last time this happened?
- **Palliative factors:** Does anything make the pain better? If so, what?
    - Improved by sitting up?
    - Leaning forward?
    - NSAIDS?
- **Provocative factors:** Is there anything that makes the pain worse? If so, what?
    - Worsened by lying down (especially on left side)?
    - Coughing? Deep inspiration?
    - Swallowing (proximity of the esophagus to the pericardium)?
- **PMH/PSH:** MI, malignancy, radiation, renal failure, or SLE
- **MEDS:** Procainamide, hydralazine, dantrolene, cromolyn sodium, or if female, OCP
- **SH:** Smoking, EtOH, and street drugs

Physical Examination

- **Vitals:** HR, BP, RR, and temperature
- **General:** Note position and posture, respiratory distress
- **Resp:** Chest expansion (symmetry), auscultation (breath sounds, adventitious sounds)
- **CVS:** Measure the JVP. Palpate peripheral pulses. Note pulse volume, contour, and rhythm. Inspect and palpate the apical impulse. Palpate for thrills, heaves, and pericardial friction rub. Auscultate the heart, looking for extra heart sounds or murmurs. Use the diaphragm to listen for the high-pitched, inconstant pericardial friction rub. It is best heard in the sitting position and is described as "Velcro-like."
- **Abdomen:** Examine for ascites and organomegaly.
- **Neuro:** Mental status (adequate brain oxygenation)

PEARL

- **Cardiac tamponade** is a life-threatening complication of pericarditis.
  - **Beck's triad:** Hypotension, jugular venous distension (JVD), and muffled heart sounds
  - **Electrocardiograph (ECG):** Electrical alternans (variation in the QRS axis seen on ECG as the heart moves within the fluid-filled pericardium)

INSTRUCTIONS TO CANDIDATE: A 56-year-old female presents to the emergency department with 3 hours of severe left-sided chest pain. The nurse hands you an ECG. Take a detailed history, exploring possible etiologies, and perform an appropriate physical examination. Interpret the ECG (Figure 1-18).

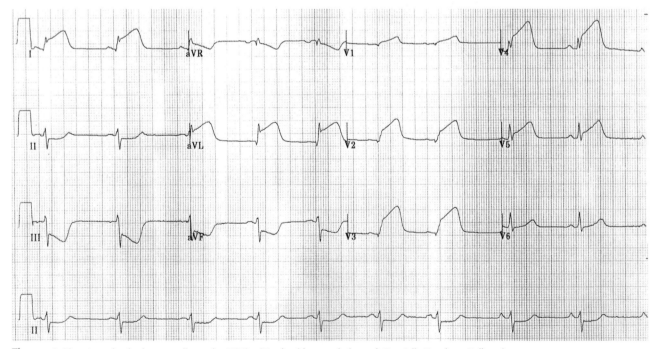

Figure 1-18   A 12-lead electrocardiograph (ECG). (Used with permission of Dr. Arik Drucker, Dalhousie University.)

ECG Interpretation
- Normal sinus rhythm (NSR), 55 bpm
- Four to 5 mm of ST elevation in leads I, aVL, and V2 to V4
- There is 2 to 3 mm of ST elevation in V5 and reciprocal ST depression in leads II, III, and aVF.
- These ECG changes are consistent with an anterolateral MI.

Definition
- An **acute myocardial infarction (AMI)** occurs with a sudden deficiency of oxygenated blood to the myocardium, usually a result of acute thrombus formation on a ruptured atheromatous plaque in a coronary vessel. As many as 20% of patients with AMI will be asymptomatic. Classic symptoms include crushing retrosternal chest pain, radiating to the left arm or jaw, lasting >20 minutes. This pain is unrelieved by nitroglycerin (NTG). Beware of atypical chest pain and nondiagnostic ECGs. Serial ECGs may be necessary. ST elevation of 1 to 2 mm in ≥2 contiguous leads is diagnostic in a patient with a compatible history.

DD$_X$ Chest Pain (VITAMINS C)
- **V**ascular: MI, aortic dissection, PE, and pulmonary infarction
- **I**nfectious: Pericarditis, pneumonia, bronchiectasis, TB, empyema, subphrenic abscess, and herpes zoster
- **T**raumatic: Pneumothorax, fractured rib, and chest wall injury
- **A**utoimmune/**A**llergic: SLE (serositis)
- **M**etabolic: DKA
- **I**diopathic/**I**atrogenic: Dressler's syndrome, esophageal spasm, PUD, and GER
- **N**eoplastic: Malignant pericarditis
- **S**ubstance abuse and **P**sychiatric: Cocaine (coronary vasospasm), other sympathomimetic ingestion, and anxiety
- **C**ongenital/genetic: Hiatal hernia

- **First evaluate A**irway, **B**reathing, and **C**irculation. It may be necessary to perform an immediate intervention, such as supplemental O$_2$, IV access, or intubation.
  - Is the patient able to talk? Swallow? Cough?
  - Are both lungs ventilated? Is the patient oxygenating (mentation, pulse oximetry)?
  - Abnormal vitals? Peripheral circulation (pulses, capillary refill)?
  - If no immediate interventions are required, proceed to take the history, and perform the physical examination.

History
- **C**haracter: Describe the pain. Crushing, squeezing, tight, heavy, or burning? Tearing? Sharp?
- **L**ocation: Where exactly is the pain?
- **O**nset: When did it start? Was it gradual or sudden? What events led up to this episode of pain?
- **R**adiation: Does the pain go anywhere else? Shoulder, neck, jaw, or arms? Back?
- **I**ntensity: How bad is it on a scale of 1 to 10, with 1 being mild pain and 10 being the worst pain? Does it hinder you from performing daily tasks?
- **D**uration: How long has the pain been there?
- **E**vents associated:
  - N/V, diaphoresis, weakness, or anxiety?
  - SOB, orthopnea, or PND?
  - PE: Hemoptysis, pleuritic chest pain, and DVT
  - Pneumonia, other infections: Fever/chills, rigors, increased sputum production, and cough

- Frequency: How often does this occur?
- **Palliative factors:** Does anything make the pain better? If so, what?
  - NTG?
  - Rest?
  - Antacids?
  - Sitting forward?
- **Provocative factors:** Does anything make the pain worse? If so, what?
  - Exercise/exertion?
  - Movement?
  - Deep inspiration?
  - Eating?
- **Risk factors** for cardiovascular disease:
  - Age (men, >55 years; women, >65 years)
  - Cigarette smoking
  - HTN
  - DM
  - Hyperlipidemia
  - Obesity (BMI, >30)
  - Physical inactivity
  - Family history of premature cardiovascular disease (men, <55 years; women, <65 years)
- **PMH/PSH:** IHD, COPD, or stroke
- **MEDS:** Antihypertensives, acetylsalicylic acid (ASA), NTG, or anticoagulants
- **FH:** IHD, stroke

Physical Examination
- **Vitals:** HR and rhythm, RR (depth, effort, and pattern), BP, and temperature
- **General:** Respiratory distress, restlessness, apprehension, diaphoresis
- **Skin:** Check capillary refill in distal extremities. Palpate for pitting edema over tibia, behind medial malleolus, dorsum of the foot, and presacral area. Note any peripheral cyanosis or pallor.
- **HEENT:** Look in the mouth for central cyanosis.
- **Resp:** Inspect for thoracic deformity and chest expansion (symmetry). Perform tactile fremitus and percussion. Decreased tactile fremitus and flat percussion may indicate pleural effusion. Auscultate the lungs, and describe the breath sounds and adventitious sounds. You may note inspiratory crackles in pulmonary edema or expiratory wheezes (cardiac asthma).
- **CVS:** Measure the JVP and hepatojugular reflux (increased venous pressure in CHF). Palpate peripheral pulses. Note pulse volume, contour, and rhythm. Pulses may be decreased, or pulsus alternans may be present. Inspect and palpate the apical impulse (enlarged, sustained, and displaced with LVH). Palpate for thrills and heaves. Auscultate the heart, looking for an S_3, S_4, or murmur. A pericardial friction rub over the infarcted area occurs in a minority. Listen for the murmur of AR and asymmetric pulses to distinguish aortic dissection.
- **Abdomen:** Inspect for ascites (bulging flanks, protuberant abdomen, umbilical herniation). Percuss the abdomen, noting any shifting dullness. Assess liver span. Palpate the liver and spleen.
- **Neuro:** Mental status (adequate brain oxygenation)

PEARLS
- Absolute contraindications (CI) for thrombolytic therapy in AMI:
  - Aortic dissection
  - Acute pericarditis
  - Active bleeding from a noncompressible site

- Relative CI for thrombolytic therapy in AMI:
  - Cerebrovascular disease
  - Diabetic retinopathy
  - Oral anticoagulation
  - HTN (SBP, ≥180 mm Hg; DBP, ≥110 mm Hg)
  - Within 10 days: GI or genitourinary hemorrhage, major surgery, or trauma

SAMPLE CHECKLISTS

> INSTRUCTIONS TO CANDIDATE: Demonstrate how you would measure blood pressure in a patient referred to you for evaluation of hypertension. Explain what you are doing, and document the patient's BP measurement.

Key Points	Satisfactorily Carried out
Introduces self to the patient	❏
Determines how the the patient wishes to be addressed	❏
Explains nature of the examination to the patient	❏
Selects correctly sized cuff	❏
Places cuff in correct position	❏
Checks systolic pressure by palpating radial or brachial pulse	❏
Arm position held at heart level with patient supine/ sitting and standing	❏
Supports the patient's arm	❏
BP auscultation: Arms	
• Stethoscope position	❏
• Inflates to 20 to 30 mm Hg above estimated systolic pressure	❏
• Rate of deflation 2 to 3 mm Hg/sec	❏
• Patient supine	❏
• Patient standing/sitting	❏
• States that BP would be measured in both arms	❏
BP reading	
• Systolic	❏
• Diastolic	❏
Makes appropriate closing remarks	❏

INSTRUCTIONS TO CANDIDATE: Examine this patient's lower extremities for evidence of peripheral arterial insufficiency. Describe your findings.

Key Points	Satisfactorily Carried out
Introduces self to the patient	❏
Determines how the patient wishes to be addressed	❏
Explains nature of the examination to the patient	❏
Inspection (compare both sides)	
• Color/pigmentation of skin	❏
• Texture of skin	❏
• Hair distribution	❏
• Skin breakdown or ulcers	❏
• Infarction of distal extremity (e.g., toes)	❏
• Nails	❏
Palpation	
• Temperature	❏
• Edema (absent or mild)	❏
• Capillary refill	❏
Auscultation	
• Bruits	❏
Palpation of pulses	
• Femoral	❏
• Popliteal	❏
• Dorsalis pedis	❏
• Posterior tibial	❏
Evaluates color of extremity	
• With elevation of leg	❏
• With leg dangling down	❏
Buerger's test	❏
Trendelenburg's test	❏
Drapes the patient appropriately	❏
Makes appropriate closing remarks	❏

INSTRUCTIONS TO CANDIDATE: A 40-year-old male with ankylosing spondylitis has been referred to the cardiology clinic for evaluation of possible aortic regurgitation. Perform a focused physical examination, and describe your findings.

Key Points	Satisfactorily Carried out
Introduces self to the patient	❏
Determines how the patient wishes to be addressed	❏
Explains nature of the examination to the patient	❏
Examines the patient in a logical fashion	❏
Pulses	
• Collapsing pulse (water-hammer pulse)	❏
• Nail bed pulsations (Quincke's sign)	❏
• Palpates carotid pulse (note upstroke and volume)	❏
• Duroziez's sign	❏
• Pistol shot sound (femorals)	❏
Measures BP	
• Comments on pulse pressure (widened)	❏
Precordium	
• Inspects precordium	❏
• Palpates the apical impulse (note location, amplitude, and diameter)	❏
• Palpation	❏
Auscultation	
• Auscultates with diaphragm and bell	❏
• Positions patient seated and leaning forward to accentuate the murmur	❏
• Describes early, blowing, decrescendo diastolic murmur	❏
• Murmur is best heard in second to fourth ICSs	❏
Drapes the patient appropriately	❏
Makes appropriate closing remarks	❏

CHAPTER 2

Respiratory System

OBJECTIVES

ANATOMY

CARDINAL SIGNS AND SYMPTOMS

ESSENTIAL CLINICAL COMPETENCIES
>   APPROACH TO THE RESPIRATORY HISTORY
>   PALPATION: TACTILE FREMITUS
>   PERCUSSION
>   AUSCULTATION: THE LUNGS
>   CHEST X-RAY INTERPRETATION

SAMPLE OSCE SCENARIOS
- A 62-year-old male presents to the emergency department with new onset of shortness of breath. Take a detailed history, exploring possible etiologies, and perform a focused physical examination.
- A 58-year-old smoker presents to his family doctor with increasing shortness of breath on exertion. Take a detailed history, exploring possible etiologies, and perform a focused physical examination.
- A 67-year-old female complains of a bothersome cough. Take a detailed history, exploring possible etiologies, and perform a focused physical examination.
- A 70-year-old male presents to the emergency department after coughing up some blood. Take a detailed history, exploring possible etiologies, and perform a focused physical examination.
- A 20-year-old female with a long history of asthma presents to her family doctor complaining of frequent exacerbations since moving out of her parents' home. Take a detailed history, exploring possible etiologies.
- A 26-year-old female presents to the emergency department with an "asthma attack." She has used her albuterol puffer several times and is still having difficulty speaking in full sentences. Treatment is initiated in the emergency department. Perform a focused physical examination.
- One of your patients recently had a "screening chest x-ray." Your assistant hands you a report saying there is a solitary nodule in the left lung. This 56-year-old male is now in your office. Perform an appropriate functional inquiry. List the differential diagnosis of a solitary pulmonary nodule.
- A 48-year-old male with unresectable bronchogenic carcinoma presents with worsening shortness of breath. Perform a focused physical examination. Interpret this patient's chest x-ray, and describe expected physical findings.
- A 32-year-old female presents with fever, rigors, and green sputum. Perform a focused physical examination. Interpret this patient's chest x-ray, and describe expected physical findings.
- A 24-year-old female presents to the emergency department with sudden onset of left-sided chest pain and mild shortness of breath. She has had two previous pneumothoraces. Perform a focused physical examination. Interpret this patient's chest x-ray, and describe expected physical findings.

SAMPLE CHECKLIST
- ❏ Demonstrate the boundaries of the right middle lobe of the lung. Auscultate the lung, and state over which lobe you are listening. Describe auscultatory findings consistent with right middle lobe consolidation.

OBJECTIVES

*The successful student should be able to take a **focused history** of the respiratory system, including:*
- Cough
- Hemoptysis
- Sputum production (color, quantity)
- Pleuritic chest pain
- Wheezing
- Shortness of breath (SOB), shortness of breath on exertion (SOBOE)
- Orthopnea, paroxysmal nocturnal dyspnea (PND)
- Exercise tolerance
- Chronic obstructive pulmonary disease (COPD), acute asthma
- Tuberculosis (TB) contacts, last chest x-ray (CXR)
- Occupational and environmental exposures (e.g., asbestos, radiation)
- Smoking history
- Sleep pattern: Snoring, apnea
- Recurrent respiratory infections
- History of thromboembolic disease
- Family history of respiratory disease (e.g., α_1-antitrypsin deficiency)

*The respiratory **examination** will include:*

Inspection
- Color (e.g., cyanosis, plethora, or pallor)
- Respiratory rate, effort, rhythm, and depth
- Symmetry of chest movement
- Accessory muscle use, retractions, tracheal tug
- Thoracic deformity
    - Pectus excavatum/carinatum
    - Scoliosis, kyphosis
    - Barrel chest
- Clubbing

Palpation
- Tactile fremitus
- Tracheal position
- Evaluation of thoracic expansion
- Palpation of chest wall for tenderness or deformity

Percussion
- Compare percussion notes from side to side, front to back, and in the axillae and supraclavicular region

Auscultation
- Note the quality and intensity of breath sounds and adventitious sounds
- Pulsus paradoxus

ANATOMY

- There are 12 ribs. The costal cartilages of the first seven ribs articulate with the sternum. The second rib articulates at the manubriosternal joint or the **angle of Louis.** Ribs 8, 9, and 10 articulate with the costal cartilages above them. The eleventh and twelfth ribs are "floating." The intercostal spaces (ICSs) are named for the rib above them.
- The trachea bifurcates into its mainstem bronchi at the angle of Louis.

- The pleurae are serous membranes that cover the outer surface of the lungs (**visceral pleura**) and line the inner rib cage and dome of the diaphragm (**parietal pleura**). A thin layer of pleural fluid lubricates the pleural space between the visceral and parietal pleura.

Surface Anatomy

- Angle of Louis: Articulation of the second costal cartilage
- Nipple: Fifth ICS
- Inferior tip of the scapula: Seventh ICS
- Spinous prominence: Spinous process of C7
- The right lung is divided into three lobes (upper, middle, and lower), whereas the left lung has just two lobes (the upper and lower lobes; Figure 2-1).
  - **Apex:** Two to 4 cm above inner third of the clavicle.
  - **Lower border:** Crosses the sixth rib at the midclavicular line (MCL) and eighth rib at the midaxillary line (MAL). Posteriorly the lower border is at T10 and on inspiration it descends further (T12).
  - **Oblique fissure:** Runs like a string connecting T3 posteriorly to the fifth rib at the MAL and to the sixth rib at the MCL.

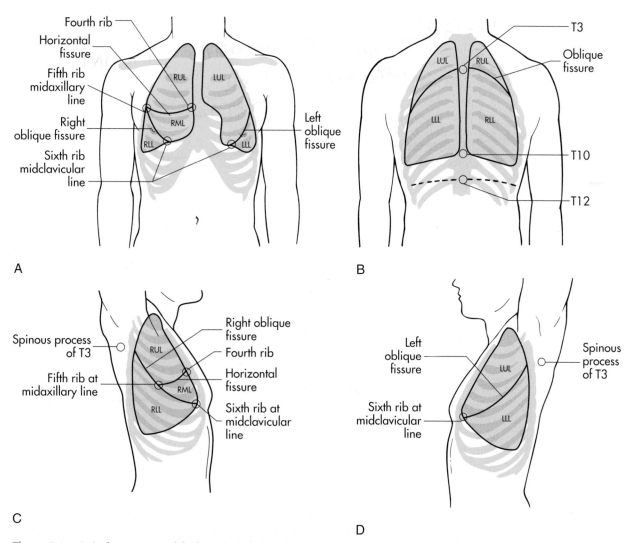

Figure 2-1   **A,** Surface anatomy of the lungs (anterior). **B,** Surface anatomy of the lungs (posterior). **C,** Surface anatomy of the lungs (right lateral). **D,** Surface anatomy of the lungs (left lateral). (From Seidel HM, Ball JW, Dains JE, Benedict GB: *Mosby's guide to physical examination*, ed 5, St. Louis, 2003, Mosby, p 361.)

- **Horizontal fissure:** Anteriorly it runs close to the fourth rib and meets the oblique fissure in the MAL near the fifth rib.
- The parietal pleura and costophrenic recesses generally extend about two ribs inferior to the lung.

Breathing

- The diaphragm is the primary muscle of inspiration. With its contraction it descends and enlarges the thoracic cavity, causing decreased intrathoracic pressure, allowing air to enter the tracheobronchial tree and expand the lungs. O_2 diffuses into blood from the alveoli to the capillary bed, and CO_2 diffuses from the blood into the alveoli. At the end of inspiration the chest wall and lungs recoil, forcing air outward. The most important accessory muscle of inspiration is the sternocleidomastoid (SCM); abdominal muscles *may* assist in forced expiration.

CARDINAL SIGNS AND SYMPTOMS

Respiratory Distress

- **Respiratory distress** is a subjective term that is poorly defined. Signs consistent with distress include:
  - Apprehension
  - Inability to speak in full sentences
  - Tachypnea
  - Pursed lips
  - Nasal flare
  - Tripod positioning: Patient holds onto an object to fix pectoral girdle
  - Tracheal tug
  - Accessory muscle use
  - Intercostal/subcostal retractions
  - Thoracoabdominal dissociation

Cyanosis

- **Cyanosis** is bluish discoloration of the skin or mucosa.
- **Central cyanosis** occurs when there is an excess of reduced hemoglobin in blood. Hence central cyanosis occurs more readily in patients with polycythemia than anemia. It is best detected by inspecting the tongue. Etiologies of central cyanosis are:
  - Inadequate O_2 transfer caused by lung disease (e.g., COPD) or hypoventilation. This is usually at least partially reversed by optimizing inspired O_2.
  - Shunting from pulmonary to systemic circulation (e.g., transposition of the great arteries). Optimizing inspired O_2 does not correct cyanosis caused by shunting.
  - Hemoglobinopathies such as methemoglobinemia.
- **Peripheral cyanosis** is detected by inspecting the lips or extremities. Because of the array of etiologies, peripheral cyanosis is a nonspecific sign. In patients with normal hemoglobin saturations, peripheral cyanosis occurs when impaired peripheral or cutaneous circulation leads to increased uptake of O_2 by the tissues, causing a localized increase in desaturated hemoglobin. Cold, anxiety, and vascular disease may contribute to peripheral cyanosis. Underlying causes of central cyanosis can also result in peripheral cyanosis.

Clubbing

- **Clubbing** is an exaggerated longitudinal curvature of the fingernail (>180 degrees) and loss of the angle between the nail and the nail bed (Figure 2-2). The distal phalanx is rounded and bulbous; the nail fold may feel "boggy." Clubbing is also known as hypertrophic peripheral arthropathy. It is a nonspecific sign because of its long list of possible etiologies (Table 2-1).

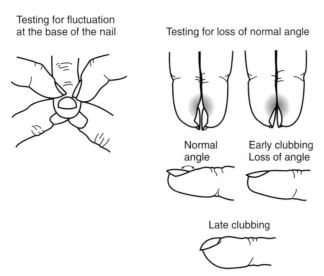

Figure 2-2   Tests for clubbing. (From Lehrer S: *Understanding lung sounds*, ed 3, Philadelphia, 2002, WB Saunders, p 39, Figure 3-4.)

Table 2-1   Etiologies of Clubbing

Malignancy	Chronic Suppurative Disease	Cyanotic Disease	Other
Bronchogenic carcinoma	Cystic fibrosis	Congenital heart disease	Inflammatory bowel disease, celiac disease
Mesothelioma	Bronchiectasis	Sequelae of infective endocarditis	Familial clubbing (often before puberty)
Gastrointestinal lymphoma	Empyema	*Unilateral clubbing* Brachial AV malformation	Chronic renal failure
Myelogenous leukemia	Abscess	Axillary artery aneurysm Thoracic outlet syndrome	Cirrhotic liver disease Thyrotoxicosis, Graves' disease

- Observe the angle between the nail bed and base of the finger. This is known as the ungual-phalangeal angle or Lovibond's angle. Place the dorsal surfaces of the right and left fingers against each other, knuckle to knuckle and tip to tip. A definite rhombus should be seen in normal individuals; no rhombus will be seen if clubbing is present.

Thoracic Deformities (Figure 2-3)
- **Pectus excavatum:** Backward displacement of the sternum (funnel chest)
- **Pectus carinatum:** Forward projection of the sternum (pigeon chest)
- **Kyphosis:** Excessive flexion of the spine (humpback)
- **Scoliosis:** Abnormal lateral curvature of the spine
- **Barrel chest:** Increased anteroposterior (AP) diameter

Patterns of Abnormal Breathing (Figure 2-4)
- **Stridor** is a high-pitched sound reflecting some degree of upper airway obstruction. Obstruction above the cords results in inspiratory stridor, whereas obstruction below the cords may produce expiratory or mixed stridor. Etiologies include foreign body (FB), tumor, edema, croup, and external compression by goiter or enlarged lymph nodes.

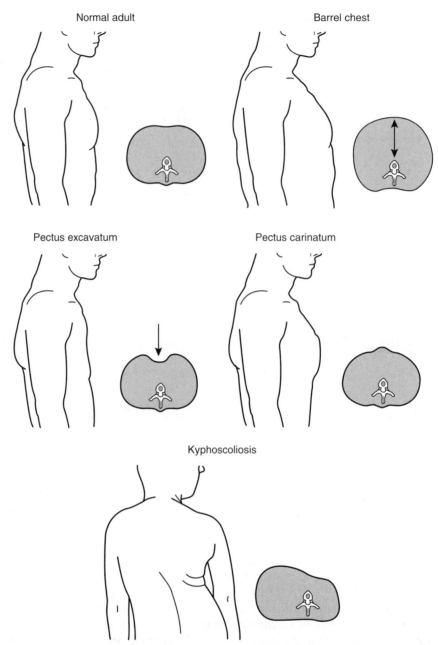

Normal adult

Barrel chest

Pectus excavatum

Pectus carinatum

Kyphoscoliosis

Figure 2-3   Thoracic deformities. (Adapted from Lehrer S: *Understanding lung sounds,* ed 3, Philadelphia, 2002, WB Saunders, p 42, Figure 3-7.)

- **Apnea** is the absence of breathing.
- **Bradypnea** is abnormal slowness of respirations (<12 breaths/min).
- **Tachypnea** is abnormal increase in frequency of respirations (>20 breaths/min).
- **Kussmaul respiration** is deep, rapid breathing characteristic of metabolic acidosis (e.g., diabetic ketoacidosis [DKA]).
- **Cheyne-Stokes respiration** is a cyclic breathing pattern with periods of increased depth of respiration, followed by decreased depth, down to a period of apnea. Etiologies include brainstem lesions, bilateral cerebral lesions, increased intracranial pressure (ICP), metabolic encephalopathy, poor cardiac output, and drug-induced respiratory depression (e.g., narcotics).
- **Biot's respiration** is an irregular breathing pattern with variable rate and depth and periods of apnea. It may result from medullary brain lesions, increased ICP, or drug-induced respiratory depression.

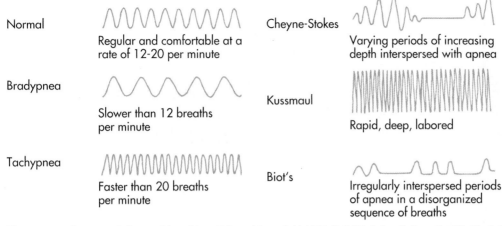

Normal — Regular and comfortable at a rate of 12-20 per minute

Bradypnea — Slower than 12 breaths per minute

Tachypnea — Faster than 20 breaths per minute

Cheyne-Stokes — Varying periods of increasing depth interspersed with apnea

Kussmaul — Rapid, deep, labored

Biot's — Irregularly interspersed periods of apnea in a disorganized sequence of breaths

Figure 2-4   Patterns of abnormal breathing. (Adapted from Seidel HM, Ball JW, Dains JE, Benedict GB: *Mosby's guide to physical examination,* ed 5, St. Louis, 2003, Mosby, p 372, Figure 12-13.)

Pathologic Transmission of Voice Sounds

- **Bronchophony** is the increased transmission of the spoken voice. On auscultation words will be noted to have increased intensity and clarity.
- If the "EE" sound is heard as an "AA" on auscultation, **egophony** is said to be present.
- **Whispering pectoriloquy** is the increased transmission of the whispered voice such that it is clearly heard on auscultation.

Pulsus Paradoxus (see Figure 1-6)

- **Pulsus paradoxus** refers to an inspiratory decrease in systolic blood pressure (SBP) that is >10 mm Hg (see Figure 1-6). The exaggerated waxing and waning in pulse volume may be detected by a palpable decrease in pulse amplitude on quiet expiration, or it may be **measured by a sphygmomanometer.** As the patient quietly breathes, lower the cuff pressure to the level of the first Korotkoff sound, which identifies the *highest systolic pressure* during the respiratory cycle. Then lower the pressure slowly until sounds can be heard throughout the respiratory cycle; note the pressure level as that of the *lowest systolic pressure.*
  - The difference between the highest and lowest systolic pressures is *normally* no greater than 3 to 4 mm Hg.
  - A difference of >10 mm Hg indicates a paradoxical pulse and may suggest severe asthma/COPD, tension pneumothorax, pulmonary embolism (PE), pericardial tamponade, or constrictive pericarditis.
  - Evaluate the jugular venous pressure (JVP), and check for **Kussmaul's sign**—a high JVP that paradoxically increases with inspiration.

ESSENTIAL CLINICAL COMPETENCIES

APPROACH TO THE RESPIRATORY HISTORY

- Use **ChLORIDE FPP** to delineate the presenting complaint.

Functional Respiratory Inquiry

- Mnemonic: **SPACED**
  - **S**moking (quantify pack-years), SOBOE, **s**putum production (mucus, pus, or blood)
  - **P**ain (pleuritic, bony/musculoskeletal [MSK], tracheobronchial), **p**igeons

Continued on p 50

Table 2-2 Signs and Symptoms: Emphysema, Atelectasis, Pulmonary Fibrosis, and Pneumonia

	Normal	Emphysema	Atelectasis	Pulmonary Fibrosis	Pneumonia
Definition		Characterized by loss of interstitial elasticity and permanent abnormal enlargement of air spaces distal to terminal bronchioles with destructive changes in alveolar walls.	A shrunken, airless state affecting all or part of a lung. May be acute or chronic. The chief cause is intraluminal bronchial obstruction.	Chronic inflammation of the alveolar walls with progressive fibrosis of unknown etiology.	An acute infection of lung parenchyma, including alveolar spaces and interstitial tissue. May affect an entire lobe or a segment (lobar pneumonia), alveoli contiguous to bronchi (bronchopneumonia), or interstitial tissue.
		Dilated alveoli with septal destruction	Bronchial obstruction with distal collapse of alveoli	Thickened and irregularly dilated alveoli	Alveoli consolidated with fluid, bacteria, and cells

Symptoms		Exertional dyspnea is the most common symptom. Chronically hypercapnia, polycythemia, and right-sided heart failure may develop.	Symptoms depend on the rate of bronchial occlusion and percentage of affected lung. Rapid occlusion with massive collapse may cause sudden pain, dyspnea, cyanosis, and shock. Slowly developing collapse may be asymptomatic.	Exertional dyspnea and nonproductive cough. In advanced disease cor pulmonale, digital clubbing, and cyanosis may occur.	Typical symptoms include cough, fever, and sputum production, usually developing over days and sometimes accompanied by pleuritic chest pain. Signs of respiratory distress may develop.
Percussion	Resonant	Hyperresonant	Absent in affected area	Resonant to hyperresonant	Dullness over consolidated area
Tactile fremitus	Normal	Decreased	Usually absent	Normal	Increased over consolidated area
Breath sounds	Vesicular	Diminished or not audible	Diminished or not audible	Bronchovesicular	Bronchial over consolidated area
Adventitious sounds	None	When audible, breath sounds are faint and harsh.	None	Velcro-type inspiratory crackles	Late inspiratory crackles over consolidated area
Other		Barrel chest, accessory muscle use, pursed lips, and tripod positioning may be present.	Decreased or delayed chest expansion on affected side	Decreased or delayed chest expansion on affected side	Bronchophony, egophony, whispered pectoriloquy, and decreased chest expansion on affected side

Adapted from Jarvis C: *Physical examination and health assessment*, Philadelphia, 1992, WB Saunders.

■ **A**sthma (wheeze, nocturnal/morning cough), **a**topy, α_1-antitrypsin deficiency
■ **C**ough (nocturnal/morning), **C**XR (known abnormalities)
■ **E**xercise tolerance (quantify: ability to dress oneself, distance walked, and climbing stairs), **e**nvironmental/occupational **e**xposure (allergies, TB, asbestos, vapors, dusts, or farms)
■ **D**yspnea (provocative/palliative factors)

- Upper respiratory tract: Nasal polyps, rhinitis, and sneezing
- Sleeping patterns: Snoring, apnea
- Constitutional symptoms: Fever, chills, night sweats, weight loss, anorexia, and asthenia
- Differentiate from cardiac etiology (see p. 7): PND, orthopnea, and peripheral edema
- Immunization status: Pneumococcal vaccine, influenza vaccine, childhood vaccinations, and Bacille bilié de Calmette-Guérin (BCG) vaccine
- Previous history of respiratory problems: TB, COPD, deep venous thrombosis/pulmonary embolism (DVT/PE), bronchiectasis, recurrent infections such as bronchitis or pneumonia, lung cancer, and cystic fibrosis (CF)

PALPATION: TACTILE FREMITUS

Definition
- **Fremitus** refers to the vibrations transmitted through the bronchopulmonary tree to the chest wall when the patient speaks.

Palpation
- Ask the patient to repeat the words "ninety-nine" or "one-to-one." Palpate the chest wall using the hypothenar aspect of your hand (the vibratory sensitivity of the bones in your hand detects the fremitus). The simultaneous use of both hands, to compare sides, may be beneficial in terms of speed and detection of asymmetry (Figure 2-5).

Decreased Fremitus
- Voice is too soft.
- Transmission of vibrations is impeded: Obstructed bronchus, COPD, pleural effusion, pleural thickening, pneumothorax, infiltrating tumor, or thick chest wall.

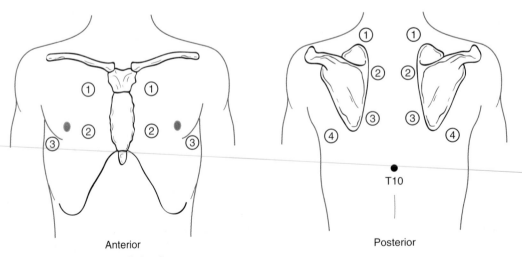

Anterior   Posterior

Figure 2-5 Sites for tactile fremitus.

Increased Fremitus
- Consolidation (pneumonia)
- Atelectasis

PEARL
- Fremitus is often more prominent on the right side, and it disappears below the diaphragm.

PERCUSSION

Definition
- **Percussion** is the act of striking a surface to determine whether underlying tissues are air filled, fluid filled, or solid. It penetrates only 5 to 7 cm and is therefore unable to detect deep lesions. The percussion note should be interpreted using sound and tactile sense (Table 2-3, Figure 2-6).

Percussion
- Percuss posteriorly with both arms of the patient crossed in front to displace the scapulae. Place the palmar surface of your left hand on the chest wall, hyperextending the distal interphalangeal (DIP) joint of your middle finger. Remember that the action of percussion is at the wrist. Using the middle finger of your right hand, strike

Table 2-3   Percussion Notes

Percussion Note	Example	Pathology
Flat	Extremity (e.g., thigh, forearm)	Large pleural effusion
Dull	Liver or spleen	Consolidation (e.g., pneumonia)
Resonant	Normal lung	
Hyperresonant	None normally (very loud, hollow sounding)	Emphysema, pneumothorax
Tympanitic	Gastric air bubble	

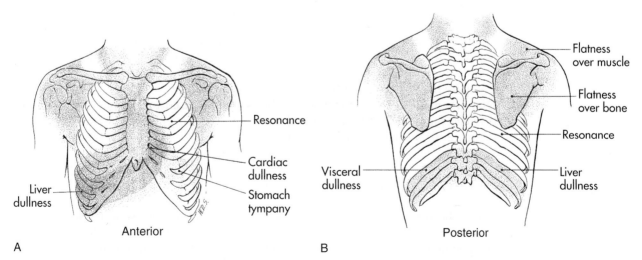

Figure 2-6   A, Expected percussion notes (anterior). **B,** Expected percussion notes (posterior). (From Barkauskas VH, Baumann LC, Darling-Fisher CS: *Health and physical assessment*, ed 3, St. Louis, 2002, Mosby, p. 326, Figure 15-15.)

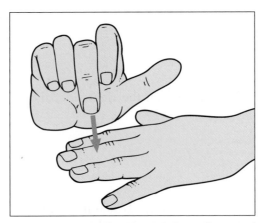

Figure 2-7   Technique for percussion. (From Munro JF, Campbell IW, editors: *Macleod's clinical examination,* ed 10. Edinburgh, 2000, Churchill Livingstone, p 134, Figure 4.16.)

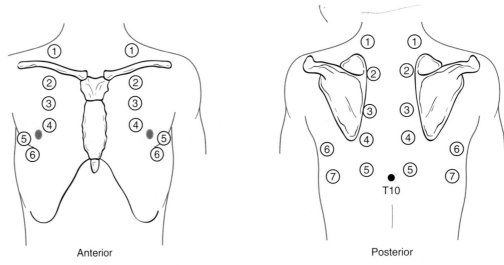

Figure 2-8   Sites for percussion and auscultation.

the DIP of your left middle finger (this requires short fingernails for your own comfort). Percussion of the chest should be performed over the ICSs (to avoid the "dullness" of percussing the ribs). This technique can be difficult to master. An alternative is to use your reflex hammer to strike the hyperextended DIP of your left middle finger (Figure 2-7).

- Compare the percussion notes for symmetry (Figure 2-8).
- **Diaphragmatic excursion** is a percussion technique used to estimate the difference between the level of dullness on inspiration and the level of dullness on expiration (Figure 2-9). Normal excursion is 5 to 6 cm.

AUSCULTATION: THE LUNGS

- Using the diaphragm of the stethoscope, listen for breath sounds, adventitious sounds, and transmitted voice sounds. Instruct the patient to breathe deeply through an open mouth. Use the same pattern suggested for percussion in Figure 2-8, moving from side to side for comparison. Listen to at least one full breath at each location (Table 2-4, Figure 2-10). Ask the patient to cross his or her arms in front when auscultating posteriorly. Beware of hyperventilation, which may cause lightheadedness.

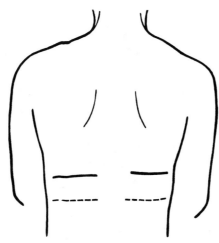

Figure 2-9   Diaphragmatic excursion: the solid line represents the level of dullness at expiration, and the dotted line indicates the level of dullness on inspiration. (From Wilkins RL, Sheldon RL, Krider SJ: *Clinical assessment in respiratory care,* ed 4. St. Louis, 2000, Mosby, p 80, Figure 4-16.)

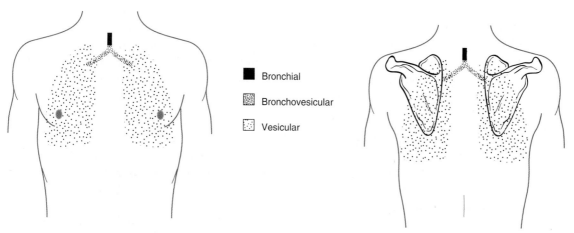

■ Bronchial

▨ Bronchovesicular

⬚ Vesicular

Figure 2-10   Distribution of breath sounds.

Table 2-4   Normal Breath Sounds

Normal Breath Sounds	Duration	Relative Intensity	Example
Vesicular	Inspiration > expiration	Soft	Over most of both lungs
Bronchovesicular	Inspiration = expiration	Intermediate	First and second ICSs anteriorly and between the scapulae
Bronchial	Inspiration < expiration	Loud	Over the manubrium if heard at all

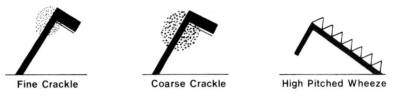

Figure 2-11   Adventitious breath sounds. (Adapted from Lehrer S: *Understanding lung sounds,* ed 3. Philadelphia, 2002, WB Saunders, p 121, Figure 5-29.)

- Breath sounds may be louder at the base posteriorly. Breath sounds are decreased when airflow is decreased (e.g., COPD) or when sound transmission is poor (e.g., pleural effusion, consolidation).

Adventitia
- Adventitious sounds are extra sounds (e.g., crackles, wheezes, and pleural rub) that are superimposed on normal breath sounds (Figure 2-11). Describe the location at which these sounds were identified and their timing within the respiratory cycle. Note the persistence of these sounds from breath to breath and any changes after cough or change in position.

Transmitted Voice Sounds
- Assess transmitted voice sounds if abnormally located bronchial or bronchovesicular sounds are identified. Increased transmission of breath sounds indicates an "airless lung" as in consolidation. Auscultate in symmetric areas over the chest wall as for percussion in Figure 2-8.
  - Ask the patient to say "ninety-nine"; sound should be transmitted as muffled and indistinct.
  - Ask the patient to say "EE"; normally you will hear a muffled long "E" sound.
  - Ask the patient to whisper "ninety-nine" or "one-two-three"; normally heard faintly if at all.

CHEST X-RAY INTERPRETATION

- Start by checking the name and date on the film.
- Note the orientation of the film and adequacy of penetration.
  - Two views are needed to localize lesions.
  - Heart size and mediastinal size should be assessed on a posteroanterior (PA) view of the chest rather than an AP view, on which they will appear larger. On a PA film the cardiothoracic ratio should not be >50%.
  - Assess rotation by looking at the relationship of the sternoclavicular joints to the midline.
  - Note patient position: Upright versus supine.

Interpretation (ABCs)
- **A**irway
  - Trachea and mainstem bronchi

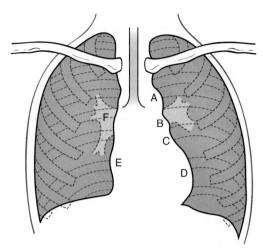

Figure 2-12   Normal chest x-ray. **A,** Aortic knuckle. **B,** Pulmonary artery. **C,** Depression over left auricle. **D,** Left ventricle. **E,** Right atrium. **F,** Position of the horizontal fissure. (Used with permission of Dr. Tom Scott, Memorial University of Newfoundland.)

- **B**reathing
  - Lung fields (apex, upper and lower lobes, right middle lobes, and lingula)
  - Fissures
  - Costophrenic angles
  - Peribronchial changes
  - Pleura: Thickening, effusion
- **C**irculation (Figure 2-12)
  - Vasculature in the lungs
  - Pulmonary artery and aortic knuckle
  - Left ventricle, heart size
  - Hila
- **S**oft tissues and **s**keleton
  - Bilateral breast shadows in females
  - Subcutaneous emphysema
  - Mediastinal enlargement
  - Ribs, clavicle, and humerus

SAMPLE OSCE SCENARIOS

> INSTRUCTIONS TO CANDIDATE: A 62-year-old male presents to the emergency department with new onset of shortness of breath. Take a detailed history, exploring possible etiologies, and perform a focused physical examination.

Definition
- **Dyspnea** is the subjective sensation of SOB that is inappropriate to the circumstances.

DD$_X$ VITAMINS C
- **V**ascular: PE, congestive heart failure (CHF; pulmonary edema, large pleural effusion, significant ascites), and acute coronary syndrome (ACS)
- **I**nfectious: Pneumonia
- **T**raumatic: Pneumothorax, FB aspiration
- **M**etabolic: DKA
- **I**diopathic/**I**atrogenic: Exacerbation of COPD/asthma, massive atelectasis
- **N**eoplastic: Large pleural effusion, significant ascites
- **S**ubstance abuse and **P**sychiatric: Anxiety (diagnosis of exclusion)

- **First evaluate A**irway, **B**reathing, and **C**irculation. It may be necessary to perform an immediate intervention, such as supplemental O$_2$, IV access, or intubation.
  - Is the patient able to talk? Swallow? Cough?
  - Are both lungs ventilated? Is the patient oxygenating (mentation, pulse oximetry)?
  - Abnormal vitals? Peripheral circulation (pulses, capillary refill)?
  - If no immediate interventions are required, proceed to take the history, and perform the physical examination.

History
- **C**haracter: Describe the nature of your breathing difficulty.
- **O**nset: How did the SOB start (sudden versus gradual)? What were you doing when you became SOB?
- **I**ntensity: How severe is your SOB right now, on a scale of 1 to 10 with 1 being mild and 10 being the worst? Has it gotten worse?
- **D**uration: How long have you been SOB?
- **E**vents associated:
  - PE: Hemoptysis, pleuritic chest pain, DVT
  - Pulmonary edema/ACS: Exertional chest pain (CP), PND, orthopnea, and peripheral edema
  - COPD: Cough, wheeze, and progressively worsening SOBOE
  - Pneumonia, other infections: Fever/chills, rigors, increased sputum production, cough
  - Ascites: Abdominal distension
  - Anxiety (diagnosis of exclusion): Lightheadedness, diaphoresis, trembling, choking sensation, palpitations, numbness or tingling in hands/feet, chest pain, nausea, abdominal pain, depersonalization/derealization, flushes or chills, fear of dying, fear of going crazy or doing something uncontrolled
  - Constitutional symptoms: Fever, chills, night sweats, weight loss, anorexia, and asthenia
- **F**requency: Has this ever happened to you before? If so, how often does it happen? When was the last time you became SOB?
- **P**alliative factors: Is there anything that makes your SOB better? If so, what?
- **P**rovocative factors: Is there anything that makes your SOB worse? If so, what?
  - Exertion?

- Position (sitting up versus lying down)?
- Exposure to cold air?
- Infection?
- Allergies?
- **Functional respiratory inquiry:** SPACED
- **Past medical history (PMH)/past surgical history (PSH):** Thromboembolic disease, ischemic heart disease (IHD), valvular disease, COPD, diabetes mellitus (DM), or systemic disease causing immunosuppression
- **Previous investigations:** Pulmonary function tests (PFTs), peak flow, electrocardiogram (ECG), or CXR. What were the results?
- **Medications (MEDS):** Bronchodilators, inhaled steroids, cardiac medications, or antihypertensives
  - Consider noncompliance with medications.
- **Social history (SH):** Smoking, EtOH
- **Immunizations:** Pneumococcal vaccine, influenza vaccine, childhood vaccinations, and BCG vaccine
- **Family history (FH):** Thromboembolic disease, premature IHD

Physical Examination
- **Vitals:** Heart rate (HR) and rhythm, respiratory rate (RR; depth, effort, and pattern), blood pressure (BP), pulsus paradoxus, and temperature
- **General:** Respiratory distress, diaphoresis
- **Skin:** Peripheral edema, cyanosis, clubbing
- **Head, eyes, ears, nose, and throat (HEENT):** Central cyanosis, tracheal position, and lymphadenopathy
- **Respiratory (Resp):** Inspect for thoracic deformity (barrel chest with COPD), chest expansion for symmetry (Figure 2-13), tactile fremitus, percussion, and auscultation (breath sounds, transmitted voice sounds, adventitious sounds); may note a prolonged expiratory phase in obstructive disease.

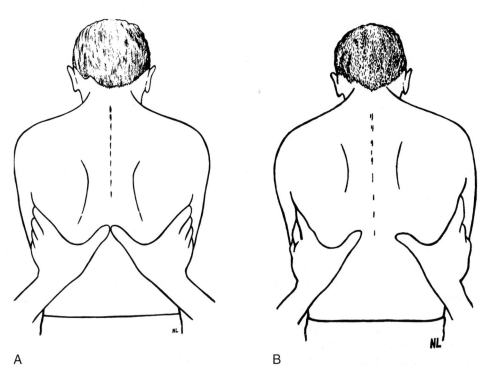

A   B

Figure 2-13 Palpating chest expansion. **A,** Exhalation. **B,** Maximal inhalation. (From Wilkins RL, Sheldon RL, Krider SJ: *Clinical assessment in respiratory care,* ed 4. St. Louis, 2000, Mosby, p 79, Figure 4-14.)

- **Cardiovascular system (CVS):** JVP and hepatojugular reflux (increased venous pressure in CHF), peripheral pulses; palpate apical impulse, and auscultate looking for S_3 or murmurs.
- **Abdomen:** Examine for ascites and organomegaly.
- **Neurologic (Neuro):** Mental status (adequate brain oxygenation)

INSTRUCTIONS TO CANDIDATE: A 58-year-old smoker presents to his family doctor with increasing shortness of breath on exertion. Take a detailed history, exploring possible etiologies, and perform a focused physical examination.

DD$_X$ VITAMINS C
- **Vascular:** CHF (pulmonary edema, pleural effusion)
- **Infectious:** TB
- **Autoimmune/Allergic:** Sarcoidosis
- **Metabolic:** Anemia, asbestosis
- **Idiopathic/Iatrogenic:** COPD, massive atelectasis, pulmonary fibrosis, and abdominal distension (ascites, organomegaly)
- **Neoplastic:** Large pleural effusion

History
- **Ch**aracter: Describe the nature of your breathing difficulty.
- **O**nset: How does the SOB start (sudden versus gradual)? In what type of activity are you engaged when you become SOB?
- **I**ntensity: How severe is your SOB? Do you need to stop and rest during activity? How far can you walk before you must rest? How many stairs can you climb? Has it gotten worse? Over what period of time has it changed?
- **D**uration: When did these episodes start? How long do these episodes last?
- **E**vents associated:
  - COPD: Cough, wheeze, and progressively worsening SOBOE
  - CHF: PND, orthopnea, peripheral edema, ± exertional CP
  - Anemia: Pallor, weakness, fatigue, palpitations
  - Hemoptysis: May be a sign of pulmonary malignancy or TB. It is highly unusual in COPD.
  - Ascites: Abdominal distension
  - Constitutional symptoms: Fever, chills, night sweats, weight loss, anorexia, and asthenia
- **F**requency: How often does it happen? When was the last time you became SOB?
- **P**alliative factors: Is there anything that makes your SOB better? If so, what?
- **P**rovocative factors: Is there anything that makes your SOB worse? If so, what?
  - Exertion?
  - Lying down?
  - Exposure to cold air?
  - Infection?
  - Allergies?
- **Functional respiratory inquiry:** SPACED
- **PMH/PSH:** COPD/asthma, IHD, valvular disease, or malignancy
- **Previous investigations:** PFTs, peak flow, ECG, or CXR. What were the results?
- **MEDS:** Bronchodilators, inhaled steroids, or cardiac medications.
  - Consider noncompliance with medications.
  - Pulmonary fibrosis: Amiodarone, sulfonamides (long-term use), IV abuse of opioids and psychotropics, antineoplastic agents such as bleomycin and chlorambucil

- **SH:** Smoking, EtOH, occupational history, and TB contacts
- **Immunizations:** Pneumococcal vaccine, influenza vaccine, childhood vaccinations, and BCG vaccine
- **FH:** α_1-Antitrypsin deficiency, atopy (eczema, allergic rhinitis, asthma), CF, or premature IHD

Physical Examination
- **Vitals:** HR and rhythm, RR (depth, effort, and pattern), BP, and temperature
- **General:** Respiratory distress, diaphoresis
- **Skin:** Peripheral edema, plethoric appearance (caused by erythrocytosis), cyanosis, clubbing
- **HEENT:** Central cyanosis, tracheal position, lymphadenopathy
- **Resp:** Inspect for thoracic deformity (barrel chest), chest expansion (symmetry), tactile fremitus, percussion, diaphragmatic excursion (low diaphragm in COPD), and auscultation (breath sounds, adventitious sounds); may note a prolonged expiratory phase in obstructive disease.
- **CVS:** JVP and hepatojugular reflux (increased venous pressure in CHF), peripheral pulses, palpate apical impulse, and auscultate, looking for S_3 or murmurs.
- **Abdomen:** Examine for ascites and organomegaly.

PEARLS
- **COPD** includes several disease entities: chronic bronchitis, emphysema, asthma, and bronchiectasis. It is characterized by progressive airway obstruction, punctuated by acute exacerbations—increasing dyspnea and sputum production or acute respiratory failure. Forced expiratory volume in 1 second (FEV_1) and FEV_1/forced vital capacity (FVC) decrease as severity of disease increases. Severe disease may result in cor pulmonale. Cigarette smoking is the major risk factor.
- Most patients have a combination of chronic bronchitis and emphysema rather than exclusively one or the other.

INSTRUCTIONS TO CANDIDATE: A 67-year-old female complains of a bothersome cough. Take a detailed history, exploring possible etiologies, and perform a focused physical examination.

Definition
- **Cough** is a sudden, noisy expulsion of air from the lungs. It is a nonspecific reaction to irritation anywhere from the pharynx to the lungs. Cough may be voluntary or stimulated by external agents (e.g., dust), internal agents (e.g., mucus, inflammation), or external pressure on air passages. Stimulation in the external auditory meatus may also precipitate cough.

DD$_X$ VITAMINS C
- **Vascular:** CHF, PE
- **Infectious:** Pneumonia, upper respiratory tract infection (URTI; pharyngitis, laryngitis, tracheitis, tracheobronchitis), pertussis, and TB
- **Traumatic:** Inhalational injury, FB aspiration
- **Autoimmune/Allergic:** Sarcoidosis

- **I**diopathic/**I**atrogenic: Postnasal drip, gastroesophageal reflux (GER), aspiration pneumonitis, COPD/asthma, and angiotensin-converting enzyme (ACE) inhibitor
- **N**eoplasm
- **C**ongenital/genetic: Anatomic abnormalities in tracheobronchial tree or compressing the tracheobronchial tree, CF

History

- **Ch**aracter: What is the cough like?
  - Clearing of the throat: GER and postnasal drip
  - Brassy cough (hard and metallic): Conditions that narrow the trachea or larynx
  - Barking cough (like a seal): Croup
  - Hacking cough: Pharyngitis, tracheobronchitis, and early pneumonia
  - Whooping cough: Pertussis
  - Any sputum production? If so, what color and how much (mucus, blood, pus, pink froth)?
- **O**nset: How did it start (sudden versus gradual)?
- **I**ntensity: At what time of day is your cough at its worst? Does it keep you awake at night (asthma and chronic bronchitis may be associated with nocturnal or morning cough)?
- **D**uration: How long has it been going on (acute versus chronic versus paroxysmal versus seasonal versus perennial)? If cough is chronic, how has it changed recently? Is it getting better, worse, or staying the same?
- **E**vents associated:
  - Pneumonia: Fever, chills, rigors, increased sputum production
  - URTI: Malaise, sore throat, rhinorrhea, myalgias, headache, ear pain
  - Tracheitis: Retrosternal pain like a hot poker
  - TB/malignancy: Hemoptysis, constitutional symptoms
  - CHF: Exertional dyspnea, orthopnea, PND
  - GER: Heartburn, epigastric pain
  - Constitutional symptoms: Fever, chills, night sweats, weight loss, anorexia, and asthenia
- **F**requency: Have you ever had a cough before? When? How often?
- **P**alliative factors: Is there anything that makes the cough better? If so, what?
- **P**rovocative factors: What brings on the cough? What makes the cough worse?
- **Functional respiratory inquiry:** SPACED
- **PMH/PSH:** Previous pneumonia, CHF, COPD/asthma, TB exposure, immuno-suppression, or previous aspiration
- **MEDS:** ACE inhibitors are known to have cough as a side effect.
- **SH:** Travel history, smoking, and EtOH (increased risk for aspiration)
- **Immunizations:** Pneumococcal vaccine, influenza vaccine, childhood vaccinations, and BCG vaccine
- **FH:** COPD, IHD, α_1-antitrypsin deficiency, CF, or TB

Physical Examination

- **Vitals:** HR and rhythm, RR (depth, effort, and pattern), BP, and temperature
- **General:** Respiratory distress, observe for coughing during the history and examination
- **Skin:** Peripheral edema, cyanosis, clubbing
- **HEENT:** Central cyanosis, tracheal position, lymphadenopathy, tympanic membranes, pharynx, and tonsils
- **Resp:** Chest expansion (symmetry), tactile fremitus, percussion, and auscultation (breath sounds, transmitted voice sounds, adventitious sounds)
- **CVS:** JVP and hepatojugular reflux (increased venous pressure in CHF), peripheral pulses; palpate apical impulse and auscultate, looking for S_3 or murmurs.
- **Abdomen:** Examine for ascites and organomegaly.

> INSTRUCTIONS TO CANDIDATE: A 70-year-old male presents to the emergency department after coughing up some blood. Take a detailed history, exploring possible etiologies, and perform a focused physical examination.

Definition
- **Hemoptysis** is the coughing or "spitting" up of blood originating from lungs or airways.

DD$_X$ VITAMINS C
- **V**ascular: PE, pulmonary hypertension (e.g., mitral stenosis), arteriovenous malformation (AVM), and vasculitis
- **I**nfectious: TB, lung abscess, pneumonia, and bronchitis
- **T**raumatic: FB aspiration
- **A**utoimmune/**A**llergic: Goodpasture's syndrome, Wegener's granulomatosis
- **M**etabolic: Coagulopathy
- **I**diopathic/**I**atrogenic: Bronchiectasis
- **N**eoplastic: Bronchogenic carcinoma

- **First evaluate A**irway, **B**reathing, and **C**irculation. It may be necessary to perform an immediate intervention, such as supplemental O_2, IV access, or intubation.
  - Is the patient able to talk? Swallow? Cough?
  - Are both lungs ventilated? Is the patient oxygenating (mentation, pulse oximetry)?
  - Abnormal vitals? Peripheral circulation (pulses, capillary refill)?
  - If no immediate interventions are required, proceed to take the history, and perform the physical examination.

History
- **Ch**aracter: Did you vomit blood or cough up blood? Was it pure blood or blood-tinged mucus? What color was it: bright red, rust, brown, pink and frothy, coffee ground appearance? Amount?
- **O**nset: What were you doing when it first happened?
- **I**ntensity: Quantify the amount of blood coughed up.
- **D**uration: How long has this been happening? Is it getting better, worse, or staying the same?
- **E**vents associated:
  - Recent infections, exposure to TB
  - Lung cancer: Pain, SOB, constitutional symptoms
  - CHF: PND, orthopnea, peripheral edema, ± exertional CP/dyspnea
  - PE: Sudden SOB, pleuritic chest pain, DVT
  - Goodpasture's syndrome: SOB, hematuria, renal failure
  - Wegener's granulomatosis: Epistaxis, sinusitis, hematuria, constitutional symptoms, skin lesions
  - Constitutional symptoms: Fever, chills, night sweats, weight loss, anorexia, and asthenia
  - Differentiate from gastrointestinal (GI) bleeding, aspirated blood from epistaxis, bleeding gums, and so on.
- **F**requency: Has this ever happened to you before? When? How often?
- **P**alliative factors: Is there anything that has helped make this better? If so, what?
- **P**rovocative factors: What brought on previous episodes, if anything?
- **Functional respiratory inquiry:** SPACED
- **PMH/PSH:** Lung cancer, bleeding diathesis, CHF, HIV, poor dental hygiene, peptic ulcer disease (PUD), or TB
- **MEDS:** Anticoagulants (warfarin, heparin), acetylsalicylic acid (ASA), or NSAIDS

- **SH:** Smoking, EtOH use (Mallory-Weiss tear caused by severe retching or esophageal varices), and occupational hazards (e.g., asbestos, coal, hay)
- **FH:** Bleeding disorders, lung cancer, other lung disease, or TB

Physical Examination
- **Vitals:** HR and rhythm, RR (depth, effort, pattern), BP (hypotension in massive hemoptysis), and temperature
- **General:** Respiratory distress
- **Skin:** Clubbing, purple plaques (Kaposi's sarcoma), rashes (paraneoplastic syndromes), petechiae, and ecchymosis
- **HEENT:** Central cyanosis, tracheal position, lymphadenopathy, nose trauma, ulceration of nasal septum and mucosa (Wegener's), dental caries, gum disease
- **Resp:** Chest expansion (symmetry), tactile fremitus, percussion, auscultation (breath sounds, transmitted voice sounds, adventitious sounds, apical crackles [TB], friction rub)
- **CVS:** JVP and hepatojugular reflux (increased venous pressure in CHF), peripheral pulses, palpate apical impulse, and auscultate looking for P_2, S_3, or murmurs.
- **Abdomen:** Palpate for organomegaly, epigastric tenderness.
- **MSK:** Peripheral edema, calf circumference, Homans's sign, and Lisker sign

PEARL
- Blood originating from the stomach is usually darker than that from the respiratory tract. Blood originating from the GI tract is sometimes aspirated and coughed up.

INSTRUCTIONS TO CANDIDATE: A 20-year-old female with a long history of asthma presents to her family doctor complaining of frequent exacerbations since moving out of her parents' home. Take a detailed history, exploring possible etiologies.

Definition
- **Asthma** is a pulmonary disease characterized by reversible airway obstruction, airway inflammation, and increased airway responsiveness to a variety of stimuli. Airway obstruction in asthma is caused by spasm of airway smooth muscle, edema of airway mucosa, increased mucus secretion, cellular infiltration of airway walls, and injury and desquamation of the airway epithelium.

History
- **Character:** How has your asthma changed since moving to your new apartment? Cough? Dyspnea? Wheezing? Chest pain? Sleep disturbance? Night cough? When are symptoms most severe (time of day, time of week)? Diurnal variation (worse in early morning)?
- **Onset:** How long have you been known to have asthma? When did you notice that your asthma was worse?
- **Intensity:** Please rate the severity of your asthma on a scale of 1 to 10 with 1 being mild and 10 being the worst.
- **Duration:** How long do your asthma attacks last?
- **Events associated:**
  - Ask about adjustment to living away from home.
  - How much time have you lost from school/work?
  - Have you had any asthma attacks that required treatment in hospital? How were you treated?
  - Have you ever been intubated?
  - Do you keep records of your peak flow? How has it changed in the past year?
  - Exercise induced?

- **Frequency:** How frequently are you having asthma attacks?
- **Palliative factors:** What improves your asthma?
- **Provocative factors:** What brings on the attacks?
  - Exposure to known allergens: Animal dander, dust mites, pollen, feathers
  - Basement apartment? Roommate with pets or stuffed animals? Carpets? Pillow?
  - Environment: Exposure to cold air, industrialized area, air pollution/smog, scented products
  - Do you smoke? Does your roommate smoke?
  - Occupational: Industrial chemicals, plastics, detergents, plush
  - Infections: URTI, pneumonia, influenza
  - Exercise: Change in exercise habits, exposure to cold air
  - Emotional stress: Crying, screaming, or hard laughing
- **Functional respiratory inquiry:** SPACED
- **PMH/PSH:** Asthma, atopy, or GER
- **MEDS:** NSAIDs, ASA, β-blockers, or sulfa drugs
  - Any increase/decrease in medication dosage? More frequent use of inhalers?
  - Noncompliance?
  - Have you been prescribed any new medications?
- **SH:** Smoking, EtOH
- **FH:** Asthma, allergic rhinitis, atopy, or eczema

PEARLS

- Symptoms of asthma are variable. Episodes may be mild and brief. Others have mild coughing and wheezing much of the time, punctuated by severe exacerbations. An attack may begin suddenly with wheezing, coughing, SOB, and chest tightness or insidiously with slowly increasing manifestations of respiratory distress. The cough during an acute attack sounds "tight" and generally does not produce sputum. Dry cough, particularly at night and during exercise, may be the sole presenting symptom.
- **Asthma triad:** Atopy, ASA sensitivity, and nasal polyps

> INSTRUCTIONS TO CANDIDATE: A 26-year-old female presents to the emergency department with an "asthma attack." She has used her albuterol puffer several times and is still having difficulty speaking in full sentences. Treatment is initiated in the emergency department. Perform a focused physical examination.

- **First evaluate A**irway, **B**reathing, and **C**irculation. It may be necessary to perform an immediate intervention, such as supplemental O_2, IV access, or intubation.
  - Is the patient able to talk? Swallow? Cough?
  - Are both lungs ventilated? Is the patient oxygenating (mentation, pulse oximetry)?
  - Abnormal vitals? Peripheral circulation (pulses, capillary refill)?
  - If no immediate interventions are required, proceed to perform an appropriate physical examination.

Physical Examination

- **Vitals:** HR and rhythm, RR (depth, effort, and pattern), BP, pulsus paradoxus, and temperature
- **General:** Respiratory distress (e.g., inability to speak), diaphoresis, anxiety
- **Resp** (Table 2-5): Inspect for thoracic deformity, chest expansion (symmetry), tactile fremitus, percussion, and auscultation (breath sounds, adventitious sounds).
- **CVS:** JVP and hepatojugular reflux (signs of venous congestion may herald a pneumothorax), peripheral pulses, palpate apical impulse, and auscultate looking for loud P_2, S_3, or murmurs.

Table 2-5 Expected Findings in an Acute Exacerbation of Asthma	
Examination	**Expected Findings**
Thoracic deformity	Barrel chest: hyperinflation
Chest movement	May be asymmetrical in case of associated pneumothorax
Trachea	Midline, may note tracheal tug
Tactile fremitus	Decreased
Percussion	Hyperresonant, flattened diaphragms
Breath sounds	Prolonged expiratory phase; localized disappearance of breath sounds can occur temporarily from bronchial plugging
Adventitious sounds	High pitched wheezes

- **Neuro:** Mental status (adequate brain oxygenation)
- If there are no signs of respiratory distress then proceed with the remainder of the examination:
- **Skin:** Peripheral edema, cyanosis, clubbing, eczema
- **HEENT:** Central cyanosis, tracheal position (tug may be noted), lymphadenopathy, nasal polyps, rhinitis

PEARLS
- A quiet-sounding chest in a patient having an asthma attack may be a *warning* of patient fatigue or obstruction of small airways. It can quickly become *life threatening*.
- The most reliable signs of a severe attack are dyspnea at rest, inability to speak, accessory muscle use, cyanosis, and pulsus paradoxus. An asthma attack may begin with cough and wheezing, rapidly progressing to dyspnea. Confusion and lethargy may indicate respiratory failure and CO_2 narcosis. A normal or increased $PaCO_2$ may indicate respiratory failure (hyperventilation should result in a decreased $PaCO_2$).

INSTRUCTIONS TO CANDIDATE: One of your patients recently had a "screening CXR." Your assistant hands you a report saying there is a solitary nodule in the left lung (Figure 2-14). This 56-year-old male is now in your office. Perform an appropriate functional inquiry. List the differential diagnosis of a solitary pulmonary nodule.

DD$_X$ VITAMINS C
- **Vascular:** Infarct, vascular lesion
- **Infectious:** TB (granuloma), histoplasmosis, aspergilloma, abscess, and consolidation
- **Traumatic:** Hematoma
- **Idiopathic/Iatrogenic:** Fluid-filled cyst, artifact
- **Neoplastic:** Bronchial carcinoma (squamous cell carcinoma, adenocarcinoma, small cell carcinoma, large cell carcinoma), metastatic disease, and benign neoplasm (bronchial adenoma, hamartoma)

History
- Use **ChLORIDE FPP** to delineate any identified symptoms.
  - Hemoptysis
  - Wheeze: Obstructing lesion
  - Chest infections: Postobstructive process, pneumonia, TB, and abscess
  - Alcoholism: Increased risk of aspiration

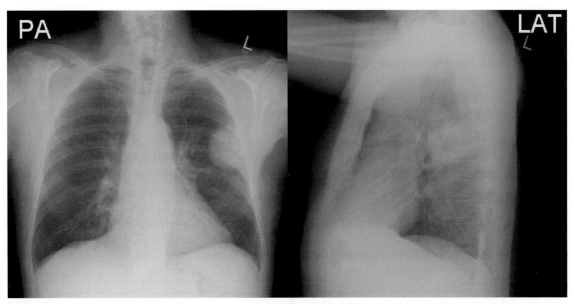

Figure 2-14   Posteroanterior and lateral views of the chest. There is a solitary mass in the left upper lobe of the lung.

- Constitutional symptoms: Fever, chills, night sweats, weight loss, anorexia, and asthenia
- **Functional respiratory inquiry:** SPACED
  - **S**moking (quantify pack-years), **S**OBOE, and **s**putum production (mucus, pus, blood)
  - **P**ain (pleuritic, bony/MSK, tracheobronchial), **p**igeons
  - **A**sthma (wheeze, nocturnal/morning cough), **a**topy, and α_1-antitrypsin deficiency
  - **C**ough (nocturnal/morning), **C**XR (known abnormalities)
  - **E**xercise tolerance (quantify: ability to dress oneself, distance walked and climbing stairs), **e**nvironmental/occupational **e**xposure (allergies, TB, asbestos, vapors, dusts or farms)
  - **D**yspnea (provocative/palliative factors)

Symptoms Associated with Malignant Spread
- Hoarseness (recurrent laryngeal nerve)
- Superior vena cava (SVC) syndrome (increased JVP, dyspnea, congestion of face and neck)
- Dysphagia (esophageal compression)
- Horner's syndrome and brachial plexus invasion (Pancoast tumor)
- Hepatomegaly and lymphadenopathy (metastasis)
- Bone pain (bone mets)
- Seizures or neurologic deficits (brain mets)

Paraneoplastic Syndromes
- **Endocrine:** Hypercalcemia (bony mets or PTH-related protein [PTHrp] secretion by squamous cell carcinoma), Cushing's syndrome (secretion of adrenocorticotropic hormone [ACTH] by small cell carcinoma), and hyponatremia (syndrome of inappropriate antidiuretic hormone [SIADH])
- **Neuromuscular:** Sensory neuropathy, cerebellar ataxia, and Eaton-Lambert myasthenic syndrome (small cell carcinoma; characterized by progressive proximal myopathy with absent reflexes brought out after brief periods of isometric contractions; bulbar muscles are unaffected)
- **Cutaneous:** Acanthosis nigricans in body folds such as in the axillae (adenocarcinoma)

- **MSK:** Hypertrophic osteoarthropathy—clubbing, arthralgias of the wrists and ankles (squamous cell carcinoma)

Risk Factors for Malignancy

- Cigarette smoking is the major risk factor for developing lung malignancy. *Adenocarcinoma is not related to cigarette smoking.* Other risk factors include increasing age and exposure to asbestos, radiation, chromium, iron, or iron oxides.

PEARL

- **Tuberculosis** is an infection caused by *Mycobacterium tuberculosis or Mycobacterium bovis*. TB is usually transmitted through inhalation of droplet nuclei from a person who has active pulmonary TB. Initial infection leaves **nodular scars** in the apex of the lung; immunity rapidly develops, and infection is walled off **(Ghon complex)**. Identification of acid-fast bacilli (AFB) in a sputum smear is strong presumptive evidence of TB; definitive diagnosis is made only on results of polymerase chain reaction (PCR) identification of *M. tuberculosis* or a sputum culture.

> INSTRUCTIONS TO CANDIDATE: A 48-year-old male with unresectable bronchogenic carcinoma presents with worsening shortness of breath. Perform a focused physical examination. Interpret this patient's CXR, and describe expected physical findings (Figure 2-15).

- **First evaluate A**irway, **B**reathing, and **C**irculation. It may be necessary to perform an immediate intervention, such as supplemental O_2, IV access, or intubation.
  - Is the patient able to talk? Swallow? Cough?
  - Are both lungs ventilated? Is the patient oxygenating (mentation, pulse oximetry)?
  - Abnormal vitals? Peripheral circulation (pulses, capillary refill)?
  - If no immediate interventions are required, proceed to take the history, and perform the physical examination.

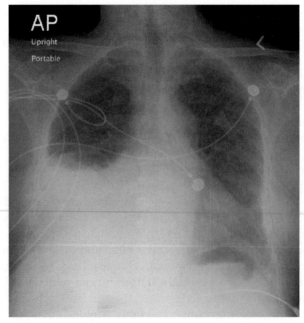

Figure 2-15   Anteroposterior view of the chest (portable).

CXR Interpretation
* Start by checking the name and date on the film. This is an AP view of the chest that is adequately penetrated. The right hemidiaphragm is not visible, and the right heart border is obliterated. There is some tracking at the pleural margin, suggesting a right-sided pleural effusion.

Definitions
* **Pleural effusion** is the accumulation of fluid in the pleural space, which lies between the chest wall and the air-filled lung. A thin layer of pleural fluid usually lines the pleural space. Types of effusions:
  * Transudate
  * Exudate
  * Pus *(empyema)*
  * Chyle *(chylothorax)*
  * Blood *(hemothorax)*
* A transudate is differentiated from an exudate using laboratory values based on the pleural fluid. This fluid is collected using **thoracentesis** (Table 2-6). The fluid should be sent for cell count, protein, albumin, lactate dehydrogenase (LDH), glucose, Gram stain, culture, and cytology.
* **Transudates** may be caused by increased venous pressure or hypoproteinemic states causing reduced capillary oncotic pressure. Transudates are often bilateral. Etiologies include:
  * Hypoproteinemia: Nephrotic syndrome, protein-losing enteropathy
  * Increased venous pressure: CHF, constrictive pericarditis, fluid overload, cirrhosis, PE, and myxedema
* **Exudates** may be caused by increased leakiness of pleural capillaries/inflammation. Effusions are unilateral in focal diseases and bilateral in systemic and diffuse lung diseases. Etiologies include:
  * Infectious: Pneumonia, TB, fungal infection, viral infection, and abscess
  * Inflammatory: Pulmonary infarction, collagen vascular disease, pancreatitis, and Dressler's syndrome
  * Neoplastic: Lung cancer, mesothelioma, lymphoma, and metastatic disease
  * Miscellaneous: Asbestos exposure, drugs, and Meige's syndrome

Physical Examination
* **Vitals:** HR and rhythm, RR (depth, effort, and pattern), BP, and temperature
* **General:** Respiratory distress, diaphoresis, anxiety
* **Skin:** Peripheral edema, cyanosis, clubbing
* **HEENT:** Central cyanosis, tracheal position, lymphadenopathy
* **Resp** (Table 2-7): Chest expansion (symmetry), tactile fremitus, percussion, and auscultation
* **CVS:** JVP, peripheral pulses, palpate apical impulse, and auscultate
* **Neuro:** Mental status (adequate brain oxygenation)

Table 2-6   Pleural Fluid

	Protein (PRO)	LDH	Fluid:Serum PRO Ratio	Fluid:Serum LDH Ratio
Transudate	<30 g/L	<200 U/L	<0.5	<0.6
Exudate	>30 g/L	>200 U/L	>0.5	>0.6

Table 2-7   Expected Findings in Pleural Effusion

Examination	Expected Findings
Chest expansion	May be decreased ipsilaterally
Trachea	Deviation toward opposite side with large effusions
Tactile fremitus	Decreased to absent; may be increased near top of a large effusion
Percussion	Dull to flat over fluid
Breath sounds	Decreased to absent; bronchial sounds may be heard near the top of a large effusion
Adventitious sounds	None except for possible pleural rub

> INSTRUCTIONS TO CANDIDATE: A 32-year-old female presents with fever, rigors, and green sputum. Perform a focused physical examination. Interpret this patient's CXR, and describe expected physical findings (Figure 2-16).

- **First evaluate A**irway, **B**reathing, and **C**irculation. It may be necessary to perform an immediate intervention, such as supplemental O_2, IV access, or intubation.
  - Is the patient able to talk? Swallow? Cough?
  - Are both lungs ventilated? Is the patient oxygenating (mentation, pulse oximetry)?
  - Abnormal vitals? Peripheral circulation (pulses, capillary refill)?
  - If no immediate interventions are required, proceed to take the history, and perform the physical examination.

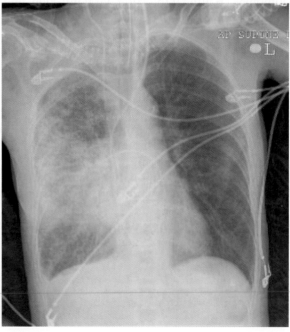

Figure 2-16   Anteroposterior view of the chest (portable).

CXR Interpretation

- Start by checking the name and date on the film. This is an AP view of the chest that is adequately penetrated. There is an infiltrate throughout the right lung with lobar

consolidation of the right middle lobe (RML). The right costophrenic angle is blunted.
- At the time of this CXR, the patient had already been admitted to the intensive care unit (ICU) because of respiratory failure and septic shock. The CXR shows that the patient is intubated. There is a right internal jugular central line and a left internal jugular line through which a pulmonary artery catheter has been inserted. Cardiac monitor leads also are visible.

Definitions
- **Pneumonia** is inflammation of the lungs causing consolidation.
- **Lobar pneumonia** is marked by inflammation of one or more lobes of the lung and an intraalveolar exudate resulting in consolidation; often caused by *Streptococcus pneumoniae*.
- **Bronchopneumonia** is a patchy distribution of inflammation that generally involves more than one lobe.
- **Atypical pneumonia** is an extensive but tenuous pulmonary infiltrate with fever, malaise, myalgia, sore throat, and a cough. Common causative agents are *Mycoplasma pneumoniae* and *Chlamydia pneumoniae*.

Physical Examination
- **Vitals:** HR and rhythm, RR (depth, effort, and pattern), BP, and temperature
  - The patient was febrile, tachypneic, tachycardic, and hypotensive.
- **General:** Respiratory distress, diaphoresis
- **Skin:** Peripheral edema, cyanosis, clubbing
- **HEENT:** Central cyanosis, tracheal position, lymphadenopathy, inspect oropharynx and tympanic membranes (TMs)
- **Resp** (Table 2-8): Chest expansion (symmetry), tactile fremitus, percussion, and auscultation (breath sounds, adventitious sounds, transmitted breath sounds). Expect positive findings in the area of the RML (some findings may be evident throughout the right lung).
- **CVS:** JVP, peripheral pulses, palpate the apical impulse, and auscultate, looking for extra heart sounds or murmurs.
- **Neuro:** Mental status (adequate brain oxygenation)

Table 2-8 Expected Findings in Consolidation

Examination	Expected Findings
Chest movement	May be asymmetrical because of pleuritic chest pain
Trachea	Midline
Tactile fremitus	Increased
Percussion	Dull over airless area
Breath sounds	Bronchial or bronchovesicular over consolidated area; breath sounds may be decreased
Adventitious sounds	Late inspiratory crackles over consolidated area
Transmitted voice sounds (ask patient to speak while you listen with stethoscope)	Spoken words: louder and clearer *(bronchophony)* Spoken "EE": heard as "AY" *(egophony)* Whispered words: louder and clearer *(whispered pectoriloquy)*

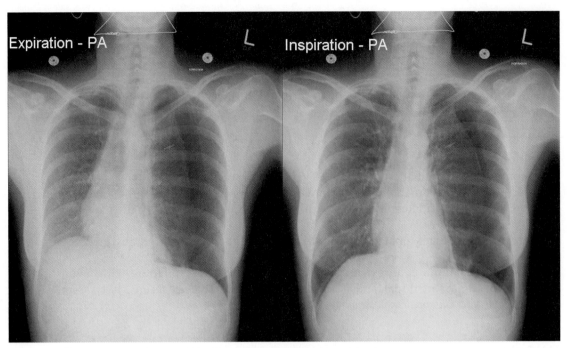

Figure 2-17   Expiratory and inspiratory posteroanterior views of the chest.

INSTRUCTIONS TO CANDIDATE: A 24-year-old female presents to the emergency depart-ment with sudden onset of left-sided chest pain and mild shortness of breath. She has had two previous pneumothoraces. Perform a focused physical examination. Interpret this patient's CXR, and describe expected physical findings (Figure 2-17).

- **First evaluate A**irway, **B**reathing, and **C**irculation. It may be necessary to perform an immediate intervention, such as supplemental O_2, IV access, or intubation.
  - Is the patient able to talk? Swallow? Cough?
  - Are both lungs ventilated? Is the patient oxygenating (mentation, pulse oximetry)?
  - Abnormal vitals? Peripheral circulation (pulses, capillary refill)?
  - If no immediate interventions are required, proceed to take the history, and perform the physical examination.

CXR Interpretation
- Start by checking the name and date on the film. These are PA expiratory and inspi-ratory films that are adequately penetrated. The pulmonary vascular markings do not extend to the left chest wall in either film, and there is increased lucency of the left hemithorax. This is enhanced on the expiratory film where there is also notable shift of the trachea and mediastinum.

Definition and Pathogenesis
- Pneumothorax is the presence of air in the pleural cavity. The pressure in the thoracic cavity is usually less than atmospheric pressure. An opening in the thoracic wall or the lung will admit air to the pleural cavity, producing a pneumothorax (Figure 2-18). If the pressure in the cavity increases to atmospheric pressure, the lung will collapse, recoiling from the chest wall. An open pneumothorax is present after puncture of the thoracic wall in which the chamber is still open to the atmosphere. A closed pneu-mothorax is present when air has been admitted to the cavity but the route is subse-quently sealed.

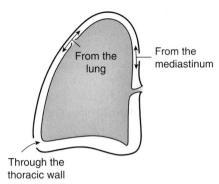

From the
lung

From the
mediastinum

Through the
thoracic wall

Figure 2-18   Pneumothorax. (Used with the permission of Dr. Tom Scott, Memorial University of Newfoundland.)

Table 2-9   Expected Findings in Pneumothorax

Examination	Expected Findings
Chest movement	May be decreased ipsilaterally
Trachea	Deviation toward the opposite side
Tactile fremitus	Decreased to absent ipsilaterally
Percussion	Hyperresonant or tympanitic over pleural air
Breath sounds	Decreased to absent ipsilaterally
Adventitious sounds	None except for possible pleural rub

DD$_x$ VITAMINS C
- **Infectious:** Abscess, pneumonia, and TB
- **Traumatic:** Puncture by a fractured rib, penetrating injury (stab wound, gunshot wound)
- **Idiopathic/Iatrogenic:** Spontaneous pneumothorax, COPD/asthma (bleb formation), central line insertion, thoracentesis, mechanical ventilation (barotrauma), thoracentesis, ascent in airplane
- **Neoplasm**
- **Congenital/genetic:** Rupture of subpleural bleb, CF

Physical Examination
- **Vitals:** HR and rhythm, RR (depth, effort, and pattern), BP, pulsus paradoxus, and temperature
- **General:** Respiratory distress, diaphoresis, anxiety
- **Skin:** Peripheral edema, cyanosis, clubbing, eczema
- **HEENT:** Central cyanosis, tracheal position, lymphadenopathy
- **Resp** (Table 2-9): Inspect for thoracic deformity (e.g., pectus excavatum associated with Marfan's syndrome), chest expansion (symmetry), tactile fremitus, percussion, and auscultation.
- **CVS:** JVP and hepatojugular reflux (signs of venous congestion consistent with pneumothorax), peripheral pulses, palpate the apical impulse, and auscultate.
- **Neuro:** Mental status (adequate brain oxygenation)

PEARLS
- A **tension pneumothorax** is an *emergency* and occurs when a pleural defect forms a one-way valve, allowing air to enter during inspiration but preventing escape of air during expiration. Positive pressure in the pleural space escalates, resulting in extreme shift of the trachea and mediastinum. Both lungs and heart are compressed,

causing severe dyspnea, decreased venous return, decreased CO, and decreased BP. This is a *clinical diagnosis* rather than a radiologic one.

- **Signs and symptoms:** Severe dyspnea, deep cyanosis, ipsilateral hyperresonance to percussion and absence of breath sounds, contralateral tracheal and mediastinal deviation, distended neck veins, hypotension, and tachycardia
- **Treatment:** Insertion of large-bore needle into the second ICS at the MCL to release pressure. Definitive management includes insertion of a chest tube.

SAMPLE CHECKLIST

INSTRUCTIONS TO CANDIDATE: Demonstrate the boundaries of the right middle lobe of the lung. Auscultate the lung, and state over which lobe you are listening. Describe auscultatory findings consistent with right middle lobe consolidation.

Key Points	Satisfactorily Completed
Introduces self to the patient	❏
Determines how the patient wishes to be addressed	❏
Explains nature of the examination to the patient	❏
Examines the patient in a logical fashion	❏
Boundaries of the RML of the lung • Oblique fissure: Like a string connecting T3 posteriorly, to the fifth rib at the MAL and the sixth rib at the MCL	❏
• Horizontal fissure: Anteriorly, runs close to the fourth rib and meets the oblique fissure in the MAL near the fifth rib	❏
Auscultation • Uses diaphragm of stethoscope	❏
• Instructs patient to breathe deeply through an open mouth	❏
• Moves from side to side for comparison	❏
• Listens for at least one full breath in each location	❏
• Auscultates posteriorly with both arms of the patient crossed in front to displace scapulae	❏
• States he or she would listen to at least five locations anteriorly and posteriorly	❏
Description of expected findings • Breath sounds: Bronchial or bronchovesicular sounds over consolidated area; breath sounds may be decreased	❏
• Adventitious sounds: Late inspiratory crackles over consolidated area	❏
Transmitted voice sounds: • Spoken "EE": Heard as "AY" (egophony)	❏
• Whispered words: Louder and clearer (whispered pectoriloquy)	❏
• Spoken words: Louder and clearer (bronchophony)	❏
Drapes the patient appropriately	❏
Makes appropriate closing remarks	❏

CHAPTER 3

Gastrointestinal System

OBJECTIVES

ANATOMY

CARDINAL SIGNS AND SYMPTOMS

ESSENTIAL CLINICAL COMPETENCIES

APPROACH TO TAKING A HISTORY OF ABDOMINAL PAIN
APPROACH TO THE GASTROINTESTINAL EXAMINATION
PERFORM A FOCUSED EXAMINATION OF THE LIVER
PERFORM A FOCUSED EXAMINATION OF THE SPLEEN
PERFORM A FOCUSED EXAMINATION FOR HERNIAS
PERFORM A DIGITAL RECTAL EXAMINATION
PERFORM A FOCUSED PHYSICAL EXAMINATION FOR ASCITES

SAMPLE OSCE SCENARIOS

- A 27-year-old male with chronic viral hepatitis presents with jaundice. Perform a focused physical examination for extrahepatic manifestations of liver disease.
- An 18-year-old female presents to the emergency department with right lower quadrant pain and loss of appetite since yesterday. Perform a focused history and physical examination, exploring possible etiologies.
- A 40-year-old female presents to the emergency department with severe right upper quadrant pain for 8 hours. She is also worried because her friend told her she looked yellow. Perform a focused history and physical examination.
- A 70-year-old male presents to the emergency department with excruciating epigastric pain and vomiting. He has been living alone since his wife died 2 years ago and admits to drinking a "flask daily." Perform a focused history and physical examination.
- A 58-year-old female presents to the emergency department with sharp left lower quadrant pain, worsening over 2 days. She has had one similar episode last year that resolved spontaneously over several days. Perform a focused history and physical examination.
- A 77-year-old female presents to the emergency department complaining of passing bright red blood with her bowel movements. Take a detailed history, exploring possible etiologies, and perform a focused physical examination.
- A 57-year-old male presents to his family doctor complaining of "trouble swallowing." He is losing weight because he is unable to eat. Take a detailed history, exploring possible etiologies.
- A 42-year-old homeless female well known to the emergency department presents complaining of vomiting for 2 days. She now notes blood in her vomitus. Take a detailed history, exploring possible etiologies.
- A 22-year-old female presents to her family doctor complaining of "greasy," foul-smelling stools. She also notes weight loss. Take a detailed history, exploring possible etiologies.
- A 33-year-old male presents to the emergency department with 6 hours of diarrhea and vomiting. He vomits twice in triage. Take a detailed history, exploring possible etiologies.
- A 64-year-old male presents to his family doctor requesting a laxative because he is always "blocked up." Take a detailed history, exploring possible etiologies.

Continued

SAMPLE CHECKLISTS
- ❏ Demonstrate examination of the liver, and describe your actions.
- ❏ Demonstrate a focused physical examination for splenomegaly.
- ❏ Inspect for visible extrahepatic stigmata of liver disease, and describe your findings.
- ❏ Perform a focused physical examination for ascites, and describe your findings.

OBJECTIVES

*The successful student should be able to take a **focused history** of the gastrointestinal (GI) system, including:*
- Appetite, weight gain/loss
- Diet and eating habits
- Dysphagia (liquids/solids), pain on swallowing
- Nausea, vomiting, hematemesis
- Hematochezia, melena, stool color
- Constipation, diarrhea, change in bowel habits/stool caliber
- Laxative use
- Heartburn
- Abdominal pain
- Jaundice
- Alcohol use
- Hemorrhoids

*The GI **examination** will include:*

Inspection
- Extrahepatic stigmata of liver disease
  - Skin and nail changes
  - Muscle wasting
  - Hypogonadism
  - Striae, scars
- Distension
- Masses
- Peristalsis
- Abdominal pulsations

Auscultation
- Identify the presence of bowel sounds in each quadrant.

Palpation
- Tenderness, guarding
- Rebound tenderness
- Liver
- Spleen
- Ascites: Fluid thrill
- Identify any masses.
- Identify any hernias: Inguinal, umbilical, incisional, and spigelian.

Percussion
- Compare percussion notes in each quadrant from side to side.
- Determine the liver span.
- Spleen: Traube's space and Castell's sign
- Ascites: Shifting dullness

ANATOMY (Figure 3-1)

- The **esophagus** is a muscular tube that extends from the pharynx to the stomach whose function is to convey food (Figure 3-2). Under normal circumstances there are four esophageal constrictions: the beginning, the arch of the aorta, the left main bronchus, and at the end where it passes through the diaphragm. It is at these points where obstructions are most likely to occur. The diaphragm acts as a sphincter, normally efficient in preventing reflux of gastric contents.
- The **stomach** comprises four parts: the cardia, fundus, body, and pylorus. The muscular pyloric sphincter controls flow of gastric contents into the duodenum.
- The **small intestine** is made up of three parts: the duodenum, the jejunum, and the ileum.
  - The **duodenum** is the first and shortest component of the small intestine and frames the head of the pancreas.
  - The duodenojejunal junction is marked by the presence of the **ligament of Treitz,** a landmark that is considered to divide the upper GI tract from the lower GI tract.
  - Most of the **jejunum** lies in the left upper quadrant (LUQ).
  - The **ileum** lies predominantly in the right lower quadrant (RLQ) and ends at the ileocecal junction.
- The **large intestine** consists of cecum; appendix; ascending, transverse, descending, and sigmoid colon; rectum; and anal canal.
  - The **appendix** is an intestinal diverticulum that usually originates from the posteromedial aspect of the cecum.
  - The **cecum** is the first part of the large intestine, continuous with the **ascending colon,** which passes to the hepatic flexure.
  - The largest and most mobile part of the large intestine, the **transverse colon,** passes from the hepatic flexure to the splenic flexure.
  - The **descending colon** passes from the splenic flexure to the sigmoid colon.

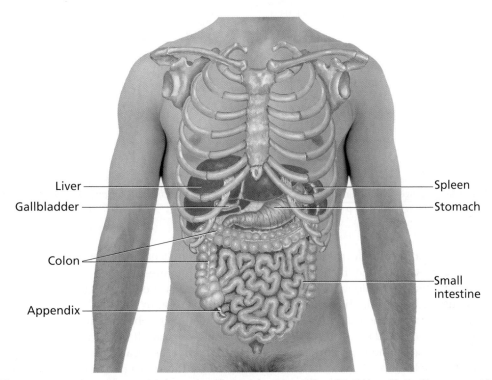

Figure 3-1   Surface anatomy of the gastrointestinal system. (From Wilson SF, Giddens JF: *Health assessment for nursing practice*, ed 2, St. Louis, 2001, Mosby, p 479, Figure 20-1.)

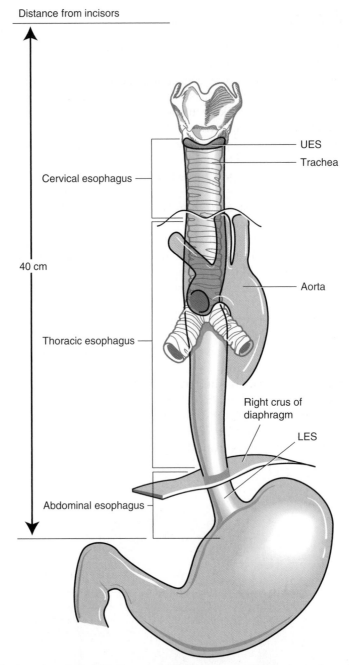

Distance from incisors

Cervical esophagus

40 cm

Thoracic esophagus

Abdominal esophagus

UES
Trachea

Aorta

Right crus of
diaphragm

LES

Figure 3-2 Esophageal anatomy. *UES,* Upper esophageal sphincter; *LES,* lower esophageal sphincter. (From Feldman M, Sleisenger MH, Scharschmidt BF: *Sleisenger & Fordtran's gastrointestinal and liver disease,* ed 6, Philadelphia, 1998, WB Saunders, p 458, Figure 31-1.)

- ▪ The **sigmoid colon** forms an S-shaped loop that connects the descending colon and **rectum,** which is the fixed terminal part of the large intestine.
- • The **pancreas** is an elongated, retroperitoneal organ with endocrine (e.g., glucagon, insulin) and exocrine (digestive enzymes) functions (Figure 3-3).
- • The falciform ligament divides the **liver** into right and left lobe and anterior quadrate and posterior caudate. It is covered by **Glisson's capsule.** It is pyramidal in shape with its base on the right and apex at the left. The liver is located in the right upper quadrant (RUQ) and is almost entirely covered by the rib cage. It moves inferiorly with inspiration, making it easier to palpate. Because of its soft consistency the liver may be difficult to feel through the abdominal wall.

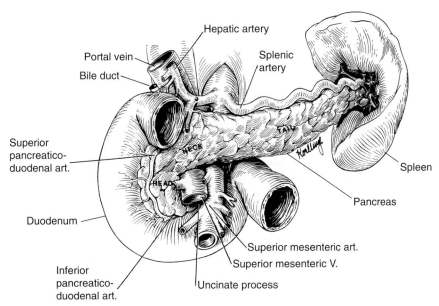

Figure 3-3   Anterior view of the pancreas and its relations. (Adapted from Feldman M, Sleisenger MH, Scharschmidt BF: *Sleisenger & Fordtran's gastrointestinal and liver disease,* ed 6, Philadelphia, 1998, WB Saunders, p 761, Figure 45-1.)

- The **gallbladder** lies on the inferior surface of the liver. Bile is produced in the liver, stored in the gallbladder, and released when fat enters the duodenum.
- The **spleen** is the largest lymphatic organ in the body and is covered by a capsule. The spleen is located in the LUQ, posterior to the stomach and anterior to the upper pole of the left kidney. It lies in the curve of the diaphragm posterior to the midaxillary line (MAL), deep to the ninth, tenth and eleventh ribs (12 cm in length and 7 cm in width). The normal spleen does not extend beyond the costal margin and is usually not palpable. Like the liver, it moves inferiorly with inspiration.

CARDINAL SIGNS AND SYMPTOMS

Jaundice
- **Jaundice** refers to the yellowish staining of skin and other tissues with bile pigment. The presence of jaundice correlates reliably with hyperbilirubinemia. Bilirubin is normally taken up by liver cells and excreted in the bile. Mechanisms of jaundice include increased production of bilirubin, decreased uptake by liver cells, decreased ability to conjugate bilirubin, and decreased excretion. Unconjugated bilirubin binds with albumin; therefore, jaundice is observed clinically in tissues rich in albumin, such as skin and eyes (**scleral icterus**). Jaundice occurs with bilirubin concentrations of 40 to 45 μmol/L. It is best observed in natural light.

Odors
- **Halitosis** is foul-smelling breath. Although it is unpleasant, it does not generally reflect GI disease.
- **Flatus** is the expulsion of GI air through the anus. The presence of flatus is rarely pathologic, although patients with malabsorption syndromes, such as lactose intolerance, may pass excessive gas. The absence of both flatus and the passage of bowel movements (BMs) is termed **obstipation,** a symptom of intestinal obstruction.

GI bleeding
- **Hematemesis** is the vomiting of blood from the upper GI (UGI) tract, proximal to the ligament of Treitz. It generally reflects brisk bleeding. **Coffee-ground emesis** also

reflects UGI bleeding, but it is generally slower, having had time for the gastric acid to convert hemoglobin (red) into hematin (brown). Hematemesis should be carefully differentiated from hemoptysis, which is the coughing up of blood from the respiratory tract.

- **Hematochezia** is the passage of bloody stools. Although hematochezia generally reflects lower GI (LGI) bleeding (distal to the ligament of Treitz), it may also reflect brisk UGI bleeding with rapid transit.
- **Melena** is the passage of dark, tarry, malodorous stools. It typically is a result of UGI bleeding, although blood in the small bowel or right colon may appear as melena with prolonged transit times. Melena stools will test positive for occult blood. Black stools caused by foods and substances, such as iron and bismuth, will test negative for occult blood.

Steatorrhea
- **Steatorrhea** is the passage of fatty stools. The stools are pale, soft, greasy, malodorous, and difficult to flush away. It is caused by malabsorption of fat, such as in pancreatic insufficiency or celiac disease. Some patients with documented steatorrhea by measurement of fecal fat are not symptomatic.

Abdominal Pain
- **Visceral pain** originates in the abdominal organs and is caused by forceful contractions or distension of hollow organs. The pain tends to be midline and poorly localized (Figure 3-4). It is described as gnawing, burning, crampy, or achy and is often associated with nausea and vomiting (N/V).

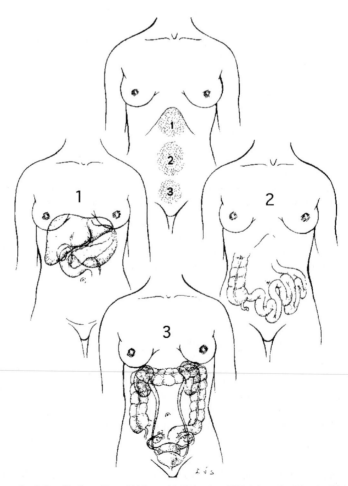

Figure 3-4   Visceral pain localization. (From Feldman M, Sleisenger MH, Scharschmidt BF: *Sleisenger & Fordtran's gastrointestinal and liver disease*, ed 6, Philadelphia, 1998, WB Saunders, p 82, Figure 5-2.)

- **Parietal pain** originates in the parietal peritoneum and is usually caused by inflammation. It may be described as a steady aching pain or a sharp intermittent pain that is aggravated by movement and coughing. Parietal pain is well localized over the involved structure.
- **Referred pain** is felt at a remote location from the involved structure. The pain is felt at the level of somatic innervation (dermatome) to which the sympathetic pain carrying nerves innervate. It tends to radiate from the original site and is well localized. Pain may be referred from abdominal to nonabdominal sites (e.g., cholecystitis may cause pain in the right shoulder because of involvement of the phrenic nerve).
- **Rebound tenderness** is abdominal tenderness when pressure is suddenly released. It is classically detected by slowly pressing over the painful area and then quickly withdrawing. However, this is a painful process and is probably unnecessary if the patient reports localized abdominal pain with coughing and rocking the pelvis back and forth (or shaking the bed). Rebound tenderness is considered a sign of peritoneal irritation.

ESSENTIAL CLINICAL COMPETENCIES

APPROACH TO TAKING A HISTORY OF ABDOMINAL PAIN

- **ID:** Age, sex
- **Character:** What is the pain like?
  - Sharp?
  - Crampy?
  - Dull?
- **Location:** Where does the pain originate (Figure 3-5)?
  - RUQ?
  - RLQ?
  - LUQ?
  - Left lower quadrant (LLQ)?
  - Suprapubic?
  - Epigastric?
  - Flank?
- **Onset:** When did the pain start? How did it come on (sudden versus gradual)?
- **Radiation:** Does the pain move anywhere?
- **Intensity:** How severe is the pain on a scale of 1 to 10, with 1 being mild pain and 10 being the worst?
  - How does it affect your activities of daily living?
  - Is it getting better, worse, or staying the same?
- **Duration:** How long has the pain been there (acute versus chronic)?
- **Events associated:**
  - Fever, chills?
  - N/V, reflux, or hematemesis?
  - Hematuria, change in color of urine, dysuria, polyuria, urinary frequency, nocturia, or anuria?
  - Appetite, weight loss or gain?
  - Diarrhea, steatorrhea, constipation, melena, or hematochezia?
  - Jaundice?
  - Last menstrual period (LMP)?
- **Frequency:** Have you ever had this pain before? How often does the pain come (intermittent versus constant)?
- **Palliative factors:** Is there anything that makes the pain better? If so, what?
  - Lying in one position?
- **Provocative factors:** Is there anything that makes the pain worse? If so, what?
  - Movement?

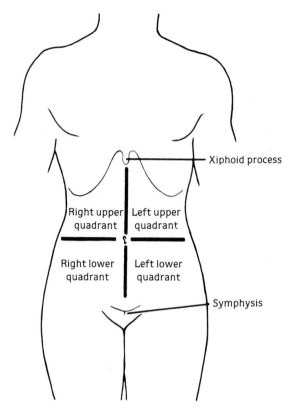

Figure 3-5 Division of the abdomen into quadrants. (From Wilkins RL, Sheldon RL, Krider SJ: *Clinical assessment in respiratory care,* ed 4, St. Louis, 2000, Mosby, p 90, Figure 4-26.)

- **Past medical history (PMH)/past surgical history (PSH):**
  - Previous surgeries?
  - Malignancy?
  - Hepatitis? Previous blood transfusions?
  - Inflammatory bowel disease (IBD)? Irritable bowel syndrome (IBS)?
  - Other medical problems?
- **Medications (MEDS):** Antacids, laxatives
- **Allergies**
- **Social history (SH):** Smoking, EtOH, street drugs, and sexual history
- **Family history (FH):** IBD, hemochromatosis

PEARL
- It is important to manage pain. If the patient is in a great deal of pain, it should be addressed early in the encounter. Getting the patient's pain under control will facilitate history taking and examination.

APPROACH TO THE GASTROINTESTINAL EXAMINATION

Inspection
- **Skin:** Scars, striae, dilated veins (caput medusae, spider nevi), excoriations, jaundice, and ulcerations
- **Umbilicus:** Contour and location, obvious herniation
- **Contour:** Flat, protuberant, scaphoid, bulging flanks, symmetry, and visible organs or masses
- **Peristalsis:** May be seen in thin patients (increased in obstruction)

- **Pulsations:** Normal aortic pulsation in epigastrium (increased in abdominal aortic aneurysm [AAA])
- **Abdominal wall movement** with respiration.

Auscultation
- **Bowel sounds:** Clicks, gurgles, and borborygmi (loud prolonged gurgles of hyper-peristalsis). Before deciding that bowel sounds are absent, listen in each quadrant for 2 to 3 minutes.
- **Friction rubs:** Listen over liver and spleen (inflammation of peritoneal surface of organ).

Palpation
- Before palpation ask the patient to cough and point to the most tender area with one finger. Palpate the most tender area last.
  - **Light palpation:** Gently palpate each quadrant to identify tenderness, muscular resistance, and superficial masses. Distinguish between voluntary guarding and involuntary muscular spasm. Voluntary guarding decreases when the patient is relaxed. To optimize relaxation place the patient supine with arms at the side, and ask the patient to mouth breathe with the jaw open. Involuntary rigidity persists despite relaxation and may indicate peritoneal inflammation.
  - **Deep palpation:** Palpate all four quadrants, using the volar surface of your fingers. Identify any masses, and describe the size, shape, consistency, tenderness, and mobility (Figure 3-6). Localize pain as accurately as possible.
  - **Rebound tenderness:** Abdominal pain on coughing or driving over bumps in the road suggests peritoneal inflammation. Press your fingers in firmly and slowly, then quickly withdraw. Watch and listen to the patient for signs of pain. Pain on withdrawal constitutes rebound tenderness.

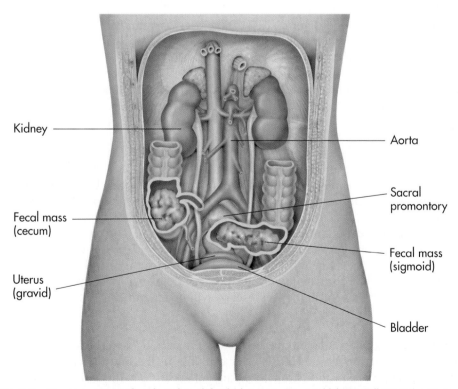

Figure 3-6   Structures commonly palpated as abdominal masses. (From Seidel HM, Ball JW, Dains JE, Benedict GB: *Mosby's guide to physical examination,* ed 5, St. Louis, 2003, Mosby, p 548, Figure 16-18.)

Percussion

- Percuss lightly in all four quadrants. Tympany usually dominates, but scattered areas of dullness are normal (feces/fluid). Note amount and distribution of gas. Identify possible masses. Estimate the size of the liver by percussing from above and below the costal margins. Percuss Traube's space and for Castell's sign. Test for shifting dullness to identify the presence of ascites.

Other Pertinent Examinations

- A pelvic examination in females may be necessary to rule out an ovarian cyst, ovarian torsion, ectopic pregnancy, or pelvic inflammatory disease (PID). Examine the groin and male genitalia for hernias (see p 86). Perform a digital rectal examination (DRE; see pp 86-88). Examine the liver and spleen (see pp 84-86).

Specific Signs

- **McBurney's point:** One-third the distance between anterior superior iliac spine (ASIS) and umbilicus
- **Psoas sign:** Ask the patient to raise the right thigh against resistance, or ask the patient to lie on his or her left side and extend the right leg at the hip. Increased abdominal pain suggests irritation of psoas muscle.
- **Obturator sign:** Flex the right thigh at the hip with the knee bent. Rotate the leg internally at the hip. Right hypogastric pain suggests irritation of the obturator muscle.
- **Murphy's sign:** Hook your fingers under the right costal margin, and ask the patient to take a deep breath. A sharp increase in tenderness or sudden stop in inspiratory effort suggests acute cholecystitis.
- **Rovsing's sign:** Pain in the RLQ during left-sided pressure/deep palpation is suggestive of peritoneal irritation.

PERFORM A FOCUSED EXAMINATION OF THE LIVER

Inspection

- **Extrahepatic stigmata** of liver disease: Dilated veins, jaundice, excoriations, and so on (see pp 91-92)
- **Skin:** Scars, striae, rashes, other lesions
- **Umbilicus:** Location, contour, herniation
- **Abdomen:** Contour (flat, protuberant, scaphoid, bulging flanks), symmetry, visible masses. Ask the patient to take a deep breath, and observe the hepatic area.

Auscultation

- Use the diaphragm of the stethoscope to auscultate the RUQ for a venous hum or **Cruveilhier's sign,** a humming noise indicative of increased collateral circulation between the portal and systemic circulation. Note any hepatic bruits (may occur in liver cancer, alcoholic hepatitis) or friction rubs (inflammation of peritoneal surface of the liver).
- If the abdomen is distended or the abdominal muscles are tense, a "scratch test" may be useful to determine the lower border of the liver. Place the diaphragm of the stethoscope over the liver, and with the finger of your other hand scratch the abdominal surface lightly, moving toward the border of the liver. When you encounter the liver, the sound you hear in the stethoscope will be magnified.

Percussion

- Start percussing in an area of tympany below the umbilicus in the RLQ, and percuss upward to the lower border of the liver dullness in the midclavicular line (MCL). Mark the area of transition from tympany to dullness with a skin marker. Now percuss in an area of lung resonance down toward the liver in the MCL. Again mark the area of transition from resonance to dullness. Measure the span between the two marks. The normal liver spans 6 to 12 cm at the right MCL and 4 to 8 cm in the mid-sternal line. Percussion typically underestimates the size of the liver.

Palpation
- **Light palpation:** Use a light gentle dipping motion in the area around the liver. Look at the patient's face for evidence of tenderness or increased resistance to palpation.
- **Bimanual palpation:** Place your left hand behind the patient, parallel to and supporting the eleventh and twelfth ribs. Remind the patient to relax on your hand. Press your left hand anteriorly. Place your right hand on the patient's right abdomen, with your fingertips well below the lower border of liver, oblique or parallel to the right costal margin. Ask the patient to take a deep breath, and press gently posteriorly and cranially to try to feel the liver edge descend to meet your fingers. If palpable, the edge of a normal liver is soft, sharp, and regular; its surface is smooth. Try to trace the liver edge laterally and medially. Note any nodules, tenderness, and irregularity.

PEARL
- Use indirect **fist percussion** to check for liver tenderness when the liver is not palpable. Place the palm of your left hand over the lower right rib cage. Gently strike the dorsal surface of your left hand with your right fist. Compare the sensation in the LUQ and RUQ of the abdomen. The healthy liver is not tender to percussion.

PERFORM A FOCUSED EXAMINATION OF THE SPLEEN

Inspection
- **Skin:** Scars, striae, dilated veins, rashes, other lesions
- **Umbilicus:** Location, contour, herniation
- **Abdomen:** Contour (flat, protuberant, scaphoid, bulging flanks), symmetry, visible masses. Ask the patient to take a deep breath, and observe the splenic area.

Auscultation
- Place the diaphragm of the stethoscope in the LUQ, tenth ICS. Listen for a splenic friction rub as in inflammation of the peritoneal surface of the spleen (splenic infarct).

Percussion
- The spleen enlarges anteriorly, caudally, and medially toward the right iliac fossa. It replaces the tympany of the colon and stomach with the dullness of a solid organ. Percuss for the spleen beginning in the right iliac fossa toward the left costal margin.
- **Castell's sign:** Percuss the lowest ICS in the left anterior axillary line (AAL); this area is usually tympanitic. Ask the patient to take a deep breath and percuss again. The percussion note should remain tympanitic if the spleen is of normal size. A change in percussion note from tympany to dullness constitutes a positive Castell's sign and suggests splenic enlargement.
- **Traube's space:** Percuss along Traube's space (lower left anterior chest wall between the area of lung resonance above and the costal margin below). Note the lateral extent of tympany, which marks the splenic border (MAL). Traube's space may also be defined as the space bordered by the left anterior sixth rib, MAL, and costal margin. Dullness in Traube's space suggests splenic enlargement.

Palpation
- The normal spleen is usually not palpable.
- **Light palpation:** Gently palpate using a light dipping motion in the LUQ. Look at the patient's face for evidence of tenderness or increased resistance to palpation.

- **Bimanual palpation:** Use your left hand to reach over the patient and support the lower left rib cage. Starting in the right iliac fossa, use your right hand to palpate across the midline toward the region below the left costal margin. Ask the patient to take a deep breath. Try to feel the tip or edge of the spleen as it comes down to meet your fingertips. Attempt to palpate the splenic notch. Note any tenderness. Assess the splenic contour, and measure the distance between the spleen's lowest point and the left costal margin. Repeat with the patient lying on his or her right side with the legs slightly flexed at the hips and knees. In this position gravity may make the spleen more easily palpable.

PERFORM A FOCUSED EXAMINATION FOR HERNIAS

Definitions
- A **hernia** is the protrusion of a structure or viscus through the tissues that normally contain it. The most common type of hernia is an inguinal hernia.
- An **indirect inguinal hernia** passes through the internal inguinal ring, lateral to the inferior epigastric artery, into the inguinal canal. With a patent processus vaginalis, this hernia can extend into the scrotum or labia majora.
- A **direct inguinal hernia** protrudes through the abdominal wall, medial to the inferior epigastric artery, and usually emerges near the superficial inguinal ring.
- A **femoral hernia** is one in which the viscus passes through the femoral ring into the femoral canal. It is palpable just inferior to the inguinal ligament. It is at high risk for strangulation.
- Hernias may also develop at the umbilicus **(umbilical hernia)** or at the site of a surgical incision **(incisional hernia)**.
- **Spigelian hernias** are rare. They occur when a viscus protrudes through the linea semilunaris at the lateral edge of the rectus sheath.

Inspection
- Inspect the anterior abdominal wall and inguinal area for obvious bulges.
- Inspect the genitalia (labia/scrotum) for any bulges or asymmetry. Use a small light source to transilluminate a scrotal mass. A hernia or tumor will fail to transilluminate.
- Ask the patient to cough or bear down. Inspect the anterior abdominal wall and inguinal wall for any sudden bulges.

Auscultation
- If bulges are identified in the groin or genitalia, it may be auscultated with the diaphragm of the stethoscope. Listen for any bowel sounds (presence of bowel within the mass).

Palpation
- Palpate any identified masses. Note the size and consistency of the mass and whether it is reducible. Note any tenderness.
- **Inguinal hernias** (Figure 3-7): Place your index finger on the scrotal skin above the testicle. Gently invaginate the skin, and follow the spermatic cord into the inguinal canal. In this position ask the patient to cough or bear down. If a hernia is present you will feel a bulge against your finger with this maneuver (performing the examination with the patient standing may facilitate hernia identification). Look at the patient's face for evidence of tenderness.

PERFORM A DIGITAL RECTAL EXAMINATION

Patient Positioning
- The patient may be positioned in a number of ways for the DRE. Consider patient comfort during this sensitive examination. Ask the patient to lie on his or her left side

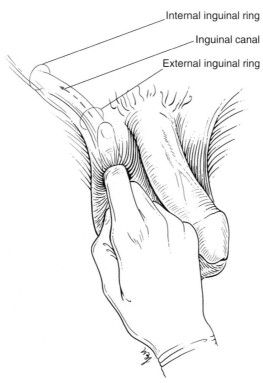

Internal inguinal ring

Inguinal canal

External inguinal ring

Figure 3-7 Examination for inguinal hernia. (From Swartz M: *Textbook of physical diagnosis: history and examination,* ed 4, Philadelphia, 2002, WB Saunders, Figure 17-33.)

and flex the knees, bringing them toward the chest. Alternatively, the patient can be examined standing, bent over the examination table. The lithotomy position (supine at the end of the examining table with knees flexed and feet in stirrups) is also useful, especially for rectovaginal examinations.

Inspection
- Spread the buttocks, and inspect the anus and perianal area for inflammation, bleeding, fistulas, fissures, or hemorrhoids. Asking the patient to strain may accentuate hemorrhoids.

Palpation
- Begin by palpating any abnormal areas detected on inspection of the anus and perianal area, noting any tenderness or induration.
- Now explain the rectal examination to the patient, and warn them about the coolness of the lubricant.
- Use your gloved, index finger to apply gentle, steady pressure at the anus. Ask the patient to take a deep breath, and insert the finger into the rectum (Figure 3-8).
- Note **sphincter tone**. This is especially important in neurologic injury.
- Palpate the **rectal walls** for polyps or masses. Ensure that you fully palpate the anterior, posterior, and lateral walls of the rectum. The sensation of external compression on the rectum or a rectal shelf is known as **Blumer's shelf** and is associated with malignancy.
- Palpate the **prostate** gland, which lies anterior to the anterior rectal wall. Note any tenderness and the size, symmetry, consistency, and nodularity of the prostate gland. Tenderness suggests prostatitis. In trauma, a "high-riding" prostate is associated with urethral disruption.
- After the examination is complete, inspect your gloved finger for blood, and note the color of the stool. Test the stool for the presence of occult blood using a guaiac test.

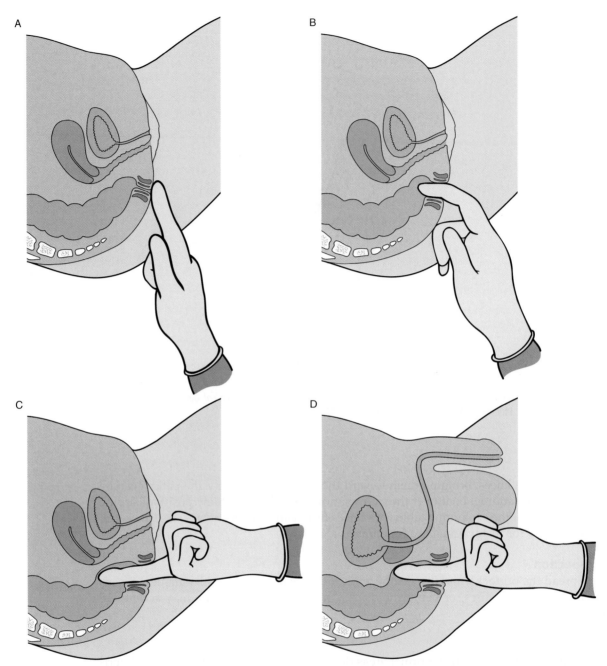

Figure 3-8 **A** to **D,** Technique for digital rectal examination. (From Munro JF, Campbell IW, editors: *Macleod's clinical examination,* ed 10, Edinburgh, 2000, Churchill Livingstone, p 175, Figure 5.22.)

- **Rectovaginal examination** (Figure 3-9) is sometimes useful, especially in gynecologic malignancy. Using a clean pair of gloves, insert your index finger into the vagina and the middle finger into the rectum. Palpate the rectovaginal septum (pouch of Douglas) between your fingers for tenderness or nodularity.

PERFORM A FOCUSED PHYSICAL EXAMINATION FOR ASCITES

Definition
- **Ascites** is the effusion and accumulation of fluid in the peritoneal cavity. It is clinically detectable when >500 ml has accumulated. The patient may notice increased

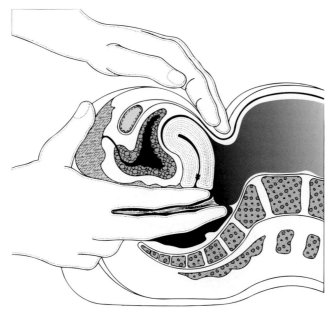

Figure 3-9   Rectovaginal examination. (From DiSaia PJ, Creasman WT: *Clinical gynecologic oncology,* ed 6, St. Louis, 2002, Mosby, p 68, Figure 3-14.)

abdominal girth or weight gain. Massive ascites may cause SOB because the ascitic abdomen prevents movement of the diaphragm and lung expansion.

Inspection
- Observe the shape of the abdomen and flanks. Suspect ascites in patients with bulging flanks (in supine position), a protuberant abdomen, and protruding umbilicus.

Palpation
- **Fluid wave** (Figure 3-10): Ask the patient or an assistant to press the hypothenar aspect of both hands firmly down the midline of the patient's abdomen. This stops transmission of a wave through fat. Tap one flank sharply with your fingertips, and feel on the opposite flank for an impulse transmitted through fluid. An easily detected fluid wave suggests ascites. This test is often not positive until ascites is obvious and is sometimes positive in patients without ascites.

Percussion
- Ascitic fluid characteristically sinks with gravity, whereas gas-filled loops of bowel float to the top. Thus percussion produces a dull note in dependent areas of the ascitic abdomen. In a supine patient look for dullness of the flanks by percussing outward in several directions from the central area of tympany. Map the border between tympany and dullness using a skin marker.
- **Shifting dullness** (Figure 3-11): Ask the patient to turn onto one side. Wait 20 to 25 seconds. Percuss from an area of tympany (upper side) to dullness (dependent side) in several places to map the border between tympany and dullness. In a normal patient the borders between tympany and dullness are relatively constant. In an ascitic abdomen the dullness will shift to the dependent portion of the abdomen.

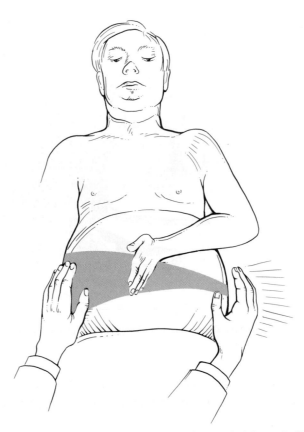

Figure 3-10   Testing for a fluid wave. (From Swartz M: *Textbook of physical diagnosis: history and examination,* ed 4, Philadelphia, 2002, WB Saunders, Figure 16-19.)

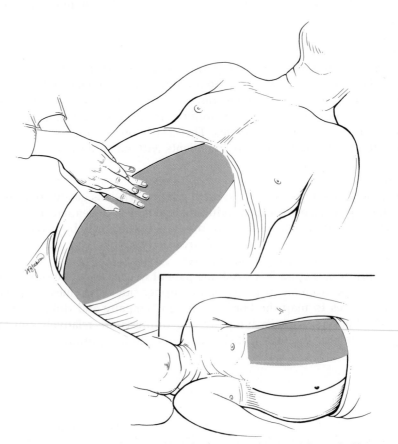

Figure 3-11   Testing for shifting dullness. (From Swartz M: *Textbook of physical diagnosis: history and examination,* ed 4, Philadelphia, 2002, WB Saunders, Figure 16-18.)

SAMPLE OSCE SCENARIOS

INSTRUCTIONS TO CANDIDATE: A 27-year-old male with chronic viral hepatitis presents with jaundice. Perform a focused physical examination for extrahepatic manifestations of liver disease (Figure 3-12).

Vitals
- Heart rate (HR), blood pressure (BP), respiratory rate (RR), and temperature
- Fever may be noted in acute viral hepatitis, alcoholic hepatitis, or infection.

General
- **Fetor hepaticus (liver breath):** Caused by volatile sulfur compounds produced by intestinal bacteria that accumulate in the blood and urine as a result of defective hepatic metabolism
- **Cirrhotic habitus:** Wasted extremities with protuberant belly
- **Muscle wasting:** Temporalis muscle, first digiti interosseous
- **Vitamin deficiency:** Beefy tongue, angular cheilosis, and koilonychia

Skin
- Xanthelasma, tendon xanthomas
- Jaundice, excoriations
- **Spider nevi:** Arterioles in the skin with radiating capillary branches simulating the legs of a spider. It blanches with diascopy (using a transparent microscope slide, apply pressure over the lesion, and you will see it blanch).

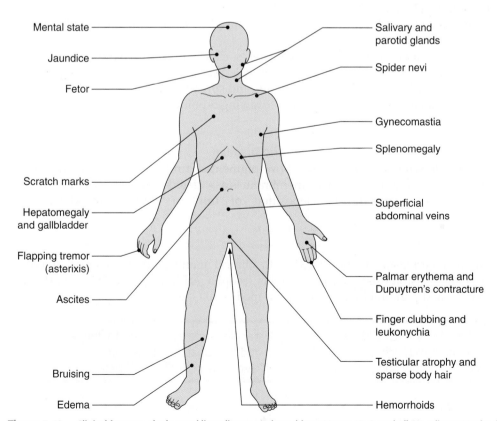

Figure 3-12 Clinical features of advanced liver disease. (Adapted from Munro JF, Campbell IW, editors: *Macleod's clinical examination,* ed 10, Edinburgh, 2000, Churchill Livingstone, p 167, Figure 5.14.)

- **Caput medusae:** Dilated cutaneous veins radiating from the umbilicus
- Petechiae, ecchymosis
- Edema caused by hypoalbuminemia
- **Hands:**
  - **Dupuytren's contracture:** Thickening and shortening of the fibrous bands in palmar fascia
  - Palmar erythema
  - **Leukonychia:** Pale nails caused by hypoalbuminemia
  - Clubbing

Head, Eyes, Ears, Nose, and Throat (HEENT)
- Parotid gland hypertrophy
- Scleral icterus
- **Virchow's node:** A firm, palpable left infraclavicular lymph node. Its presence is presumptive evidence of visceral malignancy, generally intraabdominal.

Abdomen
- Examine the spleen for splenomegaly (see pp 85-86).
- Examine for ascites (see pp 88-90).
- Pale stools caused by malabsorption (biliary obstruction)

Genitourinary (GU)
- **Hypogonadism:** Testicular atrophy, impotence, and loss of pubic hair (especially axillary)
- Gynecomastia caused by impaired estrogen conjugation
- Dark urine caused by hyperbilirubinemia

Neurologic
- Personality changes
- Confusion, altered level of consciousness caused by toxic nitrogenous substances in systemic circulation
- **Asterixis** is involuntary jerking movements, especially in the hands caused by the arrhythmic lapses of sustained posture. It is best elicited by asking the patient to extend his or her arms, extend the wrists, and spread the fingers.
- Constructional apraxia (e.g., difficulty drawing 5-point star)
- Ataxia

Findings Associated with Other Hepatic Disease
- **Kayser-Fleischer's ring:** Green-yellow pigmented ring around cornea caused by copper deposited in Descemet's membrane is associated with Wilson's disease.
- **Tanned skin appearance:** Deposition of iron in skin is associated with hemochromatosis.

PEARL
- Portal hypertension is associated with clinical manifestations at areas of portal-systemic anastomosis: esophageal veins (esophageal varices), rectal veins (hemorrhoids), and paraumbilical veins (caput medusae).

INSTRUCTIONS TO CANDIDATE: An 18-year-old female presents to the emergency department with right lower quadrant pain and loss of appetite since yesterday. Perform a focused history and physical examination, exploring possible etiologies.

DD$_x$ VITAMINS C
- **Infectious:** PID/tuboovarian abscess, psoas abscess
- **Traumatic:** MSK injury

- Idiopathic/Iatrogenic: Appendicitis, mesenteric adenitis, ascending diverticulitis, incarcerated hernia, Crohn's disease, ruptured ectopic pregnancy, ovarian torsion, and renal colic

History

- **Character:** What is the pain like? Sharp and localized? Crampy? Dull?
- **Location:** Where does the pain originate?
- **Onset:** When did the pain start? How did it come on (sudden versus gradual)?
- **Radiation:** Does the pain move anywhere?
- **Intensity:** How severe is the pain on a scale of 1 to 10, with 1 being mild pain and 10 being the worst?
  - Is it getting better/worse or staying the same?
- **Duration:** How long does it last (intermittent versus constant)?
- **Events associated:**
  - Appendicitis: Fever, N/V, anorexia, initial dull central abdominal pain that later localizes to the RLQ
  - Pregnancy: LMP, *per vaginam* (PV) bleeding
  - PID: Fever, foul vaginal discharge, intermenstrual bleeding
  - Renal colic: Hematuria, passage of stones/gritty urine
  - Intestinal obstruction/incarcerated hernia: Obstipation, feculent vomitus
  - Crohn's disease: Chronic diarrhea, weight loss, extraintestinal manifestations (e.g., uveitis, erythema nodosum, and peripheral arthritis)
- **Frequency:** Have you ever had this pain before? How often does the pain come?
- **Palliative factors:** Is there anything that makes the pain better? If so, what? Lying in one position?
- **Provocative factors:** Is there anything that makes the pain worse? If so, what? Movement?
- **PMH/PSH:** Previous surgeries, malignancy, IBD, IBS, PID, sexually transmitted infection (STI), ectopic pregnancy, or renal colic
- **MEDS:** Analgesics
- **SH:** Smoking, EtOH, street drugs, and sexual history
- **FH:** IBD, renal colic

Physical Examination

- **Vitals:** HR, BP, RR, and temperature
  - May note low-grade fever and mild tachycardia.
- **General:** Apprehension, flushed appearance. Check capillary refill. Note patient position on the stretcher and whether they are moving. Note any apparent distress.
- **HEENT:** Look at the mucous membranes to gauge hydration. Inspect the sclerae.
- **Resp:** Chest expansion (symmetry), auscultation (breath sounds, adventitious sounds)
- **CVS:** Measure the JVP. Although it is not a reliable indicator of hydration status, the JVP is a useful clinical finding. Palpate peripheral pulses. Note pulse volume, contour, and rhythm. Auscultate the heart, looking for extra heart sounds or flow murmurs associated with hyperdynamic circulation.
- **Abdomen:** Inspect the abdomen. Auscultate for bowel sounds (may be decreased in peritonitis). Before deciding that bowel sounds are absent, listen in each quadrant for 2 to 3 minutes. Percuss lightly in all four quadrants. Percussion will produce pain in a patient with appendicitis or peritonitis. Before palpation ask the patient to cough and point to the most tender area with one finger. Palpate the most tender area last. Perform light and deep palpation, and identify any masses or areas of tenderness. Check for rebound tenderness. Examine the liver and spleen. Perform a DRE. A retrocecal appendix may produce tenderness on palpation of the rectal walls.
- **GU:** It is important to perform a pelvic examination. Note any discharge, inflammation of the cervix, cervical motion tenderness, adnexal tenderness, or pelvic masses. Note uterine size.

PEARLS
- In acute appendicitis rebound tenderness is referred to **McBurney's point**.
- A patient with appendicitis may have positive **psoas, obturator,** and **Rovsing's signs.**

INSTRUCTIONS TO CANDIDATE: A 40-year-old female presents to the emergency department with severe right upper quadrant pain for 8 hours. She is also worried because her friend told her she looked yellow. Perform a focused history and physical examination.

DD$_X$ Jaundice (VITAMINS C)
- **I**nfectious: Viral hepatitis
- **T**raumatic: Resorption of a large hematoma
- **A**utoimmune/**A**llergic: Autoimmune hepatitis
- **M**etabolic: Hemolysis
- **I**diopathic/**I**atrogenic: Biliary obstruction (stone/stricture)
- **N**eoplastic: Obstructing biliary lesion
- **S**ubstance abuse and **P**sychiatric: Alcoholic or toxic hepatitis
- **C**ongenital/genetic: Gilbert's syndrome

DD$_X$ RUQ Pain (VITAMINS C)
- **V**ascular: Right heart failure (congestive hepatomegaly)
- **I**nfectious: Acute pyelonephritis, right-sided pneumonia, and viral hepatitis
- **T**raumatic: MSK injury
- **A**utoimmune/**A**llergic: Autoimmune hepatitis
- **I**diopathic and **I**atrogenic: Acute cholecystitis, duodenal ulcer/peptic ulcer disease (PUD)

History
- **Ch**aracter: What is the pain like? Sharp and localized? Crampy? Dull? Describe your current color.
- **L**ocation: Where does the pain originate?
- **O**nset: When did the pain start? How did it come on (sudden versus gradual)? When did you first notice your yellow color?
- **R**adiation: Does the pain move anywhere?
- Intensity: How severe is the pain on a scale of 1 to 10, with 1 being mild pain and 10 being the worst? Is the pain/jaundice getting better, worse, or staying the same?
- **D**uration: How long does it last (intermittent versus constant)? How long have you had jaundice (acute versus chronic)?
- Events associated:
  - Fever, chills? N/V? Appetite?
  - Last BM? Passing flatus? Diarrhea?
  - Trauma?
  - Cholelithiasis: Fatty meal intolerance, episodic RUQ pain
  - Hepatitis: Recent infection/malaise, aversion to smoking, travel, exposure to persons with hepatitis, multiple sexual partners, IV drug use, blood transfusions
  - Biliary obstruction: Pale stools, dark urine, pruritus
  - Constitutional symptoms: Fever, chills, night sweats, weight loss, anorexia, and asthenia
- **F**requency: Have you ever had this pain before? How often does the pain come (intermittent versus constant)? Have you ever had jaundice before?
- **P**alliative factors: Is there anything that makes the pain better? If so, what?
- **P**rovocative factors: Is there anything that makes the pain worse? If so, what?

- **PMH/PSH:** Cholelithiasis, hepatitis, cirrhosis, malignancy, hemolytic disorders, or Gilbert's disease
- **MEDS:** Hepatotoxic drugs (e.g., acetylsalicylic acid [ASA], isoniazid, methotrexate, anticonvulsants, antipsychotics, oral contraceptive pill [OCP], selected herbals)
- **SH:** Smoking, EtOH, street drugs, IV drugs, and sexual history
- **Immunizations:** Hepatitis
- **FH:** Wilson's disease, hemochromatosis, or Gilbert's disease

Physical Examination

- **Vitals:** HR, BP, RR, and temperature
- **General:** Check capillary refill. Note any icterus, and observe the patient's position on the stretcher and whether they are moving. Note any apparent distress.
- **HEENT:** Look at the mucous membranes to gauge hydration. Inspect the sclerae.
- **Respiratory (Resp):** Chest expansion (symmetry), auscultation (breath sounds, adventitious sounds)
- **CVS:** Measure the JVP. Although it is not a reliable indicator of hydration status, the JVP is still a useful clinical finding. Palpate peripheral pulses. Note pulse volume, contour, and rhythm. Auscultate the heart looking for extra heart sounds or flow murmurs associated with hyperdynamic circulation.
- **Abdomen:** Inspect the abdomen. Auscultate for bowel sounds (may be decreased in peritonitis). Before deciding that bowel sounds are absent, listen in each quadrant for 2 or 3 minutes. Percuss lightly in all four quadrants. Percussion will produce pain in a patient with peritoneal irritation. Before palpation ask the patient to cough and point to the most tender area with one finger. Palpate the most tender area last. Perform light and deep palpation, and identify any masses or areas of tenderness. Check for rebound tenderness. Examine the liver and spleen. Note any hepatomegaly or tenderness. Perform a DRE.
  - **Murphy's sign:** Slide your fingers under the right costal margin, and ask the patient to take a deep breath. A sharp increase in tenderness or sudden stop in inspiratory effort suggests acute cholecystitis.
- **Neurologic (Neuro):** Mental status (orientation to person, place, and time)

PEARLS

- **Charcot's triad for cholecystitis:** Fever, jaundice, and RUQ pain
- **Reynold's pentad for ascending cholangitis:** Charcot's triad plus altered mental status and hypotension

---

INSTRUCTIONS TO CANDIDATE: A 70-year-old male presents to the emergency department with excruciating epigastric pain and vomiting. He has been living alone since his wife died 2 years ago and admits to drinking a "flask daily." Perform a focused history and physical examination.

DD$_X$ Epigastric Pain (VITAMINS C)

- **V**ascular: Leaking/ruptured AAA, MI, and right-sided heart failure (congestive hepatomegaly)
- **I**nfectious: Viral hepatitis, pneumonia
- **T**raumatic: MSK injury
- **A**utoimmune/**A**llergic: Autoimmune hepatitis
- **I**diopathic/**I**atrogenic: Perforated viscus, acute cholecystitis, pancreatitis (e.g., biliary stones), and duodenal ulcer/PUD
- **S**ubstance abuse and **P**sychiatric: Alcoholic pancreatitis, alcoholic/toxic hepatitis

- **First evaluate A**irway, **B**reathing, and **C**irculation. It may be necessary to perform an immediate intervention, such as supplemental O_2, IV access, or intubation.
  - Is the patient able to talk? Swallow? Cough?
  - Are both lungs ventilated? Is the patient oxygenating (mentation, pulse oximetry)?
  - Abnormal vitals? Peripheral circulation (pulses, capillary refill)?
  - If no immediate interventions are required, proceed to take the history, and perform the physical examination.

History

- **Ch**aracter: What is the pain like? Sharp and localized? Crampy? Dull? Describe the vomitus. Is there any blood/coffee grounds?
- **L**ocation: Where does the pain originate?
- **O**nset: When did the pain start? How did it come on (sudden versus gradual)? When did the vomiting start?
- **R**adiation: Does the pain move anywhere?
- **I**ntensity: How severe is the pain on a scale of 1 to 10, with 1 being mild pain and 10 being the worst? Is it getting better, worse, or staying the same? Number of episodes of vomiting per day. Has it gotten worse? Are you able to keep anything down?
- **D**uration: How long does it last (intermittent versus constant)? How long have you been vomiting?
- **E**vents associated:
  - Trauma? Injury?
  - MI: Diaphoresis, SOB, radiation down arm or to jaw
  - Pancreatitis: Central abdominal pain radiates to the back, vomiting
  - Renal colic: Hematuria, passage of stones/gritty urine
  - Intestinal obstruction/incarcerated hernia: Obstipation, feculent vomitus
  - Constitutional symptoms: Fever, chills, night sweats, weight loss, anorexia, and asthenia
- **F**requency: Have you ever had this pain before? How often does the pain come (intermittent versus constant)?
- **P**alliative factors: Is there anything that makes the pain better? If so, what? Lying in one position?
- **P**rovocative factors: Is there anything that makes the pain worse? If so, what? Movement?
- **PMH/PSH:** Diverticular disease, previous surgeries, malignancy, IBD, IBS, PID, STI, ectopic pregnancy, or renal colic
- **MEDS:** Analgesics, antibiotics
- **SH:** Smoking, EtOH, street drugs, and sexual history
- **FH:** IBD, renal colic

Physical Examination

- **Vitals:** HR, BP, RR, and temperature
- **General:** Check capillary refill. Observe the patient's position on the stretcher and whether they are moving. Note any apparent distress.
- **Skin:** Note any painful nodules in the extremities (fat necrosis).
- **HEENT:** Look at the mucous membranes to gauge hydration. Inspect the sclerae.
- **Resp:** Chest expansion (symmetry). Auscultate the lungs, and describe the breath sounds and adventitious sounds. You may note inspiratory crackles in pulmonary edema.
- **CVS:** Measure the JVP and hepatojugular reflux (increased venous pressure in CHF). Palpate peripheral pulses. Note pulse volume, contour, and rhythm. Inspect and palpate the apical impulse. Palpate for thrills and heaves. Auscultate the heart, looking for an S_3, S_4, or murmur. Auscultate for abdominal bruits.
- **Abdomen:** Inspect the abdomen. Blue or green ecchymosis in the flank from extravasation of hemolyzed blood **(Grey Turner's sign)** and bluish discoloration at the umbilicus **(Cullen's sign)** are signs of pancreatitis. Auscultate for bowel sounds (may

be decreased in pancreatitis). Percuss lightly in all four quadrants. Percussion will produce pain in a patient with peritoneal irritation. Before palpation ask the patient to cough and point to the most tender area with one finger. Palpate the most tender area last. Perform light and deep palpation. Identify any masses (pulsatile or non-pulsatile) or areas of tenderness. Check for rebound tenderness. Examine the liver and spleen. Perform a DRE.

> INSTRUCTIONS TO CANDIDATE: A 58-year-old female presents to the emergency department with sharp LLQ pain, worsening over 2 days. She has had one similar episode last year that resolved spontaneously over several days. Perform a focused history and physical examination.

DD$_X$ LLQ Pain (VITAMINS C)
- **Infectious:** PID/tuboovarian abscess
- **Traumatic:** MSK injury
- **Idiopathic/Iatrogenic:** Sigmoid diverticulitis, incarcerated hernia, perforated colon, Crohn's disease, ulcerative colitis, ruptured ectopic pregnancy, ovarian torsion, and renal colic

History
- **Character:** What is the pain like? Sharp and localized? Crampy? Dull?
- **Location:** Where does the pain originate?
- **Onset:** When did the pain start? How did it come on (sudden versus gradual)?
- **Radiation:** Does the pain move anywhere?
- **Intensity:** How severe is the pain on a scale of 1 to 10, with 1 being mild pain and 10 being the worst? Is it getting better, worse, or staying the same?
- **Duration:** How long does it last (intermittent versus constant)?
- Events associated:
  - Fever, chills? N/V? Appetite? Change in bowel habit? Last BM?
  - Trauma? Injury?
  - Pregnancy: LMP, PV bleeding
  - PID: Fever, foul vaginal discharge, intermenstrual bleeding
  - Renal colic: Hematuria, passage of stones/gritty urine
  - Intestinal obstruction/incarcerated hernia: Obstipation, feculent vomitus
  - Crohn's disease: Chronic diarrhea, weight loss, extraintestinal manifestations (e.g., uveitis, erythema nodosum, and peripheral arthritis)
  - Ulcerative colitis: Bloody diarrhea, tenesmus, weight loss (e.g., uveitis, erythema nodosum, and peripheral arthritis)
  - Constitutional symptoms: Fever, chills, night sweats, weight loss, anorexia, and asthenia
- **Frequency:** Have you ever had this pain before? How often does the pain come (intermittent versus constant)?
- **Palliative factors:** Is there anything that makes the pain better? If so, what? Lying in one position?
- **Provocative factors:** Is there anything that makes the pain worse? If so, what? Movement?
- **PMH/PSH:** Diverticular disease, previous surgeries, malignancy, IBD, IBS, PID, STI, ectopic pregnancy, or renal colic
- **MEDS:** Analgesics, antibiotics
- **SH:** Smoking, EtOH, street drugs, and sexual history
- **FH:** IBD, renal colic

Physical Examination

- **Vitals:** HR, BP, RR, and temperature
- **General:** Check capillary refill. Observe the patient's position on the stretcher and whether he or she is moving. Note any apparent distress.
- **HEENT:** Look at the mucous membranes to gauge hydration. Inspect the sclerae.
- **Resp:** Chest expansion (symmetry), auscultation (breath sounds, adventitious sounds)
- **CVS:** Measure the JVP. Although it is not a reliable indicator of hydration status, the JVP is a useful clinical finding. Palpate peripheral pulses. Note pulse volume, contour, and rhythm. Auscultate the heart, looking for extra heart sounds or flow murmurs associated with hyperdynamic circulation.
- **Abdomen:** Inspect the abdomen. Auscultate for bowel sounds (may be decreased in peritonitis). Before deciding that bowel sounds are absent, listen in each quadrant for 2 to 3 minutes. Percuss lightly in all four quadrants. Percussion will produce pain in a patient with peritoneal irritation. Before palpation ask the patient to cough and point to the most tender area with one finger. Palpate the most tender area last. Perform light and deep palpation, and identify any masses or areas of tenderness. Check for rebound tenderness. Examine the liver and spleen. Perform a DRE, and note any blood.
- **GU:** It is important to perform a pelvic examination. Note any discharge, inflammation of the cervix, cervical motion tenderness, adnexal tenderness, or pelvic masses. Note uterine size.

INSTRUCTIONS TO CANDIDATE: A 77-year-old female presents to the emergency department complaining of passing bright red blood with her bowel movements. Take a detailed history, exploring possible etiologies, and perform a focused physical examination.

DD$_X$ Hematochezia (VITAMINS C)

- **V**ascular: Esophageal varices, aortoenteric fistula, angiodysplasia, and ischemic colitis
- **I**nfectious: Invasive diarrhea (e.g., enteroinvasive *Escherichia coli*)
- **T**raumatic: Mallory-Weiss tear, anorectal trauma, and anal fissures
- **M**etabolic: Coagulopathy
- **I**diopathic/**I**atrogenic: Diverticular disease, IBD, and proctitis
- **N**eoplasm

- **First evaluate A**irway, **B**reathing, and **C**irculation. It may be necessary to perform an immediate intervention, such as supplemental O_2, IV access, or intubation.
  - Is the patient able to talk? Swallow? Cough?
  - Are both lungs ventilated? Is the patient oxygenating (mentation, pulse oximetry)?
  - Abnormal vitals? Peripheral circulation (pulses, capillary refill)?
  - If no immediate interventions are required, proceed to take the history, and perform the physical examination.

History

- **Character:** Describe the bleeding.
  - What color are the stools (black or tarlike versus bright red blood)?
  - Blood mixed throughout stool versus streaking on the surface of the stool or toilet paper versus in the toilet water
  - Stool form (diarrhea/loose/watery stool versus well-formed/solid stool)
- **Location:** Where is the blood coming from (rectal versus vaginal versus urinary tract)?
- **Onset:** When did the bleeding start (sudden versus insidious)?

- **R**adiation: Any other bleeding (bleeding from another location)?
- **I**ntensity: How severe is the bleeding (quantify)? Has it gotten worse?
- **D**uration: How long has the bleeding been going on (acute versus chronic)?
- **E**vents associated:
  - Syncope? Chest pain? SOB?
  - Suspect food (undercooked hamburger or chicken, shellfish)?
  - Diet: Beets (red stool), iron, or bismuth (black stools)
  - Ischemic colitis: Prodrome of abdominal pain
  - Malignancy: Reduction of stool caliber, weight loss, constitutional symptoms
  - Anal fissure: Pain on defecation, perianal itching
  - IBD: Chronic diarrhea, abdominal pain, weight loss, extraintestinal manifestations (e.g., uveitis, erythema nodosum, and peripheral arthritis)
- **F**requency: How often does the bleeding happen (intermittent versus constant)?
- **P**alliative/**P**rovocative factors: Is there anything that makes it better or worse? If so, what?
- **Previous investigations:** Barium enema, UGI series, or endoscopy
- **PMH/PSH:** Hemorrhoids, diverticulosis, IBD, malignancy, polyps, PUD, varices, alcoholism, or coagulopathy
- **MEDS:** NSAID/ASA, anticoagulants, antibiotics (pseudomembranous colitis), or corticosteroids
- **SH:** EtOH, smoking, and foreign travel (enteric infection)
- **FH:** Colon/rectal cancer or polyps, IBD, or coagulopathy

Physical Examination

- **Vitals:** HR, BP, RR, and temperature
  - Beware of signs of circulatory shock: hypotension, tachycardia, thready pulses, decreased capillary refill, and tachypnea
- **General:** Apprehension, diaphoresis, pallor, apparent distress
- **HEENT:** Inspect the sclerae.
- **Resp:** Chest expansion (symmetry), auscultation (breath sounds, adventitious sounds)
- **CVS:** Measure the JVP. Although it is not a reliable indicator of hydration status, the JVP is a useful clinical finding. Palpate peripheral pulses. Note pulse volume, contour, and rhythm. Auscultate the heart, looking for extra heart sounds or murmurs.
- **Abdomen:** Inspect the abdomen. Auscultate for bowel sounds. Percuss lightly in all four quadrants. Percussion will produce pain in a patient with peritoneal irritation. Before palpation ask the patient to cough and point to the most tender area with one finger. Palpate the most tender area last. Perform light and deep palpation, and identify any masses or areas of tenderness. Check for rebound tenderness. Examine the liver and spleen. Perform a DRE. Note any fresh blood, and test for occult blood.
- **Neuro:** Mental status (orientation to person, place, and time)

INSTRUCTIONS TO CANDIDATE: A 57-year-old male presents to his family doctor complaining of "trouble swallowing." He is losing weight because he is unable to eat. Take a detailed history, exploring possible etiologies.

Definition

- **Dysphagia** is difficulty swallowing, a sense that food or liquid is sticking. The sensation of a lump in the throat that is not associated with swallowing (**globus hystericus**) is not true dysphagia.

DDx Dysphagia (VITAMINS C)

- **Traumatic:** Ingestion of a caustic substance
- **Autoimmune/Allergic:** Collagen vascular disease (e.g., scleroderma)
- **Metabolic:** Iron-deficiency anemia (Plummer-Vinson syndrome)
- **Idiopathic/Iatrogenic:** Esophageal stricture, achalasia, and neurogenic disorders (e.g., stroke, bulbar palsy, Guillain-Barré syndrome, amyotrophic lateral sclerosis [ALS])
- **Neoplastic:** Esophageal, pharyngeal
- **Congenital/genetic:** Pharyngeal pouch

History

- **Character:** Describe your difficulty with swallowing.
  - Difficulty initiating swallowing/making swallowing movement (neuromuscular disease)? Any aspiration?
  - Does food/liquid ever come out your nose (pharyngeal pouch)?
  - Do you have trouble swallowing solids, liquids, or both?
- **Location:** Where does the food get stuck? Chest? Throat?
- **Onset:** When did it start? How has it progressed (initial difficulty with solids and then liquids)? Is it getting worse? How quickly? Has the pattern changed?
- **Radiation:** Is swallowing painful? Any pain elsewhere?
- **Intensity:** If pain is a salient feature, qualify the type of pain (e.g., sharp, burning, squeezing, or cramping)? How severe is the pain on a scale of 1 to 10, with 1 being mild pain and 10 being the worst? How does your swallowing difficulty affect your daily life?
- **Duration:** How long does it last? Do you experience difficulty swallowing every time you have a meal or drink something?
- **Events associated:**
  - N/V? Reflux? Nasal/oral regurgitation?
  - Wheezing (compression of airway by mass)? Hoarseness?
  - Constitutional symptoms: Fever, chills, night sweats, weight loss, anorexia, and asthenia
- **Frequency:** How often does it happen? Is it intermittent or constant?
- **Palliative/Provocative factors:** Is there anything that makes it better or worse? If so, what?
- **PMH/PSH:** Nasogastric (NG) tube, esophageal cancer, neuromuscular disorders, collagen vascular disease, IHD/angina, DM, or caustic agent ingestion
- **MEDS:** Previous radiation therapy, taking pills without water
- **SH:** Smoking, EtOH, and street drugs
- **FH:** Esophageal cancer, neuromuscular disease

INSTRUCTIONS TO CANDIDATE: A 42-year-old homeless female well known to the emergency department presents complaining of vomiting for 2 days. She now notes blood in her vomitus. Take a detailed history, exploring possible etiologies.

DDx VITAMINS C

- **Vascular:** Esophageal varices, angiodysplasia, and aortoenteric fistula
- **Traumatic:** Mallory-Weiss tear, nose bleed (swallowed blood)
- **Metabolic:** Coagulopathy
- **Idiopathic/Iatrogenic:** Esophagitis, gastritis, and PUD
- **Substance abuse and Psychiatric**

- **First evaluate Airway, Breathing, and Circulation.** It may be necessary to perform an immediate intervention, such as supplemental O_2, IV access, or intubation.
  - Is the patient able to talk? Swallow? Cough?

- Are both lungs ventilated? Is the patient oxygenating (mentation, pulse oximetry)?
- Abnormal vitals? Peripheral circulation (pulses, capillary refill)?
- If no immediate interventions are required, proceed to take the history, and perform the physical examination.

History

- **Ch**aracter: Describe the bleeding. Bright red blood versus coffee ground appearance? Did you begin to vomit before the bleeding began (protracted retching and vomiting, Mallory-Weiss tear)?
- **L**ocation: Where is the blood coming from? Coughing up blood versus vomiting blood versus swallowed blood from a nosebleed?
- **O**nset: When was the first time this happened? How has it progressed (sudden versus insidious)?
- **R**adiation: Any other bleeding (bleeding from another location)? Nosebleed? LGI bleed?
- **I**ntensity: How severe is the bleeding? Has it gotten worse? How much blood have you vomited (quantify)?
- **D**uration: How long has the bleeding been going on (acute versus chronic)?
- **E**vents associated:
  - Abdominal pain? Quality of stool (melena, hematochezia)?
  - Weakness/fatigue (anemia)? Chest pain?
  - Palpitations/dyspnea? Postural presyncope/syncope?
  - Easy bruising? Prolonged bleeding from cuts or dental work?
  - Mallory-Weiss tear: Bleeding preceded by protracted retching/vomiting
  - Gastritis: Often painless, associated with use of NSAIDs or EtOH
  - PUD: Epigastric pain often relieved by food or antacids, may be associated with melena
  - Constitutional symptoms: Fever, chills, night sweats, weight loss, anorexia, and asthenia
- **F**requency: Has this happened before? How often does the bleeding happen (intermittent versus constant)?
- **P**alliative/**P**rovocative factors: Is there anything that makes it better/worse? If so, what?
- **Previous investigations:** UGI series, endoscopy, or previous requirement for transfusions
- **PMH/PSH:** PUD, liver disease, coagulopathy, esophageal varices, previous GI bleeding, previous GI surgery, or AAA repair (aortoenteric fistula)
- **MEDS:** NSAIDs/ASA, anticoagulants, or corticosteroids
- **SH:** EtOH, smoking
- **FH:** Coagulopathy

INSTRUCTIONS TO CANDIDATE: A 22-year-old female presents to her family doctor complaining of "greasy," foul-smelling stools. She also notes weight loss. Take a detailed history, exploring possible etiologies.

DD$_X$ Steatorrhea (VITAMINS C)

- **I**nfectious: *Giardia lamblia*, postinfectious malabsorption (villous sloughing)
- **A**utoimmune/**A**llergic: Celiac disease, Whipple's disease
- **I**diopathic/**I**atrogenic: Chronic pancreatitis, biliary obstruction
- **C**ongenital/genetic: Cystic fibrosis (CF)

History

- **Character: Describe your BMs.**
  - Are the stools large, oily, malodorous but somewhat formed?
  - Any blood, pus, or mucus in the stool? Describe the color of your stool.
  - Has there been a change in your bowel habit? Describe your usual BMs.
- **Onset:** When did the greasy stools start (sudden versus insidious)?
- **Intensity:** How severe is it? Number of stools per day and approximate volume of stool. Has it gotten worse?
- **Duration:** How long have you been passing fatty stools (acute versus chronic)?
- **Events associated:**
  - Appetite? Weight loss? N/V?
  - Abdominal pain (pancreatitis)?
  - Abdominal distension/bloating? Flatulence?
  - Edema (hypoalbuminemia)?
  - Easy bruising (vitamin K deficiency)? Bone pain (vitamin D malabsorption)?
- **Frequency:** How often do you pass greasy stools? Is every stool greasy (intermittent versus constant)?
- **Palliative factors:** Is there anything that makes it better? If so, what?
  - Fasting?
- **Provocative factors:** Is there anything that makes it worse? If so, what?
  - Fatty foods?
  - Dairy products?
- **Previous investigations:** Stool analysis, endoscopy, or biopsy
- **PMH/PSH:** Pancreatitis, DM, CF, IBD, Whipple's disease, chronic liver failure, jaundice, celiac disease, or GI surgery
- **MEDS:** Cholesterol-reducing drugs, "diet" drugs, or herbal medicines
- **SH:** EtOH, smoking, and ingestion of contaminated water (*Giardia* or "beaver fever")
- **FH:** IBD, CF, or celiac disease

INSTRUCTIONS TO CANDIDATE: A 33-year-old male presents to the emergency department with 6 hours of diarrhea and vomiting. He vomits twice in triage. Take a detailed history, exploring possible etiologies.

Definition

- **Diarrhea** is abnormally frequent passage of poorly formed or watery stool. Quantified, it is the passage of >300 ml of liquid feces in a 24-hour period.

DD$_X$ Diarrhea (VITAMINS C)

- **Vascular:** Ischemic colitis
- **Infectious:** Bacterial/parasitic/viral diarrhea, pseudomembranous colitis
- **Autoimmune/Allergic:** Celiac disease, Whipple's disease
- **Metabolic:** Drugs, carcinoid syndrome, and hyperthyroidism
- **Idiopathic/Iatrogenic:** IBD, IBS, malabsorption, and runner's diarrhea
- **Congenital/genetic:** CF, lactose intolerance

History

- **Character: Describe your BMs (Table 3-1).**
  - Are the stools frequent, voluminous, and poorly formed (diarrhea)?
  - Are the stools large, oily, malodorous but somewhat formed (steatorrhea)?
  - Are the stools frequent and formed but small?
  - Any blood, pus, or mucus in the stool? Describe the color of your stool.

Table 3-1 Localizing the Source of Diarrhea

Small Bowel	Large Bowel
Large volume stools	Frequent, small volume stools
Gross blood is infrequent	Gross blood may be present
Foul-smelling liquid stools ± undigested food (malabsorption caused by sloughed villi)	Tenesmus

- ■ Does diarrhea persist despite fasting?
- ■ Do you experience nocturnal diarrhea or fecal incontinence?
- ■ Has there been any change in your bowel habit? Describe your usual BMs.
- ■ Describe the vomitus. Is there any blood/coffee grounds?
- Location: Where were you when this started? Recent travel?
- Onset: When did the diarrhea start (sudden versus insidious)? When did the vomiting start?
- Intensity: How severe is it? Number of stools per day, approximate volume of stool. Has it gotten worse? Number of episodes of vomiting per day. Has it gotten worse? Are you able to keep anything down?
- Duration: How long has the diarrhea been going on (acute versus chronic)? How long have you been vomiting?
- Events associated:
  - ■ Fever/chills? Abdominal pain? Appetite? Orthostatic presyncope/syncope?
  - ■ Consumption of dairy or meat products in preceding 72 hours (undercooked hamburger or chicken, shellfish, lactose intolerance)? Excessive cereal, prunes, or roughage?
  - ■ Periods of constipation (IBS)?
  - ■ Travel to tropical/subtropical regions? Infectious contacts? Contaminated water ingestion?
  - ■ Sexual habits (anal penetration)? Increased urge to defecate (tenesmus)?
  - ■ IBD: Chronic diarrhea, abdominal pain, weight loss, extraintestinal manifestations (e.g., uveitis, erythema nodosum, and peripheral arthritis)
  - ■ Constitutional symptoms: Fever, chills, night sweats, weight loss, anorexia, and asthenia
- Frequency: Has this ever happened to you before? Is every BM like diarrhea (intermittent versus constant)?
- Palliative factors: Is there anything that makes it better? If so, what?
  - ■ Fasting?
- Provocative factors: Is there anything that makes it worse? If so, what?
  - ■ Dairy products?
  - ■ Solid foods?
- **Previous investigations:** Stool analysis, endoscopy
- **PMH/PSH:** IBD, celiac disease, hyperthyroidism, previous GI surgery, CF, HIV/AIDS, or malignancy
- **MEDS:** Laxatives, antidiarrheal agents, antibiotics (pseudomembranous colitis), corticosteroids, quinidine, or antihypertensives
- **SH:** EtOH, smoking, diet, and sexual habits (anal penetration)
- **FH:** IBD, CF, GI malignancy, or celiac disease

INSTRUCTIONS TO CANDIDATE: A 64-year-old male presents to his family doctor requesting a laxative because he is always "blocked up." Take a detailed history, exploring possible etiologies.

Definition
- **Constipation** is the difficult or infrequent evacuation of feces.

DD$_X$ VITAMINS C
- **V**ascular: Stroke (atonic colon)
- **T**raumatic: Spinal cord injury (atonic colon), anal fissure
- **M**etabolic: Hypothyroidism, hypercalcemia, drugs (e.g., chronic laxative use), and diet
- **I**diopathic/**I**atrogenic: IBS, fecal impaction, bowel obstruction (e.g., adhesions), and rectal stricture
- **N**eoplastic: Bowel tumor (benign or malignant)
- **C**ongenital/genetic: Hirschsprung's disease

History
- **Character:** Describe your current BMs.
  - Is stool too hard? Is defecation painful (fissures or perianal disease)? Do you defecate too infrequently?
  - Describe the color and shape of your stool.
  - Has there been any change in your bowel habit? Describe your usual BMs.
  - When was your last BM?
- **Onset:** When did the constipation start (sudden versus insidious)?
- **Intensity:** How severe is the constipation? Number of stools per day and per week. Has it gotten worse?
- **Duration:** How long has the constipation been going on (acute versus chronic)?
- **Events associated:**
  - Change in bowel habits or caliber of stool? Abdominal pain?
  - Diet: Decreased fiber or roughage intake, decreased fluid intake
  - IBS: Periods of diarrhea alternating with periods of constipation
  - Intestinal obstruction: Obstipation, colicky abdominal pain, feculent vomitus
  - Hypothyroidism: Cold intolerance, weight gain
  - HyperPTH: Bone pain/fractures, renal stones, abdominal pain, anxiety/depression
  - Constitutional symptoms: Fever, chills, night sweats, weight loss, anorexia, and asthenia
- **Frequency:** Has this happened to you before? How often does the constipation happen (intermittent versus constant)?
- **Palliative factors:** Is there anything that makes it better? If so, what?
- **Provocative factors:** Is there anything that makes it worse? If so, what?
- **PMH/PSH:** IBS, stroke, GI malignancy, rectal stricture, perianal disease, hyperPTH, hypothyroidism, or DM
- **MEDS:** Opioids, atropine, tricyclic antidepressants (TCAs), long-term use of cathartics, or use of enemas
- **SH:** EtOH, smoking, and diet
- **FH:** GI malignancy, hypothyroidism

SAMPLE CHECKLISTS

> INSTRUCTIONS TO CANDIDATE: Demonstrate examination of the liver, and describe your actions.

Key Points	Satisfactorily Carried out
Introduces self to the patient	❏
Determines how the patient wishes to be addressed	❏
Explains nature of the examination to the patient	❏
Examines the patient in a logical fashion	❏
Inspection	
• Looks for fullness/masses in RUQ	❏
• Asks the patient to take a deep breath and observes the RUQ	❏
Percussion	
• From resonance to dullness	❏
• From below and above costal margin	❏
Palpation	
• From RLQ toward the RUQ	❏
• On inspiration	❏
• Describes the quality of the liver edge, if palpable	❏
• Indicates direction of hepatic movement on inspiration	❏
Drapes the patient appropriately	❏
Makes appropriate closing remarks	❏

INSTRUCTIONS TO CANDIDATE: Demonstrate a focused physical examination for splenomegaly.

Key Points	Satisfactorily Carried out
Introduces self to the patient	❏
Determines how the patient wishes to be addressed	❏
Explains nature of the examination to the patient	❏
Examines the patient in a logical fashion	❏
Inspection • Notes visible signs of splenomegaly • Asks patient to take a deep breath and observes splenic area	❏ ❏
Percussion • Lower border of spleen • Traube's space • Castell's sign	❏ ❏ ❏
Palpation • Supports left rib cage with left hand • Starts palpation with right hand in RLQ toward the LUQ • Attempts to palpate splenic tip as patient inspires • Turns patient to right lateral decubitus position and palpates as above • Indicates direction of splenic movement on inspiration	❏ ❏ ❏ ❏ ❏
Indicates direction of splenic enlargement and differentiates from enlarged kidney	❏
Drapes the patient appropriately	❏
Makes appropriate closing remarks	❏

INSTRUCTIONS TO CANDIDATE: Inspect for visible extrahepatic stigmata of liver disease, and describe your findings.

Key Points	Satisfactorily Carried out
Introduces self to the patient	❏
Determines how the patient wishes to be addressed	❏
Explains nature of the examination to the patient	❏
Examines the patient in a logical fashion	❏
Face	
• Scleral icterus	❏
• Kayser-Fleischer rings	❏
• Xanthelasma	❏
• Parotid enlargement	❏
Hands	
• Clubbing	❏
• Leukonychia	❏
• Palmar erythema	❏
• Dupuytren's contracture	❏
• Tendinous xanthoma	❏
Chest (in males)	
• Gynecomastia	❏
• Axillary hair loss	❏
Abdomen	
• Caput medusae	❏
• Distension (ascites)	❏
Wasting	
• Arms and legs	❏
• First interosseous muscle in the hand	❏
• Temporalis muscle	❏
Other	
• Excoriations	❏
• Bruising	❏
• Spider nevi	❏
• Peripheral edema	❏
• Testicular atrophy	❏
Drapes the patient appropriately	❏
Makes appropriate closing remarks	❏

INSTRUCTIONS TO CANDIDATE: Perform a focused physical examination for ascites, and describe your findings.

Key Points	Satisfactorily Carried out
Introduces self to the patient	❏
Determines how the patient wishes to be addressed	❏
Explains nature of the examination to the patient	❏
Examines the patient in a logical fashion	❏
Inspection • Looks for protuberant abdomen • Looks for bulging flanks • Looks for herniated umbilicus	❏ ❏ ❏
Percussion • Tests for shifting dullness	❏
Feels for fluid wave or thrill • Uses the hands of the patient/assistant in midline • Feels with one hand while tapping with the other	❏ ❏
Drapes the patient appropriately	❏
Makes appropriate closing remarks	❏

CHAPTER 4

Genitourinary System

OBJECTIVES

ANATOMY

CARDINAL SIGNS AND SYMPTOMS

ESSENTIAL CLINICAL COMPETENCIES
PERFORM A FOCUSED EXAMINATION OF THE KIDNEY
USE PHYSICAL EXAMINATION TO DIFFERENTIATE SPLENOMEGALY FROM AN ENLARGED KIDNEY
PERFORM A FOCUSED EXAMINATION OF THE TESTICLE

SAMPLE OSCE SCENARIOS
- A 22-year-old female presents to the emergency department with a burning sensation with urination. She is concerned that she may have an infection. Perform a focused history and physical examination.
- A 70-year-old male presents with difficulty "making his water." Perform a focused history and physical examination.
- A 48-year-old male presents to the emergency department with the "worst pain" he has ever had. It radiates into his groin. The triage nurse asks him for a urine sample. Much to the patient's alarm, he passes "bloody" urine into the sample bottle. Perform a focused history and physical examination.
- A 69-year-old male presents to his family doctor complaining of blood in his "water." Perform a focused history, exploring possible etiologies.
- A 56-year-old female presents to her family doctor with a history of leaking urine. This limits her activities outside of the home. Take a detailed history, exploring possible etiologies.

SAMPLE CHECKLIST
- ❑ Demonstrate an examination of this patient's left kidney. Explain how to clinically differentiate an enlarged kidney from splenomegaly.

OBJECTIVES

*The successful student should be able to take a **focused history** of the genitourinary (GU) system, including:*
- Dysuria
- Hematuria
- Nocturia
- Urinary frequency, polyuria
- Decreased force of urination
- Urinary hesitancy
- Urinary incontinence
- Flank pain
- Testicular masses, testicular pain
- Penile/vaginal discharge, genital sores
- Sexual dysfunction

*The GU **examination** will include:*

Inspection
- Discharge
- Ulcerations
- Urethral meatus
- Scrotum
- Transillumination of scrotal masses
- Penis
- Vulva: Labia, clitoris, and vaginal introitus

Auscultation
- Scrotal mass (differentiate from indirect inguinal hernia)

Percussion
- CVA tenderness

Palpation
- Kidney
- Testicle
- Vulva: Labia, Bartholin's glands
- Digital rectal examination (DRE): Examination of the prostate

ANATOMY

- The **kidneys** are retroperitoneal organs that are often impalpable in normal adults. Shaped like a bean, the kidneys lie on either side of the vertebral column (Figure 4-1). Because of the presence of the liver on the right side, the right kidney is positioned more caudally than the left kidney. The twelfth rib protects the superior pole of the kidneys. The adrenal glands are encased on the superior poles of the kidneys.
- The **ureters** originate at the renal pelvis and insert into the urinary bladder. The peristaltic movements of the ureters convey urine from the kidney to the bladder. Its diameter is just 5 mm wide, which has clinical significance in the passage of renal stones.
- The **urinary bladder** is a distensible, muscular, pelvic organ that functions to store urine until it can be voided. When full the bladder can extend out of the pelvis and may be palpated in the abdomen as high as the level of the umbilicus. Be careful not to mistake the overly distended bladder for an abdominal mass.
- The **urethra** is a muscular tube that conveys urine from the bladder to the exterior. The male urethra is four to five times longer than the female urethra. The male urethra is also the exit tract for semen.
- The **prostate** is a walnut-sized gland that is located inferior to the urinary bladder and encapsulates part of the male urethra (Figure 4-2). Its relationship with the urethra accounts for the changes in urinary function that accompany prostatic enlargement. It is considered an accessory sex gland and contributes secretions to semen. Because of its proximity to the anterior rectal wall, the prostate can be palpated on DRE.
- The **penis** is the male sex organ, through which the urethra extends. Made of erectile tissue, its engorgement is essential for the performance of sexual intercourse. Formation of an erection is a complex orchestration of anatomic, physiologic, and psychological processes. The head of the penis is known as the **glans penis** and may or may not be covered in foreskin, depending on whether the patient has been circumcised.
- The **scrotum** is a sac that encases the testicles. It functions to regulate the temperature of the testes, necessary for the delicate process of spermatogenesis. The scrotum is

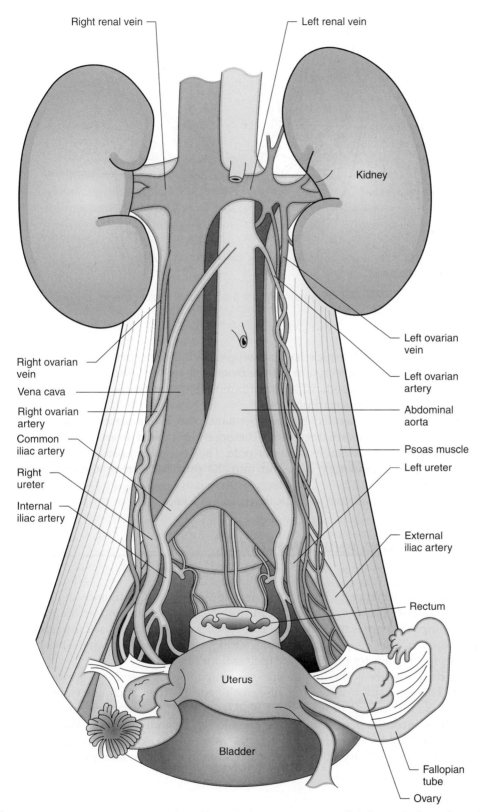

Figure 4-1 Genitourinary anatomy. (Adapted from DiSaia PJ, Creasman WT: *Clinical gynecologic oncology,* ed 6, St. Louis, 2002, Mosby, p 73, Figure 3-18.)

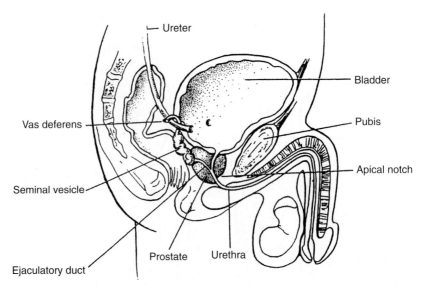

Figure 4-2   Cross-sectional anatomy of the male pelvis. (From Lepor H: *Prostatic diseases*. Philadelphia, 2000, WB Saunders, p 18, Figure 2-2.)

divided such that each testicle has its own pouch. It is important to note that the lymphatic drainage of the scrotum differs from that of the testes. The scrotal lymph vessels drain to the superficial inguinal lymph nodes, whereas the testicular lymph vessels drain to the retroperitoneum.

- The **testicles** are suspended by the spermatic cord in the scrotum. Their primary function is that of spermatogenesis. The sperm is passed from the testicle to the **epididymis,** which lies on its superior pole. The sperm then passes through the vas deferens to the ejaculatory duct and into the prostatic part of the urethra to the exterior.
- The female genital anatomy will be discussed in Chapter 10.

CARDINAL SIGNS AND SYMPTOMS

Incontinence

- **Urinary incontinence** is involuntary leakage of urine. Continence depends on a normal urinary bladder and competent sphincters (voluntary and involuntary).
- **Stress incontinence** is the leakage of urine associated with increased intraabdominal pressure, such as coughing, laughing, lifting, or increased activity. This typically results from sphincter insufficiency (pelvic floor laxity).
- **Urge incontinence** is the loss of urine accompanied by a sudden, strong desire to void. This typically results from diseases of the bladder, such as cystitis, bladder cancer, bladder calculi, or neurogenic bladder.
- **Overflow incontinence** occurs in the chronically distended bladder. When pressure inside the bladder exceeds sphincteric resistance, leakage occurs. This is usually associated with urinary obstruction, chronic anticholinergic therapy, or spinal cord injury.

Difficulty Urinating

- **Dysuria** is pain or other difficulty in urination.
- **Strangury** is the difficult passage of small amounts of urine accompanied by pain and an urgency to void.
- **Hesitancy** is an involuntary delay in starting the urinary stream. Difficulty "making urine" may refer to hesitancy or to increased force required to pass urine or the inability to empty the bladder completely.

Blood in the Urine

- **Hematuria** is blood in the urine. It is classified as microscopic (grossly normal) or macroscopic (red to brown discoloration). The dipstick reagents are sensitive to hemoglobin and myoglobin. A positive dipstick with no red blood cells (RBCs) on microscopy suggests myoglobinuria. On microscopy 2 to 3 RBC/high-powered field (HPF) is considered to be within normal limits.

ESSENTIAL CLINICAL COMPETENCIES

PERFORM A FOCUSED EXAMINATION OF THE KIDNEY

- A normal kidney in a normal person is not palpable. A normal right kidney may be palpable in an especially thin person with poor abdominal musculature. The left kidney is rarely palpable. Causes of kidney enlargement include tumors, cysts, and hydronephrosis.

Palpation

- **Right kidney:** Place your left hand under the patient parallel to the twelfth rib with your fingertips just reaching the costovertebral angle (CVA). Lift your left hand to displace the kidney anteriorly. Place your right hand on the right upper quadrant (RUQ) lateral and parallel to the rectus muscle. Ask the patient to take a deep breath. At the peak of inspiration place your right hand deep into the RUQ to "catch" the right kidney between your hands. Ask the patient to exhale and to stop breathing briefly. Release the pressure of your right hand, and feel the kidney slide back into its expiratory position. Note the size, shape, contour, consistency, and any tenderness. The lower pole of the kidney is rounded, whereas the liver edge is sharper, extends further medially and laterally, and cannot be "captured."
- **Left kidney** (Figure 4-3): Move to the patient's left side. Use your right hand to lift from below at the twelfth rib. Use your left hand to feel deep in the left upper quadrant (LUQ), and proceed as above. Because the left kidney is more superior in its position than the right kidney, it is less often palpable.

Fist Percussion

- Ask the patient to sit up. Place your left hand in the CVA, and strike your hand using the hypothenar aspect of your right fist (Figure 4-4). Use enough force to produce a

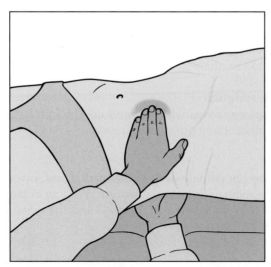

Figure 4-3 Bimanual palpation of the left kidney. (From Munro JF, Campbell IW, editors: *Macleod's clinical examination*, ed 10, Edinburgh, 2000, Churchill Livingstone, p 166, Figure 5.13, *A*.)

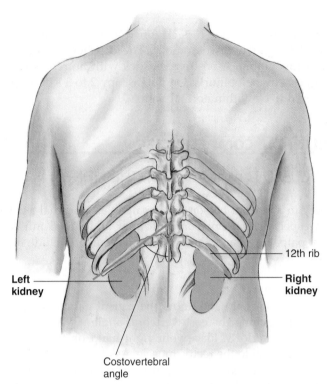

Figure 4-4   Costovertebral angle. (From Jarvis C: *Physical examination and health assessment,* ed 3, Philadelphia, 1996, WB Saunders, p 602, Figure 19-5.)

painless but audible thud. CVA tenderness suggests pyelonephritis or a musculoskeletal (MSK) problem.

USE PHYSICAL EXAMINATION TO DIFFERENTIATE SPLENOMEGALY FROM AN ENLARGED KIDNEY

Border
• The spleen has a notched medial border; the kidney does not.

Extension
• The spleen enlarges inferiorly and anteriorly toward the right lower quadrant (RLQ) and may extend beyond the midline of the abdomen. The kidney enlarges inferiorly and does not cross the midline.

Movement During Respiration
• Like the liver the spleen moves with respiration. The kidney is retroperitoneal and should not move substantially during respirations.

Palpation
• In splenomegaly one can palpate deep to the medial and lower borders of the mass but not between the mass and the costal margin. With an enlarged kidney an examiner should be able to palpate between the mass and the costal margin but not deep to its medial and lower borders.

Percussion
• In splenomegaly the LUQ will be dull to percussion; with an enlarged kidney it will be tympanitic because of the interposing bowel.

PERFORM A FOCUSED EXAMINATION OF THE TESTICLE

Patient Positioning
- The patient may be positioned supine or standing for the examination of the testicle. Consider patient comfort during this sensitive examination.

Inspection
- The scrotum is best inspected with the patient standing. Observe the lie of the testicles within the scrotum. The left testicle is often lower than the right testicle, although the opposite is true in many. Note any asymmetry or masses (Figure 4-5). Use a small light source to transilluminate a scrotal mass. A hernia or tumor will fail to transilluminate. Inspect the skin for excoriations, rashes, ulcerations, or other abnormality.

Auscultation
- Masses in the scrotum may be auscultated with the diaphragm of the stethoscope. Listen for any bowel sounds indicating the presence of bowel within the mass as in indirect inguinal hernia.

Palpation
- Begin by confirming the presence of two testicles within the scrotum. Palpate each testicle separately.
- Use your gloved index finger and thumb to gently grasp the anterior and posterior aspects of the testicle. Use your other gloved hand to similarly grasp the superior and inferior poles of the testicle.
- Note the size, shape, contour, consistency, and any tenderness in each testicle. Note any asymmetry.
- Palpate the epididymis at the superior pole of each testicle, and follow the spermatic cord into the inguinal canal. Palpate both spermatic cords simultaneously by rolling the scrotal skin between the thumb and index finger of each hand, superior to the testicles. Again note any asymmetry, masses, or tenderness.

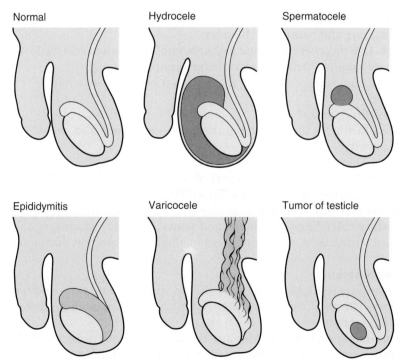

Normal   Hydrocele   Spermatocele

Epididymitis   Varicocele   Tumor of testicle

Figure 4-5   Causes of scrotal asymmetry. (From Munro JF, Campbell IW, editors: *Macleod's clinical examination*, ed 10, Edinburgh, 2000, Churchill Livingstone, p 172, Figure 5.19.)

SAMPLE OSCE SCENARIOS

> INSTRUCTIONS TO CANDIDATE: A 22-year-old female presents to the emergency department with a burning sensation with urination. She is concerned that she may have an infection. Perform a focused history and physical examination.

DD$_x$ VITAMINS C
- Infectious: Urinary tract infection (UTI), meatal or genital ulcer (e.g., herpes)
- Traumatic: Passage of a stone (trauma to the urethra)
- Idiopathic/Iatrogenic: Urethral syndrome

History
- **Character:** Describe the pain. Does pain occur at the beginning, middle, end, or throughout the stream? Is there any change in the quality of your urine (color, odor, quantity)?
- **Location:** Where is the pain?
- **Onset:** How did it start? Was the onset sudden or gradual?
- **Radiation:** Does the pain move anywhere? Where? To groin? To back?
- **Intensity:** How bad is the pain on a scale of 1 to 10, with 1 being mild pain and 10 being the worst? Is it getting better, worse, or staying the same?
- **Duration:** How long has it been going on (acute versus chronic)?
- Events associated: Urinary frequency?
  - Pain: Suprapubic, flank, groin, external genitalia
  - Genital ulcers or sores?
  - Vaginal discharge?
  - Any grit or stones in your urine?
  - UTI: Urinary frequency, dysuria, hematuria, urinary retention, urgency, strangury, incontinence, pain
  - Risk factors for UTI: Female (short urethra), pregnancy, urinary obstruction, GU malformation, and neurogenic bladder
- **Frequency:** Has this ever happened to you before? If so, when was the last time? Does it hurt every time you urinate (intermittent versus constant)?
- **Palliative factors:** Is there anything that makes it better? If so, what?
  - Analgesics?
  - Increased fluid intake?
- **Provocative factors:** Is there anything that makes it worse? If so, what?
  - Sexual activity?
  - Type of clothing?
- **Past medical history (PMH)/past surgical history (PSH):** STIs, UTI, GU malformations, nephrolithiasis, or diabetes mellitus (DM)
- **Medications (MEDS):** Antibiotics, analgesics, or antivirals (herpes)
- **Social history (SH):** Smoking, EtOH, and sexual history (including number of partners in past 6 months, new partners, and methods of protection during intercourse)

Physical Examination
- **Vitals:** Heart rate (HR), blood pressure (BP), respiratory rate (RR), and temperature
- **Respiratory (Resp):** Chest expansion (symmetry), auscultation (breath sounds, adventitious sounds)
- **Cardiovascular system (CVS):** Measure the jugular venous pressure (JVP). It is not a reliable indicator of hydration but is still a useful clinical finding. Palpate peripheral pulses. Note pulse volume, contour, and rhythm. Auscultate the heart, looking for extra heart sounds or murmurs.

- **Abdomen:** Inspect the abdomen. Auscultate for bowel sounds. Percuss lightly in all four quadrants. Before palpation ask the patient to cough and point to the most tender area with one finger. Palpate the most tender area last. Perform light and deep palpation, and identify any masses or areas of tenderness. Check for rebound tenderness. Examine the liver and spleen.
- **GU:** Percuss the CVA for tenderness. Palpate the kidneys. Inspect the external genitalia and urethral meatus for ulcerations. Depending on the history, you may wish to perform a pelvic examination. Note any discharge, inflammation of the cervix, cervical motion tenderness, adnexal tenderness, or pelvic masses. Note uterine size.

PEARL
- **Urethral syndrome** is characterized by urinary urgency, frequency, and dysuria in the absence of an identifiable cause such as infection or obstruction.

INSTRUCTIONS TO CANDIDATE: A 70-year-old male presents with difficulty "making his water." Perform a focused history and physical examination.

DD$_X$ VITAMINS C
- **Infectious:** UTI
- **Traumatic:** Posttraumatic urethral stricture
- **Idiopathic/Iatrogenic:** Bladder calculi
- **Neoplastic:** Prostatic enlargement (benign prostatic hypertrophy [BPH] or malignancy), bladder tumor
- **Congenital/genetic:** Urethral stricture (may also be a result of scarring)

History
- **Character:** Describe your difficulty with "making your water."
  - Difficulty initiating the stream despite the urge to void? Increased force needed to pass urine?
  - Sense of incomplete emptying? Continued urge to void despite termination of urinary flow?
  - Changes in the caliber of the stream (e.g., dribbling)?
- **Location:** In what setting do you notice this problem? At home or in public places (psychological component)?
- **Onset:** When did this trouble begin? How has it come about (sudden versus gradual)?
- **Intensity:** How severe is this trouble? Is it getting better, worse, or staying the same? Does it cause constant discomfort (full bladder)? Incontinence?
- **Duration:** How long has this been going on?
- **Events associated:**
  - Nocturia (urinary frequency at night)? Urinary urgency?
  - Abdominal distension? Incontinence (overflow from distended bladder)?
  - Strangury (bladder calculi)?
  - Pain: Abdominal, flank, groin
  - Hematuria (bladder tumor, bladder calculi)?
  - Fever/chills?
  - Renal colic: Hematuria, passage of stones/gritty urine
- **Frequency:** Have you ever had this trouble before? If so, when? Does it happen every time you try to urinate (intermittent versus constant)?
- **Palliative factors:** Is there anything that makes it better? If so, what?
  - Pressing on your abdomen while urinating?
- **Provocative factors:** Is there anything that makes the pain worse? If so, what?
  - Increased fluid intake?

- **PMH/PSH:** Malignancy, BPH, renal colic, previous surgeries
- **MEDS:** Anticholinergics
- **SH:** Smoking, EtOH, street drugs, and sexual history
- **Family history (FH):** Prostate cancer, renal colic

Physical Examination

- **Vitals:** HR, BP, RR, and temperature
- **General:** Cachexia, patient position on the stretcher, any apparent distress
- **Resp:** Chest expansion (symmetry), auscultation (breath sounds, adventitious sounds)
- **CVS:** Measure the JVP. It is not a reliable indicator of hydration, but it is still a useful clinical finding. Palpate peripheral pulses. Note pulse volume, contour, and rhythm. Auscultate the heart, looking for extra heart sounds or murmurs.
- **Abdomen:** Inspect the abdomen. Auscultate for bowel sounds. Percuss lightly in all four quadrants. If the urinary bladder is distended, there may be dullness in the suprapubic area to percussion that extends as far as the umbilicus. Before palpation ask the patient to cough and point to the most tender area with one finger. Palpate the most tender area last. Perform light and deep palpation, and identify any masses or areas of tenderness. Check for rebound tenderness. Examine the liver and spleen.
- **GU:** Percuss the CVA for tenderness. Palpate the kidneys. Examine the prostate gland by DRE (see pp 86-88). Use your gloved index finger to apply gentle, steady pressure at the anus. Ask the patient to take a deep breath, and insert the examining finger into the rectum. Palpate the prostate gland, which lies anterior to the anterior rectal wall (see Figure 4-2). Note any tenderness and the size, symmetry, consistency, and nodularity of the prostate gland.

INSTRUCTIONS TO CANDIDATE: A 48-year-old male presents to the emergency department with the "worst pain" he has ever had. It radiates into his groin. The triage nurse asks him for a urine sample. Much to the patient's alarm, he passes "bloody" urine into the sample bottle. Perform a focused history and physical examination.

DD$_x$ VITAMINS C

- **Vascular:** Ruptured/leaking abdominal aortic aneurysm (AAA)
- **Infectious:** UTI
- **Metabolic:** Coagulopathy, sickle cell crisis
- **Idiopathic/Iatrogenic:** Renal colic, hemorrhagic cystitis, incarcerated/strangulated hernia, appendicitis, and diverticulitis

History

- **Character:** What is the pain like? Sharp and localized? Crampy? Dull? What color is the urine? Bright red? Any clots?
- **Location:** Where does the pain originate?
- **Onset:** When did the pain start? How did it come on (sudden versus gradual)? When did you first notice blood in your urine?
- **Radiation:** Does the pain move anywhere? Groin? Penis? Testicle? Any pain with urination? Any other bleeding?
- **Intensity:** How severe is the pain on a scale of 1 to 10, with 1 being mild pain and 10 being the worst? Is it getting better, worse, or staying the same?
- **Duration:** How long does it last (intermittent versus constant)?
- **Events associated:**
  - Any grit or stones in your urine? Dysuria? Strangury?
  - N/V? Fever/chills?
  - Abdominal pain? Change in bowel habit?

- **Frequency:** Have you ever had this pain before? How often does the pain come? Any previous episodes of hematuria? Is there blood every time you micturate?
- **Palliative factors:** Is there anything that makes the pain better? If so, what?
  - Analgesics?
  - Particular position?
- **Provocative factors:** Is there anything that makes the pain worse? If so, what?
  - Movement?
- **PMH/PSH:** Renal colic, sickle cell anemia, AAA, previous surgeries
- **MEDS:** Analgesics, anticoagulants, chemotherapy (hemorrhagic cystitis), or anticoagulation
- **SH:** Smoking, EtOH, and street drugs
- **FH:** Sickle cell anemia, renal colic, or AAA

Physical Examination
- **Vitals:** HR, BP, RR, and temperature
- **General:** Check capillary refill. Note patient position on the stretcher and whether he or she is moving. Note any apparent distress, pallor, or diaphoresis.
- **Resp:** Chest expansion (symmetry), auscultation (breath sounds, adventitious sounds)
- **CVS:** Measure the JVP. It is not a reliable indicator of hydration but is still a useful clinical finding. Palpate peripheral pulses. Note pulse volume, contour, and rhythm. Auscultate the heart, looking for extra heart sounds or flow murmurs associated with hyperdynamic circulation. Auscultate for abdominal bruits.
- **Abdomen:** Inspect the abdomen. Note any bulges or obvious hernias. Auscultate for bowel sounds. Percuss lightly in all four quadrants. Before palpation ask the patient to cough and point to the most tender area with one finger. Palpate the most tender area last. Perform light and deep palpation, and identify any masses (pulsatile or nonpulsatile) or areas of tenderness. Check for rebound tenderness. Examine for hernias (see p 86). Examine the liver and spleen. Perform a DRE. A retrocecal appendix may produce tenderness on palpation of the rectal walls.
- **GU:** Percuss the CVA for tenderness (see Figure 4-4). Palpate the kidneys. Note any asymmetry. Examine the external genitalia for signs of trauma, ulcerations, or masses in the scrotum.

PEARLS
- Rebound tenderness is referred to **McBurney's point** in appendicitis.
- A patient with appendicitis may have positive **psoas, obturator,** and **Rovsing's signs.**

> INSTRUCTIONS TO CANDIDATE: A 69-year-old male presents to his family doctor complaining of blood in his "water." Perform a focused history, exploring possible etiologies.

DD$_X$ Painless Hematuria (VITAMINS C)
- **Infectious:** UTI
- **Autoimmune/Allergic:** Goodpasture's syndrome
- **Metabolic:** Sickle cell anemia, coagulopathy, and drugs
- **Idiopathic/Iatrogenic:** Glomerulonephritis, stones (bladder, renal)
- **Neoplastic:** Bladder or kidney tumor

History
- **Character:** Describe the color of your urine. Are there any clots?
- **Location:** Do you notice blood at the beginning, middle, or end of the stream?
- **Onset:** When did you first notice blood in your urine? How did this start (sudden versus insidious)?

- **Intensity:** How much blood is there? Is it getting better, worse, or staying the same?
- **Duration:** How long has this been going on (acute versus chronic)?
- **Events associated:**
  - Recent trauma? Instrumentation of the urethra?
  - Pain: Abdominal, flank, penile
  - Stones: Grit/stones in urine, strangury
  - UTI: Dysuria, urinary frequency, incontinence
  - Renal-pulmonary syndrome: Hemoptysis, shortness of breath on exertion (SOBOE)
  - Constitutional symptoms: Fever, chills, night sweats, weight loss, anorexia, and asthenia
- **Frequency:** How often does this happen? Is there blood every time you urinate (intermittent versus constant)?
- **Palliative factors:** Is there anything that makes it better? If so, what? Increased fluid intake?
- **Provocative factors:** Is there anything that makes it worse? If so, what?
- **PMH/PSH:** Bladder/kidney cancer, stones, sickle cell anemia, bleeding diathesis, Goodpasture's syndrome, or Wegener's granulomatosis
- **MEDS:** Chemotherapy (hemorrhagic cystitis), rifampin (discolors urine), or anticoagulation
- **SH:** Smoking, EtOH, and occupational or recreational exposures such as industrial dyes and solvents increase risk of bladder cancer.
- **FH:** Sickle cell anemia, coagulopathy

INSTRUCTIONS TO CANDIDATE: A 56-year-old female presents to her family doctor with a history of leaking urine. This limits her activities outside of the home. Take a detailed history, exploring possible etiologies.

DD_X

- Stress incontinence
- Urge incontinence
- Overflow incontinence

History

- **Character:** Describe the trouble you are having with urine leakage.
  - Does it occur with coughing, laughing, sneezing, or lifting?
  - Is there any urinary urgency?
  - Sense of incomplete emptying? Continued urge to void despite termination of urinary flow?
- **Onset:** When did this trouble start? Has it come about suddenly or gradually?
- **Intensity:** Do you lose small amounts of urine (dribbling)? Or large quantities? Is it getting better, worse, or staying the same? Do you need to wear an incontinence pad or diaper? How often must you change it? How does it impact on your daily life?
- **Duration:** How long has this been going on (acute versus chronic)?
- **Events associated:**
  - Pain: Abdominal, flank, groin
  - Irritative symptoms: Dysuria, strangury, urgency, and frequency
  - Obstructive symptoms: Hesitancy, increased force needed for urination, and sense of incomplete emptying
- **Frequency:** Have you ever had this trouble before? Do you have it every day (intermittent versus constant)?
- **Palliative factors:** Is there anything that makes it better? If so, what?
  - Frequent voiding?
  - Decreased fluid intake?
  - Kegel's exercises?

- **Provocative factors:** Is there anything that makes it worse? If so, what?
  - Exercise?
  - Lifting?
  - Laughing?
  - Coughing or sneezing?
  - Increased fluid intake?
- **PMH/PSH:** Malignancy, pelvic radiation, neurologic disease, previous surgeries on the GU tract (urethropexy, vaginal repair, resection of malignancy), GU trauma, or pregnancy (method of delivery and complications such as urethral injury)
- **MEDS:** Anticholinergics, diuretics
- **SH:** Smoking, EtOH, and sexual history

SAMPLE CHECKLIST

> INSTRUCTIONS TO CANDIDATE: Demonstrate an examination of this patient's left kidney. Explain how to clinically differentiate an enlarged kidney from splenomegaly.

Key Points	Satisfactorily Carried out
Introduces self to the patient	❏
Determines how the patient wishes to be addressed	❏
Explains nature of the examination to the patient	❏
Examines the patient in a logical fashion	❏
Inspection • Looks for signs of fullness (posteriorly)	❏
Auscultation • Listens for abdominal bruits	❏
Palpation • Uses bimanual technique • Palpates upper border • Palpates lower border • Asks patient to inhale while palpating	❏ ❏ ❏ ❏
Differentiates between an enlarged kidney and splenomegaly • Direction of enlargement • Palpation of upper border of kidney • Splenic notch • Presence of splenic hum	❏ ❏ ❏ ❏
Drapes the patient appropriately	❏
Makes appropriate closing remarks	❏

CHAPTER 5

Nervous System

OBJECTIVES

ANATOMY

CARDINAL SIGNS AND SYMPTOMS

ESSENTIAL CLINICAL COMPETENCIES
PERFORM A CRANIAL NERVE EXAMINATION
PERFORM A FOCUSED NEUROLOGIC EXAMINATION, LOOKING FOR SIGNS OF CEREBELLAR
     DYSFUNCTION
PERFORM A COMPREHENSIVE EXAMINATION OF THE REFLEXES
PERFORM A FOCUSED NEUROLOGIC EXAMINATION TO DIFFERENTIATE AN UPPER MOTOR
     NEURON LESION FROM A LOWER MOTOR NEURON LESION

SAMPLE OSCE SCENARIOS
- A 68-year-old female presents with complaint of "ringing" in her ears. Perform a focused history and physical examination.
- A 76-year-old female presents with left arm and leg weakness. Perform a focused history and physical examination.
- A 50-year-old female presents with lower back pain. Perform a focused history and physical examination.
- A 38-year-old male with a 20-year history of diabetes presents for a routine visit. Perform a neurologic examination on this patient, looking for signs of diabetic neuropathy.
- A 65-year-old male is referred with a complaint of tremor. Perform a focused physical examination.
- A 48-year-old female presents to your office complaining of headache. Take a detailed history, exploring possible etiologies.
- A 23-year-old female is brought to the emergency department after a witnessed fall to the ground with repetitive jerks. Take a detailed history, exploring possible etiologies.
- A 57-year-old male presents to the emergency department complaining of dizziness. Take a detailed history, exploring possible etiologies.
- A 53-year-old male presents to the emergency department via ambulance with a decreased level of consciousness.
  - Assess the level of consciousness.
  - Take a detailed history, exploring possible etiologies.

SAMPLE CHECKLISTS
- ❏ Perform a focused neurologic examination on the lower limbs, looking for evidence of an **upper motor neuron lesion.** State what you expect to find.
- ❏ Perform a comprehensive examination of reflexes in the upper and lower limbs of this patient.
- ❏ Perform a physical examination on a patient presenting with ataxia.
- ❏ Assess the function of this patient's fifth cranial nerve.

OBJECTIVES

*The successful student should be able to take a **focused history** of the neurologic system, including:*
- Syncope, blackouts (loss of consciousness)
- Seizures
- Weakness, paralysis
- Numbness, tingling (sensory changes)
- Involuntary movements, tremors
- Headache
- Visual loss or change, diplopia
- Dysphagia, dysarthria, and dysphonia
- Tinnitus, hearing loss
- Vertigo

*The neurologic **examination** will include the following:*

The student should be able to demonstrate examination of:
- Central and peripheral visual fields and visual acuity
- Extraocular movements
- Presence or absence of nystagmus
- Pupillary responses to light and convergence
- Facial sensation for light touch and pinprick
- Corneal reflex and nasal tickle
- Strength of masseter and temporalis muscles
- Jaw jerk
- Power of upper and lower facial muscles
- Auditory acuity: Weber's and Rinne's test if auditory acuity is diminished
- Speech, voice quality, and gag reflex
- Strength of sternocleidomastoid and trapezius muscles
- Strength, movement, and bulk of tongue

The student should be able to:
- Identify major muscle groups, and inspect limbs for muscle bulk and fasciculations
- Demonstrate the effective methods for testing tone and eliciting rigidity or spasticity
- Test strength of major muscle groups
- Demonstrate an understanding of innervation of major muscle groups with respect to peripheral nerves and nerve roots
- Differentiate between an upper motor neuron lesion (UMNL) and lower motor neuron lesion (LMNL)

The student should be able to demonstrate testing of:
- Pinprick
- Temperature
- Light touch
- Vibration sense
- Proprioception
- Stereognosis/graphesthesia
- Two-point discrimination
- Sensory extinction
- Romberg's test

The student should be able to elicit the following reflexes:
- Biceps
- Triceps
- Brachioradialis

- Finger
- Knee jerk
- Ankle jerk
- Plantar responses: Babinski's sign, Chaddock's maneuver, and Oppenheim's maneuver
- Abdominal

The student should be able to test coordination and cerebellar function using the following techniques:
- Observe the patient's gait and speech.
- Finger-to-nose test: Intention tremor, dysmetria
- Rapid alternating movements (finger and hands)
- Pronator drift, Holmes' rebound phenomenon
- Nystagmus
- Tandem gait
- Heel-knee-shin test

The student should be able to:
- Verify orientation to person, place, and time
- Perform basic tests of attention (serial 7s, spelling WORLD backward)
- Assess memory with three-item recall
- Assess basic elements of speech, including comprehension, repetition, fluency, and naming

The student should be able to assess the following in the context of a neurologic examination:
- Carotid bruits
- Straight leg raising
- Neck flexion

ANATOMY

Brainstem
- The brainstem is divided into three sections: midbrain, pons, and medulla. There are 12 cranial nerves (CNs) that originate from the brainstem. They control motor, sensory, and autonomic functions in the head and neck.
- Additional structures that run through the brainstem include corticospinal tracts, sensory tracts, cerebellar tracts, sympathetic tracts, and the reticular formation. Lesions involving these structures can give rise to crossed weakness, sensory loss, ataxia, Horner's syndrome, and decreased level of consciousness, respectively.
- The location of a brainstem lesion can be identified by focusing on the associated cranial nerve deficit (Figure 5-1):
  - Lateral brainstem lesions affect CNs IV, V, VII, VIII, IX, X, and XI.
  - Medial brainstem lesions affect CNs II, III, VI, and XII.
  - Midbrain lesions are identified by CN II, III, or IV involvement.
  - Pontine lesions are identified by CN V, VI, VII, or VIII involvement.
  - Medullary lesions are identified by CN IX, X, XI, or XII involvement.

Vision
- **CN II (optic nerve):** Light enters the eye and hits the retina, sending a signal along the optic nerve to the optic chiasm. At the optic chiasm a crossing over occurs such that nerve fibers originating from the left visual field go to the right hemisphere and those on the right go to the left hemisphere. From the optic chiasm the optic tract forms and relays to the thalamus. A radiation from the thalamus projects to the occipital cortex, the superior visual field via the temporal lobe (Meyer's loop), and the inferior visual field via the parietal lobe (Figure 5-2).

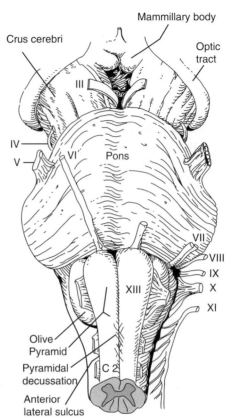

Figure 5-1   The ventral brainstem and cranial nerve anatomy. (From Marshall RS, Mayer SA: *On call neurology*, ed 2, Philadelphia, 2001, WB Saunders, p 395, Appendix A-9.)

- **Lateral conjugate gaze:** Frontal eye fields (middle frontal gyrus) regulate saccadic eye movement via brainstem nuclei and the medial longitudinal fasciculus.

Motor
- Motor output originates from the frontal lobe in the premotor cortex and primary motor strip (area 4, precentral gyrus). The motor strip is somatotopically arranged as the motor homunculus, in ascending order for face, arms, trunk, and legs (Figure 5-3).
- Fibers descend as the corticospinal tract (pyramidal tract) through the internal capsule and brainstem. Fibers cross in the lower medulla at the pyramidal decussation and run down the spinal cord on the lateral aspect as the corticospinal tract. As fibers branch off they synapse with large alpha anterior horn cells and exit the spinal cord ventrally to innervate the muscle groups at the neuromuscular junction.

Reflex Arcs
- Every muscle contains stretch receptors, which monitor the length of the muscle. A tap on the tendon stretches the muscle, causing the stretch receptors to send a signal via fast conducting Ia afferent fibers. These fibers enter the spinal cord dorsally and innervate the alpha motor neuron of the stretched muscle group. This neuron then fires, sending a signal to cause a brief contraction in the stretched muscle.
- Reflex arcs are generally limited to one or two spinal cord segments. Cortical influences tonically inhibit reflex activity, a loss of which causes hyperreflexia.

Sensory
- Sensory input originates from sensory receptors and free nerve endings. Sensory distribution can be organized by peripheral nerve innervation or dermatome

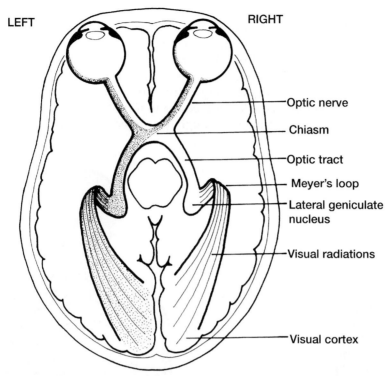

Figure 5-2   The visual pathway from retina to visual cortex. (From Bradley WG, Daroff RB, Fenichel GM, Jankovic J: *Neurology in clinical practice: principles of diagnosis and management,* ed 4, Philadelphia, 2003, Butterworth-Heinemann Medical, p 728, Figure 40.1.)

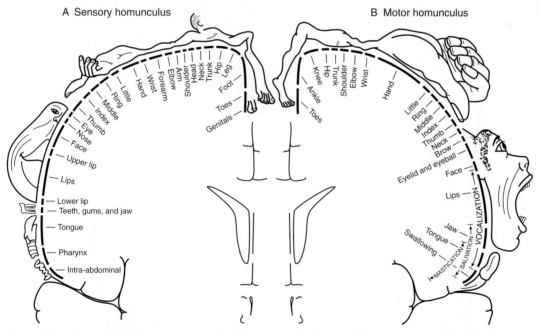

Figure 5-3   The sensory and motor homunculi. (Redrawn from Fix JD: *High-yield neuroanatomy,* ed 2, Philadelphia, 2000, Lippincott Williams & Wilkins, p 123, Figure 23-2.)

(Figure 5-4). Somatic sensation can be divided into two pathways: the posterior column–medial lemniscus pathway and the spinothalamic tract.

- The posterior columns conduct input regarding vibration, pressure, touch, joint position, and two-point discrimination. When receptors are stimulated a signal is transmitted to the posterior spinal cord. Lower extremity input travels up the spinal cord in the gracile fasciculus, upper extremity via the cuneate fasciculus. The fibers ascend the spinal cord and cross in the lower medulla to form the medial lemniscus. Fibers further ascend via the thalamus through the internal capsule to the primary

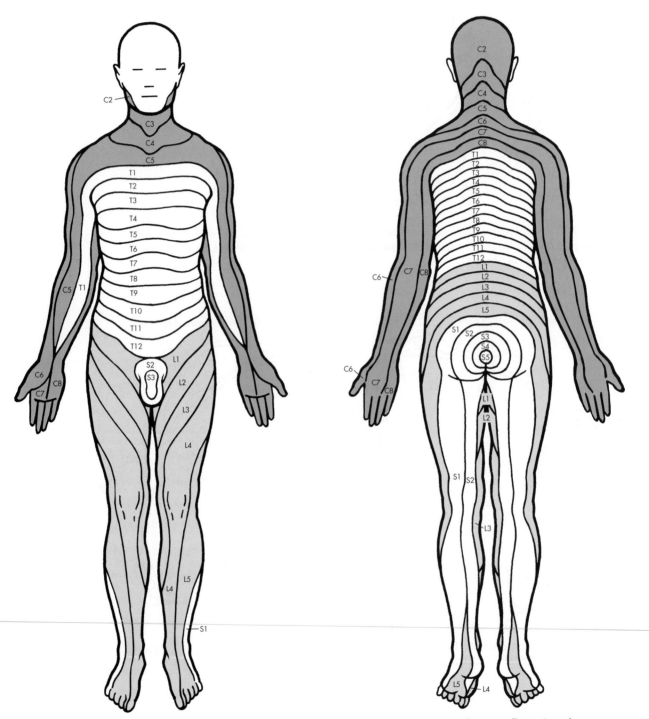

Figure 5-4 Sensory dermatomes. (From Marx JA, Hockberger RS, Walls RM, editors: *Rosen's emergency medicine: concepts and clinical practice*, ed 5, St. Louis, 2002, Mosby, p 347, Figure 36-22.)

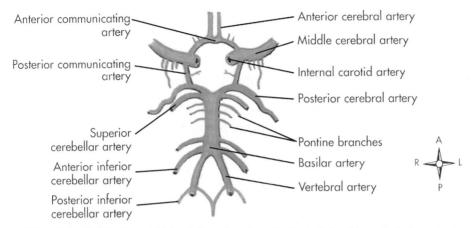

Figure 5-5   Circle of Willis. (From Seidel H, Ball J, Dains J, Benedict G: *Mosby's guide to physical examination,* ed 4, St. Louis, 1999, Mosby, p 758, Figure 20-3.)

somatosensory cortex (postcentral gyrus). Like the motor cortex the primary somatosensory cortex is arranged in a homunculus (see Figure 5-3). Sensory input is interpreted in the parietal lobe. Agraphesthesia, astereognosis, and neglect are cortical interpretation deficits.
- The spinothalamic tract conducts input for pain and temperature. Stimulated receptors send fibers to the spinal cord where they cross to the contralateral side. Once crossed, fibers ascend in the lateral funiculus to the primary somatosensory cortex via the thalamus and internal capsule.

Coordination
- Motor output is regulated by striatal and cerebellar input. The striatal (extrapyramidal) motor system includes the basal ganglia (caudate nucleus, putamen, and globus pallidus), subthalamic nucleus, substantia nigra, thalamus, and cortex. A complex interaction between these structures serves to regulate movement initiation, execution, and stereotyped reflex activity such as gait. The cerebellum connects to the thalamus, red nucleus, and cortex. It has three primary functions: maintenance of posture and balance, maintenance of muscle tone, and coordination of voluntary motor activity.

Vascular Anatomy
- The blood supply to the brain can be divided into anterior circulation and posterior circulation. The circle of Willis joins the two circulation systems (Figure 5-5).
- The anterior circulation has two main arteries: the middle cerebral arteries, which supply the lateral convexity of the hemispheres, and the anterior cerebral arteries, which supply the medial aspect of the hemispheres. The carotid artery is the main blood supply.
- The posterior circulation supplies the brainstem, cerebellum, and occipital lobe. The vertebral arteries are the primary blood supply.

CARDINAL SIGNS AND SYMPTOMS

Cerebellar Dysfunction
- **Ataxia** refers to uncoordinated, inaccurate movement not caused by paresis, tone change, loss of postural sense, or involuntary movements.
- **Dysmetria** is the inability to control distance, power, and speed of an act.
- **Dysdiadochokinesia** refers to rapid alternating movements that are fragmented, inaccurate, and worse with increasing speed.

Tremors

- **Resting tremor** is present when the body part is at rest and supported but disappears with activity.
- **Postural tremor** is present when the body part is held in a fixed posture.
- **Intention (kinetic) tremor** is present during movement and is caused by cerebellar disease.
- **Action tremor** refers to either a postural or intention tremor.
- **Static tremor** refers to either a postural or resting tremor.

Reflexes

- **Inverted reflex** refers to a scenario in which the tested reflex is absent but the response spreads to a lower or higher level (e.g., the biceps reflex is absent but the triceps reflex is elicited).
- A **pendular reflex** continues to swing after the tendon is struck. It is considered to be a cerebellar sign.

Diabetic Neuropathies

- **Distal axonal sensorimotor neuropathy** refers to distal, symmetric sensory loss in the lower extremities more so than the upper extremities and involving small fibers (pain and temperature perception) more so than large fibers. The patient may have painful dysesthesia, numbness, decreased vibration sense in his or her legs, and decreased tendon reflexes.
- **Autonomic neuropathy** may be characterized by anhidrosis, orthostatic hypotension, impotence, gastroparesis, or urinary hesitancy/incontinence.
- **Mononeuropathy** occurs from nerve infarction or entrapment (e.g., carpal tunnel syndrome, CN III palsy with pupillary sparing, CN VI palsy).
- **Mononeuropathy multiplex** is a neuropathy involving multiple peripheral nerves.
- **Diabetic amyotrophy** is an asymmetric proximal motor neuropathy or radiculoplexopathy characterized by proximal muscle pain, weakness, and atrophy.

Miscellaneous

- **Tinnitus** is the perception of buzzing, ringing, or roaring in the ears.
- **Vertigo** is the false sensation of rotation of the subject (subjective) or his or her environment (objective).

ESSENTIAL CLINICAL COMPETENCIES

PERFORM A CRANIAL NERVE EXAMINATION

CN I Olfactory Nerve

- CN I is not generally tested.
- Ask the patient to close his or her eyes, and test each nostril separately with coffee or mint.

CN II Optic Nerve

- Visual acuity: Test each eye separately using a Snellen eye chart.
- Assess color vision and red desaturation (dullness of red color in one eye compared with the other).
- Visual fields: Test each eye separately. Ask the patient to fixate on your nose, and hold your fingers equidistant between yourself and the patient. Assess when your finger can be seen, moving centrally in each of four quadrants.
- Pupillary response: Record pupil size and shape at rest. Illuminate one pupil, and note the direct and consensual responses (constriction of opposite pupil). Assess for relative afferent pupillary defect (RAPD) using the swinging flashlight test. Test

pupillary response to accommodation by asking the patient to look at an object as you bring it closer to the patient's nose.
- Funduscopy: Begin by noting the presence of the red reflex. Absence of this reflex indicates corneal or lens opacity.
  - Optic disc: Comment on color, cup-to-disc ratio, symmetry, and sharpness of the borders.
  - Retinal vessels: Arteries are light red and smaller compared with veins (dark red, larger, and pulsatile).
  - Retina: Note flame hemorrhages and white, gray, or black spots.
  - Papilledema: Look for optic disc congestion. An early sign of increased intracranial pressure (ICP) is loss of venous pulsations.

CN III Oculomotor Nerve, CN IV Trochlear Nerve, and CN VI Abducens Nerve
- Extraocular movements: Test all positions of gaze, horizontal and vertical. Inquire about double vision.
- Look for nystagmus on extremes of gaze.
- Assess saccadic eye movement by asking the patient to quickly shift gaze from one target to another.
- Observe smooth pursuit by asking the patient to follow a slow moving target.
- Opticokinetic nystagmus: Ask the patient to fixate on a moving strip with parallel lines.
- A CN III palsy will give a fixed, dilated pupil that is "down and out." Ptosis may be present (medial, superior, and inferior rectus muscles and the inferior oblique muscle).
- A patient with a CN IV palsy will be unable to look down and in. The patient may complain of difficulty walking downstairs (superior oblique muscle).
- A CN VI palsy will impair ability to move the affected eye laterally (lateral rectus muscle).
- **Horner's syndrome:** Ptosis, miosis, and facial anhidrosis

CN V Trigeminal Nerve
Motor
- Inspect for temporal wasting and jaw deviation.
- Palpate the masseter and temporalis muscle. To accentuate the temporalis muscle, ask the patient to clench his or her teeth.
- Ask the patient to open his or her mouth against resistance, and move the jaw from side to side (pterygoids).
- **Jaw jerk:** Tap on the chin with the mouth slightly open. Look for a jerk of the jaw.

Sensory
- Light touch: Touch cotton wool to the patient's face, comparing sensation in both sides (V1 forehead, V2 medial aspect of cheek, V3 chin).
- Pain: Use a sharp object to test sensory distributions V1, V2, and V3, comparing sensation in both sides.
- **Corneal reflex:** Approach the patient with a piece of tissue from the lateral side. Touch the cornea, and look for a blink response (afferent V1 division, efferent CN VII).

CN VII Facial Nerve
Motor
- Inspect the nasolabial folds for flattening, the palpebral fissures for sagging and drooping of the mouth.
- Ask the patient to raise his or her eyebrows (frontalis), close the eyes tightly (orbicularis oculi), show the teeth (buccinator), puff out the cheeks (orbicularis oris), and tense the neck muscles (platysma).

Sensory
* Test taste on the anterior two-thirds of the tongue using sugar, salt, and vinegar.

CN VIII Vestibulocochlear Nerve
* Auditory acuity: Whisper in one ear while making a distracting noise in the other ear.
* **Weber's test** (lateralization): Place a vibrating tuning fork (512 Hz or 1024 Hz) firmly on top of the patient's head. Ask the patient whether he or she hears it in one or both ears. Normally the sound is heard midline. In conductive hearing loss, sound will be lateralized to the impaired ear. In sensorineural hearing loss, the sound lateralizes to the good ear.
* **Rinne's test** (compare air conduction with bone conduction): Place a vibrating tuning fork (512 Hz or 1024 Hz) on the mastoid bone, behind the ear, level with the external auditory canal. When the patient can no longer hear the sound, move the tuning fork to the air close to the ear canal, and ask whether the sound is now audible. In conductive hearing loss, sound is best transmitted by bone conduction. In sensorineural hearing loss, sound is best transmitted through air.
* Vestibular tests: Dix-Hallpike's test (noting positional nystagmus), Romberg's test, and caloric testing

CN IX Glossopharyngeal Nerve and CN X Vagus Nerve
* Palate elevation: Look in the patient's mouth, and ask him or her to say "ahhhh." Look for symmetric elevation of the palate. If one side fails to elevate, the lesion is located ipsilaterally.
* Gag reflex: Touch the posterior pharynx with a tongue depressor. Look for symmetric elevation of the palate.
* Swallowing: Assess swallowing by asking the patient to swallow water or another beverage.
* Dysarthria: Abnormal pronunciation of speech can be caused by lesions of CNs IX and X and CNs V, VII, and XII, the motor cortex, cerebellum, or basal ganglia.
* Test taste on the posterior one-third of the tongue using sugar, salt, and vinegar.

CN XI Accessory Spinal Nerve
* Ask the patient to shrug his or her shoulders against resistance (trapezius).
* Ask the patient to turn his or her head to each side against resistance (sternocleidomastoid).

CN XII Hypoglossal Nerve
* Ask the patient to stick out his or her tongue and move it from side to side. Deviation to one side on attempted straight protrusion indicates a lesion on the side to which the tongue is pointing.
* On inspection of the tongue note any fasciculations or atrophy.

PERFORM A FOCUSED NEUROLOGIC EXAMINATION, LOOKING FOR SIGNS OF CEREBELLAR DYSFUNCTION

Head
* Inspect for nystagmus. Describe the direction of the nystagmus based on its fast phase.
* Note oscillations in saccades or impaired smooth tracking (overshooting or undershooting the visual target).
* Listen to the patient's speech. Remark on qualities such as scanning, explosiveness, or staccato.
* Note whether the head is carried with a tilt to one side.

Trunk
- **Truncal ataxia:** Ask the patient to sit up and look for truncal instability.
- **Truncal tremor:** Note any jerking movements of the head or body.

Arms
- Observe the patient's hands and arms at rest. Note any tremor, and comment on frequency.
- Ask the patient to stretch out the arms, palms up. Note whether the tremor gets better or worse.
- Perform **finger-to-nose testing**, commenting on worsening of tremor as the finger approaches the target (intention tremor) and the presence of past-pointing (dysmetria). Finger-to-nose testing is done at arms' length away by having the patient touch his or her fingertip to the nose and then to the examiner's finger repeatedly.
- **Holmes' rebound phenomenon:** Ask the patient to stretch out his or her arms, with palms up and eyes closed. Push down on the hand and then release it. Note whether the arm flies out of control, oscillating up and down.
- Ask the patient to perform **rapid alternating movements,** such as repeated pronation and supination of one hand over the other or tapping the fingers on a table.
- Instruct the patient to write a few sentences, and note whether the writing becomes larger (cerebellar) or smaller (parkinsonian).
- Motor: Expect to find decreased tone and normal power.
- Reflexes: Expect hyporeflexia, possibly with a pendular quality.

Legs
- **Heal-knee-shin:** Ask the patient to run his or her heel up and down the entire length of the shin, keeping the heel directly on the shin bone. Note any chaotic movements of the heel.
- **Patellar tap:** Ask the patient to tap his or her heel on the opposite patella repeatedly. Look for incoordination.
- Ask the patient to tap his or her foot on the ground, looking for dysdiadochokinesia.
- Motor: Expect to find decreased tone and normal power.
- Reflexes: Expect hyporeflexia and a pendular quality to the reflexes. To observe a pendular reflex, assess the knee jerk with the patient sitting up, legs dangling at the bedside.

Gait
- Expect a wide-based gait, with irregular steps and veering or falling to one side.
- **Romberg's test:** The patient with cerebellar dysfunction will lose balance with eyes open (negative Romberg).

PERFORM A COMPREHENSIVE EXAMINATION OF THE REFLEXES

Patient Positioning
- Ensure adequate exposure of the muscles to view reflex contraction.

Eliciting Deep Tendon Reflexes
- Relax the limb in question. Strike the tendon briskly. Compare reactivity of both sides.
- Use reinforcement if the reflexes are absent:
  - **Arms:** Clench teeth, or push down on bed with legs.
  - **Legs:** Lock hands, and try to pull them apart (Jendrassik's maneuver).

Grading
- 0, None
- 1+, Diminished

- 2+, Normal
- 3+, Increased
- 4+, Hyperactive, clonus

Nerve Roots
- Count from leg up: S1, 2; L3, 4; L5; C5, 6; C5, 6; and C7
    - S1, 2: Heel
    - L3, 4: Knee
    - L5: Hamstring
    - C5, 6: Brachioradialis
    - C5, 6: Biceps
    - C7: Triceps
- **Achilles (ankle jerk) S1, 2:** Dorsiflex the ankle with your hand, and strike the Achilles tendon. Look for plantar flexion at the ankle and contraction of calf muscles. Examine for clonus by rapid dorsiflexion of the ankle, followed by sustained dorsiflexion. Feel for repetitive plantar flexion.
- **Patellar (knee jerk) L3, 4:** Bend the knee, and relax the quadriceps muscles. Strike the patellar tendon firmly. Look for quadriceps contraction and extension at the knee.
- **Brachioradialis C5, 6:** Pronate the forearm, slightly flexed at the elbow. Strike the brachioradialis tendon 3 to 5 cm above the wrist on the stylus process. Look for flexion at the elbow and forearm supination.
- **Biceps C5, 6:** Pronate the forearm with elbow flexed to 45 degrees. With your thumb on the tendon, strike your thumb, and look for biceps contraction and further flexion at the elbow.
- **Triceps C7:** Flex the elbow, and pull the forearm across the patient's chest. Strike the tendon above its insertion at the olecranon process (2 to 3 cm above the elbow). Look for triceps contraction with elbow extension.

Plantar Reflex
- **Babinski's sign:** Stroke the sole of the foot, starting at the heel, following up the lateral margin across the ball of the foot to the base of the big toe. The normal response is flexion of the big toe. Extension of the big toe with fanning of toes indicates an UMNL.
- **Chaddock's sign:** Stroke the lateral aspect of the foot. Extension of the big toe with fanning of the other toes indicates an UMNL.
- **Oppenheim's sign:** Exert downward pressure on the shin. Extension of the big toe with fanning of other toes suggests an UMNL.

Primitive Reflexes (Signs of Frontal Release)
- **Glabellar tap:** Tap with a finger midline between the eyes while asking the patient to keep his or her eyes open. Persistence of blinking after three or four taps is a positive glabellar tap.
- **Snout, suck, and root:** Tap the side of the patient's mouth or upper lip, and look for a quiver in the lips.
- **Palmomental reflex:** Scraping the hypothenar eminence causes ipsilateral contraction of the mentalis muscle of the chin.
- **Grasp-place:** Place two of your fingers in the patient's palm, and look for involuntary grasping.
- **Hoffmann's sign:** Flick the volar surface of the distal portion of one of the patient's fingers, and look for flexion of the thumb, index, and middle fingers.

Cutaneous Reflexes
- **Abdominal:** Stroke the abdomen with a stick in a lateral to medial direction. A normal response is contraction of the abdominal muscles. Above the umbilicus this is mediated by T8 and T9; below the umbilicus it is mediated by T11 and T12 (**Beevor's**

sign: paralysis of the lower portions of the rectus abdominis muscle allows the umbilicus to move upward).
- **Cremasteric reflex:** Stroke the medial thigh (L1, 2), and look for scrotal retraction (S1).
- **Bulbocavernosus reflex:** Squeeze the glans of the penis, or apply traction on a Foley catheter, and look for external anal sphincter contraction (S2 to S4).
- **Anal wink:** Apply a sharp stimulus to the perianal area, and look for contraction of the anal sphincter (S2 to S4).

Other Reflexes
- **Jaw jerk:** Tap on the patient's chin with the mouth slightly open. Look for a jaw jerk forward, indicating a lesion above the level of the mid-pons.
- **Corneal reflex:** Stroke the cornea with a cotton swab, and look for a blink response. If this response is absent, suspect a trigeminal or facial nerve lesion.

PERFORM A FOCUSED NEUROLOGIC EXAMINATION TO DIFFERENTIATE AN UPPER MOTOR NEURON LESION FROM A LOWER MOTOR NEURON LESION

Definition
- **Upper motor neurons** project from the cerebral cortex to lower motor neurons in the anterior horn of the spinal cord. Signs of UMLN include muscle weakness, increased tone, and hyperreflexia (Table 5-1). An acute UMNL may initially give flaccid paralysis with decreased tone and decreased reflexes.
- **Lower motor neurons** project via peripheral nerves to skeletal muscle. LMNL signs include muscle weakness, atrophy, fasciculations, and hyporeflexia.

Table 5-1   Using Physical Examination to Differentiate an UMNL from a LMNL

	UMNL	LMNL
Cranial nerves	Facial paralysis, forehead spared Horner's syndrome with anhidrosis	Facial palsy involving forehead Horner's syndrome without anhidrosis
Motor bulk	None or slight atrophy	Focal atrophy, pronounced
Motor tone	Increased Rigidity (lead pipe, cogwheel) Spasticity (clasp knife)	Decreased Flaccidity
Motor power	Weak or absent (groups of muscles) Pronator drift	Weak or absent (focal) Fasciculations
Reflexes	Increased Plantar upgoing Hoffmann's sign Posturing	Decreased Plantar downgoing
FURTHER EXAMINATION THAT MAY ASSIST DIFFERENTIATION OF AN UMNL FROM A LMNL		
Sensory	Decreased Stereoagnosis Agraphesthesia Neglect	Decreased focally (root or peripheral nerve distribution)
Coordination	Ataxia Dysmetria Intention tremor	Not affected
Gait	Romberg positive (vestibular)	Romberg positive (sensory)

SAMPLE OSCE SCENARIOS

INSTRUCTIONS TO CANDIDATE: A 68-year-old female presents with complaint of "ringing" in her ears. Perform a focused history and physical examination.

DD$_x$ VITAMINS C
- **V**ascular: Arteriovenous malformation (AVM), bruits, and hypertension (HTN)
- **I**nfectious: Suppurative infection of middle ear or labyrinth
- **T**rauma: Foreign body (FB) in the external canal, head injury
- **M**etabolic: Anemia, drugs (e.g., quinine, salicylates, aminoglycosides, loop diuretics)
- **I**diopathic/**I**atrogenic: Cerumen occluding the external canal, temporal mandibular joint disease, hearing loss (20%), and Ménière's disease
- **N**eoplastic: Polyp in the external canal, acoustic neuroma/tumor (unilateral tinnitus)
- **S**ubstance abuse and **P**sychiatric: Psychogenic

History
- **Ch**aracter: Describe the sound. Is it pulsatile?
- **L**ocation: Is the noise heard in one or both ears?
- **O**nset: When did you first notice the ringing?
- **I**ntensity: How severe is this (on scale of 1 to 10)? How is it affecting your life?
- **D**uration: How long has it been going on?
- **E**vents associated:
  - Hearing loss? Vertigo?
  - Exposure to loud noise (gun fire, loud music, heavy machinery)?
  - Pain? Fever/chills? Weight loss?
  - Neurofibromas? Axillary freckling? Café au lait spots?
  - Psychiatric issues? EtOH use?
  - History of head injury?
- **F**requency: How often does the ringing occur? Is it constant or intermittent?
- **P**alliative factors: Is there anything that makes the ringing better? If so, what?
- **P**rovocative factors: Is there anything that makes the ringing worse? If so, what?
- **Past medical history (PMH)/past surgical history (PSH):** Aneurysms, neurofibromatosis, Ménière's disease, head injury, ear disease, or HTN
- **Medications (MEDS):** Quinine, salicylates, aminoglycosides (ototoxic), or loop diuretics
- **Family history (FH):** Neurofibromatosis, Ménière's disease

Physical Examination
- **Vitals:** Heart rate (HR), respiratory rate (RR), blood pressure (BP), and temperature (may find low-grade fever)
- **General:** Cachexia, neurofibromas, café au lait spots
- **Ears:**
  - Inspect the external ear (auricle, tragus) and auditory canal.
  - Examine the tympanic membrane, and identify landmarks (Figure 5-6). Grasp the auricle, and pull it upward, backward, and slightly away from the head. Gently insert the speculum of the otoscope into the ear canal (hold otoscope between thumb and fingers and brace your hand against the patient's face). Describe any abnormalities such as discharge, erythema, swelling, or loss of landmarks.
  - Check auditory acuity, testing one ear at a time. Occlude one ear with a finger, and whisper softly into the other ear using words or numbers of equally accented syllables.
  - **Weber's test:** Lateralization (Box 5-1)
  - **Rinne's test:** Compare air conduction with bone conduction (see Box 5-1).

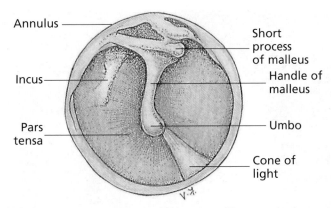

Figure 5-6   Tympanic membrane. (From Wilson SF, Gidden JF: *Health assessment for nursing practice*, ed 2, St. Louis, 2001, Mosby, p 289, Figure 15-3.)

Box 5-1   Differentiating Conductive from Sensorineural Hearing Loss

WEBER'S TEST
- Lateralization means ipsilateral conductive hearing loss or contralateral sensorineural losses.

RINNE'S TEST
- Conductive hearing loss: bone conduction > air conduction
- Sensorineural hearing loss: air conduction > bone conduction

---

- **Neurologic (Neuro):** Inspect for nystagmus. Perform Dix-Hallpike's test by bringing the patient from a seated position to lie horizontally with the head hanging 45 degrees off the end of the bed with the head turned to one side. This test may provoke vertigo and vomiting. It should be performed with the patient's eyes open to observe for the development of nystagmus.

INSTRUCTIONS TO CANDIDATE: A 76-year-old female presents with left arm and leg weakness. Perform a focused history and physical examination.

DD$_X$ VITAMINS C
- **Vascular:** Stroke (cardioembolic, atheroembolic, dissection, vasculitis), migraine
- **Infectious:** Central nervous system (CNS) abscess
- **Trauma:** Epidural hematoma (Figure 5-7), subdural hematoma
- **Autoimmune/Allergic:** Multiple sclerosis (MS)
- **Idiopathic/Iatrogenic:** Seizure (Todd's paresis)
- **Neoplastic:** CNS tumor

History
- **Character:** How much movement do you have on your weak side?
- **Location:** What body parts feel weak? Is your leg, arm, or face weak on the left or right side?
- **Onset:** When did the weakness start? Did the weakness come on suddenly or gradually?
  - Sudden onset: Stroke
  - Gradual, progressive onset: Tumor, subdural hematoma
  - After trauma: Epidural hematoma, subdural hematoma, and cervical spine injury

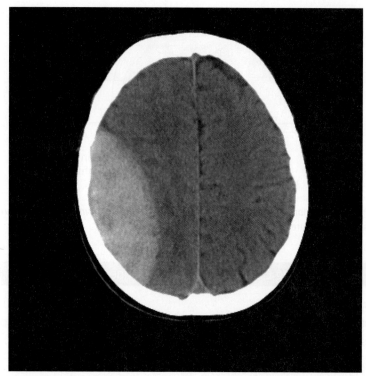

Figure 5-7 Epidural hemorrhage that presented nearly 1 week after a fall with left-sided weakness.

- Intensity: How severe is your weakness? Are you able to walk? Are you able to accomplish activities of daily living (ADLs)?
- Duration: How long has the weakness been present?
- Events associated:
  - Head trauma?
  - Neck trauma associated with headache and eye pain (dissection)?
  - Headache (atypical migraine)?
  - Changes in vision, speech, or swallowing?
  - Palpitations? Atrial fibrillation (embolic stroke)?
- **PMH/PSH:** Stroke, stroke risk factors (HTN, diabetes mellitus [DM], hyperlipidemia, smoking, previous stroke, previous myocardial infarction [MI], atrial fibrillation), brain injury, seizures, optic neuritis, or MS
- **MEDS:** acetylsalicylic acid (ASA), nonsteroidal antiinflammatory drugs (NSAIDs), Plavix, warfarin, steroids, antiepileptics, and migraine prophylaxis
- **Social history (SH):** Smoking, EtOH use, recreational drug use, and previous mobility/use of limbs
- **FH:** Stroke, MI, or migraine

> INSTRUCTIONS TO CANDIDATE: A 50-year-old female presents with lower back pain. Perform a focused history and physical examination.

DD$_X$ VITAMINS C
- **Vascular:** Spinal infarct, spinal hemorrhage, abdominal aortic aneurysm (AAA), and aortic dissection
- **Infectious:** Osteomyelitis, spinal abscess, viral myalgia, urinary tract infection (UTI), and pyelonephritis

- **Trauma:** Disk herniation, vertebral fracture, osteoarthritis, and muscle/ligament strain
- **Autoimmune/Allergic:** Rheumatoid arthritis, ankylosing spondylitis
- **Metabolic:** Paget's disease, osteomalacia, and osteoporosis
- **Idiopathic/Iatrogenic:** Pancreatitis, renal stone
- **Neoplastic:** Metastatic or primary (extradural, extramedullary, intramedullary)
- **Psychiatric**
- **Congenital:** Spina bifida, spondylolysis

History
- **Character:** Describe the pain (aching, sharp, dull, cramping, burning).
- **Location:** Where is the pain? Is the pain in the middle of your back or off to one side? Is the pain deep or superficial?
- **Onset:** How did the pain start (sudden versus gradual)? Did anything initiate the pain?
- **Radiation:** Does the pain move anywhere?
  - From abdomen to back: pancreatitis, AAA, cholecystitis, pregnancy
  - From back into groin: renal stone, pyelonephritis, UTI
  - From back into lower limb: radiculopathy
- **Intensity:** How severe is the pain on a scale of 1 to 10, with 1 being mild pain and 10 being the worst?
- **Duration:** How long has the pain been there (acute versus chronic)?
  - Minutes-hours: Trauma, infarct
  - Hours-days: Infection
  - Days-weeks: Neoplasm, arthritic
- **Events associated:**
  - Weight loss, bone pain (neoplasm, osteomyelitis)?
  - Fever/chills (infection)? Urinary symptoms such as dysuria, frequency (UTI, pyelonephritis)?
  - Trauma?
  - Urinary retention, urinary or fecal incontinence (cord compression)?
  - Unilateral weakness, sensory loss (radiculopathy)?
  - Bilateral weakness, sensory loss (myelopathy)?
  - Joint stiffness, inflammation, and pain (arthritis)?
- **Frequency:** Have you ever had this pain before? How often does the pain come (intermittent versus constant)? How long does it last?
- **Palliative factors:** Is there anything that makes the pain better? If so, what? Does rest make it better?
- **Provocative factors:** Is there anything that makes the pain worse? If so, what? Does activity, leaning forward, backward, or sideways make it worse? Does coughing, sneezing, or straining evoke the pain?
- **PMH/PSH:** Back trauma, surgery, cancer (myeloma, breast, lung), arthritis, pancreatitis, AAA
- **MEDS:** Ibuprofen, NSAIDS, or opioids
- **SH:** Smoking, EtOH use, recreational drug use, occupation (lifting, manual labor), pending lawsuits, or intent to seek compensation

Physical Examination
- Ensure stability of the spine in acute traumatic injury.
- **Vitals:** HR and rhythm, RR (depth, effort, and pattern), BP, pulsus paradoxus, and temperature
  - Neurogenic shock: Autonomic instability
  - Hypovolemic shock (ruptured AAA): Hypotensive, tachycardic
- **Respiratory (Resp):** Auscultate the chest, noting the quality of the breath sounds and any adventitious sounds.

- **Cardiovascular system (CVS):** Palpate peripheral pulses. Auscultate the heart, looking for extra heart sounds or murmurs.
- **Abdomen:** Inspect the abdomen. Auscultate for bowel sounds. Percuss lightly in all four quadrants. Perform light and deep palpation, and identify any masses (e.g., pulsatile mass) or areas of tenderness. Check for rebound tenderness. Examine the liver and spleen. Perform a digital rectal examination (DRE). Note rectal tone.
- **Neuro:** Assess for CN deficits. Examine for lower limb weakness and atrophy. Test upper and lower limb reflexes. Expect hyporeflexia at the level of a spinal cord injury and hyperreflexia below the injury with upgoing plantars (Babinski). Assess all sensory modalities, including light touch, pinprick, joint position, and vibration. Demonstrate any sensory level, and describe the pattern of distribution.
- **Musculoskeletal (MSK):** Watch the patient walk, commenting on limp, shortening of step, tilt, and ability to bear weight. Note ability to stand on toes and on heels. Inspect the curvature and alignment of the spine. Look for any pelvic tilt or asymmetry of gluteal musculature. Palpate the spine. Note any tenderness or step deformities that may indicate spondylolisthesis. Palpate the paraspinal muscles for bulk, tenderness, mass, or spasm. Percuss each vertebra with the hypothenar aspect of your closed fist. Deep pain to percussion is nonspecific but may indicate degenerative disease, malignancy, or infection. Inspect the active range of motion (ROM) in the back (flexion, extension, lateral bending). With the patient standing instruct him or her to touch the toes (forward flexion). With the patient in flexion palpate the spinous processes, noting the normal increased interspinous distance. **Finger-to-floor distance** can be used to measure the extent of flexion. The normal range varies considerably, but this measurement is useful to follow disease progression in ankylosing spondylitis. Also test ROM in the hips and knees. Assess leg-length discrepancy by measuring from the anterior superior iliac spine to the ipsilateral medial malleolus. Radicular pain from L5 or S1 roots can be reproduced by several techniques that stretch the sciatic nerve roots:
  - **Straight leg raising** is usually performed with the patient supine and legs extended. The symptomatic leg is passively raised off the bed (knee extended). A positive test is indicated by worsened pain in the affected leg at hip flexion <60 to 70 degrees.
  - The **bowstring sign** is elicited by passively raising the patient's symptomatic leg off the bed with the knee in slight flexion until just below the threshold for radicular pain. The bowstring sign is said to be present when pain is then elicited through firm compression of the popliteal fossa (pain radiates from the knee to the back).
  - **Lasègue's sign** is elicited by passively raising the patient's symptomatic leg off the bed with the knee in slight flexion until just below the threshold for radicular pain. Lasègue's sign is said to be present when passive dorsiflexion of the ankle worsens pain.

INSTRUCTIONS TO CANDIDATE: A 38-year-old male with a 20-year history of diabetes presents for a routine visit. Perform a neurologic examination on this patient, looking for signs of diabetic neuropathy.

Physical Examination
- **Vitals:** Perform orthostatic vitals to identify any postural changes.
- **CN:** Examine the fundi for evidence of hemorrhage, exudates, and neovascularization. Inspect the extraocular movements for signs of CN III, IV, or VI palsy. Diabetics with CN III palsy should have pupillary sparing.
- **Motor:** Look for atrophy and weakness in the distribution of a peripheral nerve (e.g., median, ulnar, radial, femoral, or peroneal nerves). Assess for pelvic girdle and thigh muscle atrophy.

- **Reflexes:** Examine the deep tendon reflexes (DTRs) in the upper and lower limbs. Expect decreased reflexes and an absent knee jerk.
- **Sensory:** Assess all sensory modalities, comparing symmetry and distribution. Expect decreased pain and temperature perception, two-point discrimination, and proprioception in a symmetric distribution affecting legs more so than arms, distally more so than proximally. Asymmetric sensory loss may be caused by a peripheral neuropathy (ulnar, median, radial, lateral femoral cutaneous, sciatic, or peroneal).
- **Coordination** is usually normal. If sensory modalities are severely impaired, the finger-to-nose test also may be impaired.
- **Gait:** Inspect the gait. Depending on the affected peripheral nerves and sensation, a variety of gaits may be noted:
  - Sensory-ataxic gait: Short, uneven gait with high steps, slapping feet to the ground and eyes cast downward
  - High steppage gait: Exaggerated hip and knee elevation to allow the affected foot to clear ground. This type of gait is caused by a peroneal palsy, impairing the ability to dorsiflex the foot (foot drop).
  - Dystrophic gait: Waddling gait with lordotic posture from pelvic muscle weakness

---

INSTRUCTIONS TO CANDIDATE: A 65-year-old male is referred with a complaint of tremor. Perform a focused physical examination.

DD$_X$ VITAMINS C (Table 5-2)
- **Trauma:** Posttraumatic syndrome
- **Metabolic:** Hyperthyroidism, hypoglycemia, Wilson's disease, and metabolic encephalopathy (asterixis)
- **Idiopathic/Iatrogenic:** Benign essential tremor, cerebellar disease, Parkinson's disease, Shy-Drager syndrome, Benedikt's syndrome, epilepsia partialis continua, and myoclonus
- **Substance abuse and Psychiatric:** EtOH withdrawal, caffeine withdrawal, drug intoxication, dystonic tremor, and psychogenic tremor
- **Congenital/genetic:** Huntington's chorea

Physical Examination
- **Arms:** Observe the patient at rest. Look for rhythmic movement in the hands and arms. Note the frequency of any tremor. It may be helpful to distract the patient by asking him or her to recite the months of the year. Ask the patient to hold his or her arms stretched out in front. Note any change in tremor and frequency. Perform finger-to-nose testing, and look for worsening of the tremor as his or her finger approaches the target (intention tremor) and for past pointing suggesting dysmetria. Valuable data can be gathered by watching the patient write a sample paragraph. Look for large shaky writing characteristic of postural or intention tremor or small writing (micrographia) associated with parkinsonism.
- **Head:** Note any head tremor and its direction (horizontal or vertical). Head tremor is suggestive of postural or intention tremor. Voice tremor may also be associated with postural tremors. Observe the face, jaw, lip, and tongue for tremors suggestive of parkinsonism.

Table 5-2 Classification of Common Tremors

Resting Tremor	Postural Tremor	Intention Tremor
Parkinsonism Midbrain (rubral) tremor	Enhanced physiologic tremor Essential tremor	Cerebellar disease

- **Trunk:** Ask the patient to sit unsupported. Truncal tremor in this position suggests cerebellar disease.
- **Legs:** Assess the legs at rest, during heel-knee-shin testing, and while standing and walking. Note the tremor frequency at rest and with activity such as tapping the foot on the floor. Leg tremor suggests parkinsonism, and gait ataxia suggests cerebellar disease.

Associated Features of Parkinsonism
- **Vitals:** Postural changes in BP and HR
- **Mental status:** Dementia, depression
- **CN:** Masklike facies
- **Motor:** Bradykinesia, rigidity, and cogwheeling

INSTRUCTIONS TO CANDIDATE: A 48-year-old female presents to your office complaining of headache. Take a detailed history, exploring possible etiologies.

DD$_X$ VITAMINS C
- **V**ascular: Subarachnoid hemorrhage (SAH), intracerebral hemorrhage, temporal arteritis, and migraine
- **I**nfectious: Meningitis, encephalitis, and sinusitis
- **T**rauma: Posttraumatic headache (concussion syndrome)
- **I**diopathic/**I**atrogenic: Tension headache, cluster headache, and trigeminal neuralgia
- **N**eoplastic: CNS tumor (increased ICP)
- **S**ubstance abuse and **P**sychiatric: Drug intoxication/withdrawal

History
- **C**haracter: What does the pain feel like? Is there a sensation of tightness, pressure, sharpness, stabbing, throbbing, or pulsation?
  - Tension headache: Steady sensation of tightness, pressure
  - Migraine: Pulsating, throbbing pain, and aura (scintillation, scotoma)
  - Cluster headache: Ice pick–like, stabbing pain
  - Intracranial mass: Steady, dull pain
  - Trigeminal neuralgia: Sharp, lancinating pain
- **L**ocation: Where is the pain? Is there a focus in the front, side, back of head, or in the eyes, ears, or throat?
  - Tension headache: Bilateral frontal/occipital
  - Migraine: Unilateral, ocular pain
  - Cluster headache: Unilateral, ocular pain
  - Optic neuritis, glaucoma, and iritis: Ocular pain
  - Sinusitis, nasal infection: Paranasal pain (maxillary, frontal)
  - Postherpetic neuralgia: Burning pain in a division of the trigeminal nerve
  - Trigeminal neuralgia: Lancinating pain, second or third division of the trigeminal nerve
- **O**nset: When did the pain start? How suddenly did the pain start?
  - Thunderclap: SAH
  - On awakening, worse in morning: Mass lesion, sinus headache
  - Awaken from sleep: Cluster headache, mass lesion
  - At end of the day, develop with stress: Tension headache
  - Episodic, worse during menses or weather changes: Migraine
- **R**adiation: Where does the pain go?
  - Neck pain: Occipital neuralgia (cervical osteoarthritis)
- **I**ntensity: How severe is the pain? Does the pain stop you from working or awaken you from sleep?
  - Worst headache of lifetime: SAH

- **Duration:** How long does the pain last?
  - Minutes-hours: Trigeminal neuralgia, tension headache
  - Days: Migraine, cluster headache
- **Events associated:**
  - Weight loss: Cancer, giant cell arteritis, depression
  - Fever/chills: Systemic infection, meningitis, endocarditis resulting in brain abscess
  - Visual change: Glaucoma, migraine, intracranial mass, temporal arteritis
  - N/V: Migraine, posttraumatic headache, mass lesion
  - Photophobia: Migraine, meningitis, SAH
  - Myalgias: Tension, viral syndromes, giant cell arteritis
  - Ipsilateral rhinorrhea, lacrimation: Cluster headache
  - Loss of consciousness: Migraine, glossopharyngeal neuralgia, mass lesion
- **Frequency:** How often do you have a headache?
  - Continuous, most days of the month (tension headache)?
  - Episodic (migraine, cluster headache)?
  - Progressive worsening (intracranial mass)?
- **Palliative factors:** Is there anything that makes your headache better? If so, what? Does sleep or a quiet, dark room improve your headaches?
- **Provocative factors:** Is there anything that makes your headache worse? If so, what?
  - Recent eye or dental surgery, sinusitis, hay fever, systemic viral infection, tension, emotional stress, or fatigue
  - Triggers: Menses, hunger, ice cream, nitrite-containing foods (e.g., hot dogs, salami, ham), chocolate, cheddar cheese, bright lights, OCP, intense emotion, exercise, eye strain, weather changes, or yawning
  - Cluster headache: EtOH
  - Giant cell arteritis, trigeminal neuralgia, and glossopharyngeal neuralgia: Chewing, eating
  - Coughing in patients with a structural lesion in the posterior fossa
- **PMH/PSH:** Headache, migraine, travel sickness as a child, intracranial lesion, and surgery
- **MEDS:** Withdrawal from ibuprofen, NSAIDs, opioids, monoamine oxidase inhibitors (MAOIs), or addition of a new medication
- **SH:** EtOH withdrawal, caffeine use, and diet (e.g., chocolate, cheese, wine)
- **FH:** Migraine, travel sickness

INSTRUCTIONS TO CANDIDATE: A 23-year-old female is brought to the emergency department after a witnessed fall to the ground with repetitive jerks. Take a detailed history, exploring possible etiologies.

DD$_X$ VITAMINS C
- **V**ascular: Complicated migraine
- **M**etabolic: Hypoglycemia
- **I**diopathic/**I**atrogenic: Seizure (primary or secondary), syncope, and myoclonus
- **S**ubstance abuse and **P**sychiatric: Pseudoseizure, hyperventilation, narcolepsy, panic attack, and drug intoxication/withdrawal

Collateral History
- Describe what happened. Did she fall?
- What led up to it (what was happening at the time)?
- Were there any movements? Was there any eye deviation or head deviation? Describe any other movements. Was she able to talk to you during the event?
- What was she like afterward? How long did it take to get back to normal (postictal period)?

History

- **Character:** What was the event like (break down into preictal, ictal, and postictal phases)?
  - **Preictal:** Was there any warning before the event, such as behavior change, tingling sensation, unusual smell, vision change, or sound? How long did this last? What were you doing before the event?
  - **Ictal:** Describe the event. Was there loss of consciousness, tonic or clonic activity? How long did the event last?
  - **Postictal:** After the event were you fatigued or confused? How long did it take to return to normal? Was one side weak (Todd's paralysis)?
- **Location:** Where did the event occur? What body parts were first affected?
- **Onset:** When did the event occur?
- **Radiation:** Did seizure begin in one part of the body before generalizing and affecting the entire body? What movements were present before consciousness was lost?
- **Duration:** How long did the ictal event last?
  - <15 seconds: Absence seizure
  - 30 seconds to 3 minutes: Generalized tonic-clonic seizure, simple partial seizure, or myoclonic seizure
  - 2 to 3 minutes: Complex partial seizure
- **Events associated:**
  - Incontinence or tongue biting? Can you remember the event?
  - Headache (migraine)?
  - Fever/chills (CNS infection)?
  - Palpitations (dysrhythmia, syncope)? Hyperventilation (panic)?
  - Drug use? Drug withdrawal?
- **Frequency:** Has this ever happened to you before? How often?
- **Palliative factors:** Is there anything that makes it better? If so, what? Anticonvulsants?
- **Provocative factors:** Is there anything that makes it worse? If so, what?
  - Triggers: Sleep deprivation, EtOH use, exposure to flashing lights, hyperventilation, pain, sight of blood, coughing, micturition, or Valsalva maneuver
- **PMH/PSH:** Seizure disorder, syncope, depression, or brain injury
- **MEDS:** Antiepileptics, antidepressants, or antipsychotics
- **SH:** EtOH, recreational drugs, and sleep patterns
- **FH:** Seizure disorder, syncope

INSTRUCTIONS TO CANDIDATE: A 57-year-old male presents to the emergency department complaining of dizziness. Take a detailed history, exploring possible etiologies.

DD$_X$ VITAMINS C

- **Vascular:** Stroke, postural hypotension, vasovagal, and cardiac arrhythmia
- **Infection:** Meningitis, labyrinthitis/vestibular neuropathy, and cerebellitis
- **Trauma:** Head trauma
- **Autoimmune:** MS
- **Metabolic:** Hypoglycemia, medications (antibiotics, anticonvulsants, antidepressants)
- **Idiopathic/Iatrogenic:** Benign paroxysmal positional vertigo (BPPV), Ménière's disease, and migraine
- **Neoplastic:** Primary or metastatic brainstem or posterior fossa neoplasm, cerebello-pontine angle (CPA) tumor
- **Psychiatric**

History

- **Character:** Describe what you mean by dizziness (lightheadedness, sense of passing out, vertigo).

- **O**nset: How did it start (sudden versus gradual)?
  - Acute onset: Stroke, transient ischemic attack (TIA), BPPV, Ménière's disease
  - Gradual onset: Toxicity, infection, CPA tumor, MS
- **I**ntensity: Describe the severity of your dizziness on a scale of 1 to 10, with 1 being mild dizziness and 10 being the worst. Does the dizziness stop you from participating in your daily activities?
  - Mild: Medication-related, hypoglycemia, orthostatic hypotension
  - Severe (nausea, diplopia): BPPV, Ménière's disease, CPA tumor
- **D**uration: How long does the dizziness last?
  - Minutes-hours: Labyrinthitis, BPPV, TIA
  - Days: Tumor, stroke, AVM, MS, and medication
- **E**vents associated:
  - Any difficulty walking? Are you falling to one side?
  - Nausea or vomiting? Visual changes?
  - Tinnitus (BPPV, Ménière's disease, labyrinthitis, medication)?
  - Hearing loss (Ménière's disease, CPA tumor)? Is one ear affected more than the other?
  - Chest palpitations (dysrhythmia, syncope)?
  - Headache (tumor, migraine)?
  - Upper respiratory tract infection (labyrinthitis)?
- **F**requency: Has this happened to you before? How often?
  - Daily: Medication, tumor
  - Episodic: BPPV, Ménière's disease
- **P**alliative factors: Is there anything that makes the dizziness better? If so, what? Is there a position of comfort?
- **P**rovocative factors: Is there anything that makes the dizziness worse? If so, what?
  - Turning head to one side (BPPV, labyrinthitis)?
  - Standing (orthostatic hypotension)?
- **PMH/PSH:** Ear problems, arrhythmia, stroke, brain injury, MS, Ménière's disease, or tumors
- **MEDS:** Any new medications or antibiotics (e.g., aminoglycosides)?
- **SH:** EtOH, smoking, occupational and recreational activities (any risk of falls such as climbing ladders or working at a height)
- **FH:** Ménière's disease (progressive hearing loss, tinnitus, vertigo)

INSTRUCTIONS TO CANDIDATE: A 53-year-old male presents to the emergency department via ambulance with a decreased level of consciousness.
- Assess the level of consciousness.
- Take a detailed history, exploring possible etiologies.

ASSESS THE LEVEL OF CONSCIOUSNESS

- **First evaluate A**irway, **B**reathing, and **C**irculation. It may be necessary to perform an immediate intervention, such as supplemental O_2, IV access, or intubation.
  - Is the patient able to talk? Swallow? Cough?
  - Are both lungs ventilated? Is the patient oxygenating (mentation, pulse oximetry)?
  - Abnormal vitals? Describe any abnormal patterns of breathing (e.g., Cheyne-Stokes respirations). Peripheral circulation (pulses, capillary refill)?
  - If no immediate interventions are required, proceed to take the history, and perform the physical examination.

Level of Consciousness (LOC)
- The Glasgow Coma Scale (GCS) can be used to characterize the LOC (Table 5-3). Instead of writing a simple score out of 15, it is more informative to write the score

Table 5-3 Glasgow Coma Scale

Eye Opening	Best Verbal Response	Best Motor Response	Score
Never	No response	No response	1
To pain	Incomprehensible sounds	Extension (decerebrate rigidity)	2
To verbal stimuli	Inappropriate words	Abnormal flexion (decorticate rigidity)	3
Spontaneously	Disoriented and converses	Withdraws to pain	4
	Oriented and converses	Localizes pain	5
		Obeys commands	6

Total scored out of 15

for each category: Eyes, Verbal, and Motor ($E_4V_5M_6$). The minimum achievable score is 3.

- If the patient is intubated and thus unable to speak, the verbal score is quantified by a "T" ($E_4V_TM_6$).
- If the GCS is ≤8 the LOC is such that the patient may not be able to protect his or her own airway, and endotracheal intubation is indicated.

Head, Eyes, Ears, Nose, and Throat (HEENT)
- Note any neck stiffness or meningism (CNS infection, SAH). In trauma cases note any rhinorrhea or otorrhea (may indicate a cerebrospinal fluid [CSF] leak).

Cranial Nerves
- Visual acuity: Assess whether the patient blinks to visual threat.
- Pupils: Assess the pupillary size and reactivity to light (direct and consensual).
- Perform funduscopy, and comment on presence of papilledema or hemorrhage.
- Extraocular movements: Look for any gaze deviation. Assess the oculocephalic reflex by turning his head side to side briskly (ensure the cervical spine is cleared before undertaking this maneuver). The eyes should roll to the opposite direction of the head movement. If the patient is unresponsive, perform cold caloric testing.
- **Corneal reflex:** Approach the patient with a piece of tissue from the lateral side. Touch the cornea, and look for a blink response (afferent V1 division of CN V, efferent CN VII).
- To assess the gag reflex in an intubated patient, gently pull on the endotracheal tube, and watch for a response. Be cautious about eliciting a gag reflex in a patient with decreased LOC who is not intubated because this may precipitate vomiting and aspiration.

Motor
- Inspect for spontaneous movements, looking for symmetry and purpose.
- Tone: Assess symmetry of tone in the upper and lower extremities.
- Power: Assess ability to open eyes, protrude tongue, raise arms, and show fingers.
- If the patient is not moving spontaneously and does not respond to verbal stimuli, apply a noxious stimulus (e.g., sternal rub, nail bed pressure). Comment on pattern of response (localizes, withdraws, abnormal flexion or extension, no response).

Reflexes
- Check DTRs and plantars. Note any abnormal reflexes (e.g., Babinski) and any asymmetry.

Sensory
- Note any asymmetry in response to noxious stimuli.

TAKE A DETAILED HISTORY, EXPLORING POSSIBLE ETIOLOGIES

DD$_X$ VITAMINS C

- **V**ascular: Intracranial hemorrhage, infarction
- **I**nfection: Meningitis, encephalitis, and abscess
- **T**raumatic: Head injury
- **A**utoimmune: Vasculitis
- **M**etabolic: Electrolyte abnormality, hyperthyroidism, uremia, and drugs (e.g., EtOH, cocaine, phencyclidine, amphetamines)
- **I**diopathic: Seizure, syncope, and catatonia
- **N**eoplastic: Brain metastasis or primary brain tumor

Collateral History (Obtain History From the Patient When Possible)

- **C**haracter: When was the patient last normal? What were the events leading up to the decreased LOC? Was the change in consciousness witnessed, or was he found like this?
- **L**ocation: Were there any focal deficits noted before the decreased LOC (e.g., weakness, facial droop)?
- **O**nset: How did this come on (sudden versus gradual)?
  - Sudden onset: Stroke, intracranial hemorrhage, and trauma
  - Progressive deterioration: Infection, vasculitis, and tumor
- **D**uration: How long has the patient had a decreased LOC? Has there been any improvement, or has he deteriorated further?
- **E**vents associated: What were the events leading up to the decreased LOC? How did the patient seem beforehand? Did he fall? Were there any movements? Was there any trauma or seizure activity? Did the patient complain of any headache or vision changes?
- **F**requency: Do you know whether this has happened before?
- **P**alliative factors: Is there anything that has seemed to help? If so, what?
- **P**rovocative factors: Is there anything that seems to make the patient worse? If so, what?
- Do you know of someone we can contact on the patient's behalf (e.g., family)?
- **PMH/PSH:** Head trauma, stroke, AVM, cerebral aneurysm, meningitis, seizure, tumors, renal failure, or psychiatric problems
- **MEDS:** New medications, benzodiazepines, or narcotics
- **SH:** EtOH, smoking, recreational drug use, and occupation (workplace exposures)

SAMPLE CHECKLISTS

INSTRUCTIONS TO CANDIDATE: Perform a focused neurologic examination on the lower limbs, looking for evidence of an upper motor neuron lesion. State what you expect to find.

Key Points	Satisfactorily Carried out
Introduces self to the patient	❏
Determines how the patient wishes to be addressed	❏
Explains nature of the examination to the patient	❏
Examines the patient in a logical fashion	❏
Inspection (differentiate from LMNL) • Muscle bulk, pattern of atrophy • Fasciculations	 ❏ ❏
Tone (increased)	❏
Power (decreased) • Pronator drift	 ❏
Deep tendon reflexes (increased) • Biceps • Knee jerks • Ankle jerks	 ❏ ❏ ❏
Plantar responses (upgoing)	❏
Gait (spastic)	❏
Drapes the patient appropriately	❏
Makes appropriate closing remarks	❏

INSTRUCTIONS TO CANDIDATE: Perform a comprehensive examination of reflexes in the upper and lower limbs of this patient.

Key Points	Satisfactorily Carried out
Introduces self to the patient	❑
Determines how the patient wishes to be addressed	❑
Explains nature of the examination to the patient	❑
Examines the patient in a logical fashion	❑
Positions the patient properly	❑
Compares biceps reflexes	❑
Compares brachioradialis reflexes	❑
Compares triceps reflexes	❑
Compares finger reflexes	❑
Compares knee jerks	❑
Compares ankle jerks	❑
Compares plantar responses • One method: Babinski's sign • Second method: Chaddock's maneuver • Optional method: Oppenheim's maneuver	❑ ❑ ❑
Drapes the patient appropriately	❑
Makes appropriate closing remarks	❑

INSTRUCTIONS TO CANDIDATE: Perform a physical examination on a patient presenting with ataxia.

Key Points	Satisfactorily Carried out
Introduces self to the patient	❏
Determines how the patient wishes to be addressed	❏
Explains nature of the examination to the patient	❏
Examines the patient in a logical fashion	❏
Extraocular movements (look for nystagmus)	❏
Hearing	❏
Finger-to-nose test	❏
Heel-knee-shin test	❏
Rapid alternating movements • Upper extremities • Lower extremities	❏ ❏
Proprioception in lower extremities	❏
Observes natural gait	❏
Tandem gait	❏
Romberg's test	❏
Drapes the patient appropriately	❏
Makes appropriate closing remarks	❏

INSTRUCTIONS TO CANDIDATE: Assess the function of this patient's fifth cranial nerve.

Key Points	Satisfactorily Carried out
Introduces self to the patient	❏
Determines how the patient wishes to be addressed	❏
Explains nature of the examination to the patient	❏
Examines the patient in a logical fashion	❏
Sensation to touch with patient's eyes closed	
• Ophthalmic	❏
• Maxillary	❏
• Mandibular	❏
• Compares both sides	❏
Pinprick	
• Ophthalmic	❏
• Maxillary	❏
• Mandibular	❏
Motor by palpation	
• Masseters (opens mouth)	❏
• Pterygoids (moves mandible laterally)	❏
• Temporalis (closes mouth)	❏
Corneal reflexes	
• Bilateral	❏
Bonus	
• Jaw jerk	❏
• Nose tickle	❏
Makes appropriate closing remarks	❏

CHAPTER 6

Musculoskeletal System

OBJECTIVES

ESSENTIAL CLINICAL COMPETENCIES

APPROACH TO TAKING A HISTORY OF MUSCULOSKELETAL PAIN

APPROACH TO THE MUSCULOSKELETAL EXAMINATION

PERFORM AN EXAMINATION OF THE CERVICAL SPINE

PERFORM AN EXAMINATION OF THE THORACIC SPINE

PERFORM AN EXAMINATION OF THE LUMBAR SPINE AND SACROILIAC JOINTS

PERFORM AN EXAMINATION OF THE SHOULDER

PERFORM AN EXAMINATION OF THE ELBOW

PERFORM AN EXAMINATION OF THE WRIST

PERFORM AN EXAMINATION OF THE HAND

PERFORM AN EXAMINATION OF THE HIP

PERFORM AN EXAMINATION OF THE KNEE

SAMPLE OSCE SCENARIOS

- A 33-year-old administrative assistant complains of tingling and pain in her right hand that wakes her up from sleep at night. Perform a focused physical examination.
- A 29-year-old male with a known diagnosis of ankylosing spondylitis presents to your office for a recheck. Perform an appropriate physical examination.
- A 62-year-old male complains of "terrible" knee pain. Take a detailed history, exploring possible etiologies.
- An 85-year-old female presents after a "broken arm" with concerns about osteoporosis. Take a detailed history, focusing on risk factors.

SAMPLE CHECKLISTS

- ❑ Perform an examination of the cervical spine. Describe your actions.
- ❑ Perform an examination of the lumbar spine. Describe your actions.
- ❑ Perform an examination of the right shoulder. Describe your actions.
- ❑ Perform an examination of the left elbow. Describe your actions.
- ❑ Perform an examination of the right hand and wrist. Describe your actions.
- ❑ Perform an examination of the left knee. Describe your actions.
- ❑ Perform an examination of the left ankle and foot. Describe your actions.
- ❑ Perform a focused physical examination of the hand in this patient with a history of rheumatoid arthritis. Describe your actions and expected findings.
- ❑ Examine this patient with a suspected right L4-L5 or L5-S1 disk protrusion causing root compression.

OBJECTIVES

*The successful student should be able to take a **focused history** of the musculoskeletal (MSK) system, including:*

- Joint pain or stiffness
  - Swelling, redness
  - Monoarticular versus polyarticular
  - Interference with activities of daily living (ADLs)
  - Treatments
- Joint clicking or locking
- Arthritis
- Gout
- Muscle pain (myalgia)
  - Exertional versus rest pain, limitation of movement, and associated numbness/tingling
- Muscle wasting
- Weakness
- Back pain
- Bone pain
- Overuse syndromes
  - Carpal tunnel syndrome (CTS)
  - Tennis elbow
  - Golfer's elbow
- Trauma: Mechanism of injury
- Compartment syndrome

*The MSK **examination** will include:*

Inspection
- Swelling, color (redness, bruising)
- Skin changes
- Muscle bulk
- Deformity
- Compare with contralateral joint
- Gait, posture, and position of comfort

Palpation
- Temperature, tenderness
- Muscle bulk
- Joint effusion
- Crepitus
- Edema
- Power
- Compare with contralateral joint
- Examine the joint above and below the joint in question to identify referred pain.

Range of Motion
- Active range of motion (ROM)
- Passive ROM

Percussion
- Fist percussion of the spine for tenderness

The student should be able to demonstrate examination of:

Upper Extremity Joints
- Shoulder
- Elbow

- Wrist
- Metacarpophalangeal (MCP) joints
- Proximal interphalangeal (PIP) joints
- Distal interphalangeal (DIP) joints

Lower Extremity Joints
- Hip
- Knee
- Ankle and foot
- Metatarsophalangeal (MTP) joints

Spine
- Cervical
- Thoracic
- Lumbar
- Sacral

Special Tests
- Occiput to wall distance
- Finger to floor distance
- Schober's test
- Straight leg raising
- Bowstring sign
- Lasègue's sign
- True leg length

ESSENTIAL CLINICAL COMPETENCIES

APPROACH TO TAKING A HISTORY OF MUSCULOSKELETAL PAIN

- **ID:** Age, sex
- **Character:** What is the pain like?
  - Sharp?
  - Dull?
- **Location:** From where does the pain originate? From which joint(s) or region(s)?
- **Onset:** When did the pain start? How did it come on (sudden versus gradual)?
- **Radiation:** Does the pain move anywhere?
- **Intensity:** How severe is the pain on a scale of 1 to 10, with 1 being mild pain and 10 being the worst?
  - How does it affect your ADLs (dressing, getting to bathroom, taking care of yourself, cooking, cleaning, shopping, getting around)?
  - Is it getting better, worse, or staying the same?
- **Duration:** How long has the pain been there (acute versus chronic)?
- **Events associated:**
  - Falls (especially important in the elderly population)?
  - Morning stiffness? Swelling? Redness?
  - Joint clicking or locking?
  - Muscle pain (cramps)? Wasting?
  - Is there limitation of movement? Weakness?
  - Is there any numbness or tingling associated with the pain?
  - Fever, chills?
  - Trauma? Describe the mechanism of injury.
  - Occupational activities? Sports? Repetitive movements (e.g., typing)?
- **Frequency:** Have you ever had this pain before? How often does the pain come (intermittent versus constant)?

- Palliative factors: Is there anything that makes the pain better? If so, what?
  - Rest?
  - Activity?
  - Pain medication?
  - Application of heat or cold?
- Provocative factors: Is there anything that makes the pain worse? If so, what?
  - Rest?
  - Activity? Particular movements?
- **Past medical history (PMH)/past surgical history (PSH):**
  - Arthritis? Gout?
  - Osteoporosis?
  - Connective tissue disease?
  - Past injuries? Previous surgeries?
  - Other medical problems?
- **Medications (MEDS):** Nonsteroidal antiinflammatory drugs (NSAIDs), acetaminophen, narcotics, acetylsalicylic acid (ASA), steroids, or immunosuppressants
- **Allergies**
- **Social history (SH):** Smoking, EtOH, street drugs, sexual history, use of mobility aids (e.g., wheelchair, walker, cane), and occupation
- **Family history (FH):** Arthritis, osteoporosis, or connective tissue disease

APPROACH TO THE MUSCULOSKELETAL EXAMINATION

Inspection
- Begin inspecting the patient's gait, posture, and movements from the time you enter the room.
- When examining a joint it is always important to examine the contralateral joint for comparison. While inspecting note SEADS (mnemonic below) and any asymmetry.

Mnemonic: SEADS
- Swelling
- Erythema, ecchymosis
- Atrophy
- Deformity
- Skin changes

Palpation
- It is important to examine above and below the joint in question because pain and other symptoms may be referred. This is especially important in trauma when further injuries might be overlooked in the face of an "obvious" fracture. It is equally important in those with neurologic conditions that alter pain perception or in those who cannot communicate their symptoms accurately (e.g., very young children, patients with dementia or altered level of consciousness).
- When palpating examine the contralateral joint for comparison. Note TEST CA (mnemonic below) and any asymmetry.

Mnemonic: TEST CA
- Tenderness
- Effusion
- Swelling
- Temperature
- Crepitus
- Atrophy

Range of Motion
- **Active ROM:** While immobilizing the joint proximal to the joint being examined, instruct the patient to move the joint in question (Figure 6-1). ROM should be symmetric with the contralateral joint. If there appears to be limitation in active ROM, also test the passive ROM.
- **Passive ROM:** The examiner performs these maneuvers, eliminating the patient's efforts. Move the joint in question through the same range of movement as in active ROM. Passive and active ROM should be nearly equal (passive ROM often exceeds active ROM slightly).

Power
- Grading power **(Oxford scale)**
  - 5, Normal
  - 4, Completely moves body part against gravity and some resistance
  - 3, Completely moves body part against gravity
  - 2, Partially moves body part with gravity eliminated
  - 1, A flicker or trace of movement without joint motion
  - 0, No movement

Neurovascular Assessment
- It is important to perform a neurovascular assessment on injured extremities.
- Check distal pulses and capillary refill. Assess the skin color (cyanosis, erythema, pallor) and temperature using the dorsum of your hand and compare with the contralateral limb.
- Test sensation, and map areas of decreased sensation.
- **Compartment syndrome** is a limb-threatening emergency resulting from increased pressure in an anatomic compartment that compromises associated nerves and circulation. It is characterized by pain disproportionate to the injury or clinical findings, paresthesias, and increased pain on passive stretch of involved muscles.

Special Tests
- These are specific to the joint being examined (e.g., Tinel's sign and occiput to wall distance).

PERFORM AN EXAMINATION OF THE CERVICAL SPINE

Patient Positioning
- Cooperative patients with *acute* injuries to the cervical spine should be examined in the supine position with the head and neck immobilized. Examination should be limited to light palpation of the cervical spine and soft tissues of the neck until the spine is clinically or radiographically cleared of injury.
- Patients without acute injury should be examined while sitting with the neck, upper back, and shoulders exposed.

Inspection
- Inspect the neck in a resting position, noting its normal lordotic curve (Figure 6-2). Observe any resting rotation or lateral flexion.

Palpation
- Palpate the cervical spine for tenderness, spasm, or mass starting at the base of the skull down to spinous prominence (C7). Palpate the trapezius, sternocleidomastoid (SCM), and paraspinal muscles.

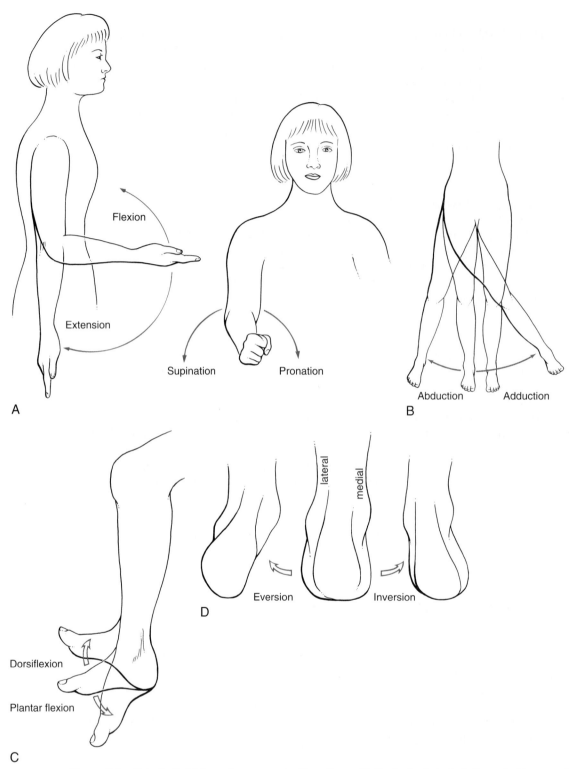

Figure 6-1 **A** to **D,** Skeletal muscle movements. (From Swartz M: *Textbook of physical diagnosis: history and examination*, ed 4, Philadelphia, 2002, WB Saunders, p 539, Figures 19-14, *B*, and 19-18.)

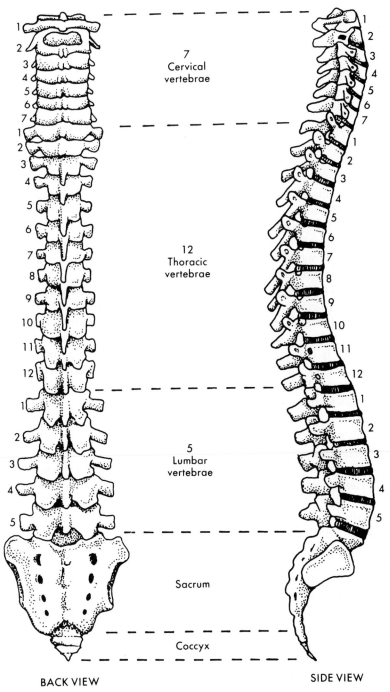

7
Cervical
vertebrae

12
Thoracic
vertebrae

5
Lumbar
vertebrae

Sacrum

Coccyx

BACK VIEW SIDE VIEW

Figure 6-2   Vertebral column. (From Marx JA, Hockberger RS, Walls RM, editors: *Rosen's emergency medicine: concepts and clinical practice,* ed 5, St. Louis, 2002, Mosby, p 330, Figure 36-1, *A*.)

Range of Motion

- Begin by inspecting the patient's active ROM. Instruct the patient to put his or her chin to the chest (flexion), look up at the ceiling (extension), turn the head from side to side (rotation), and touch ear to shoulder (lateral flexion).
- Range may be specifically measured using the central axis of the torso and a line through the vertex of the skull as a reference.
  - Flexion: 45 degrees
  - Extension: 50 degrees

- ▪ Rotation: 70 degrees
- ▪ Lateral flexion: 45 degrees
- If there is limitation in the active ROM, test the passive ROM by placing your hands on either side of the head and guiding the neck through the same motions (flexion, extension, rotation, and lateral bending).

Power
- Repeating the motions elicited for ROM, apply an opposing force. Grade the muscle power according to the Oxford Scale.

Special Tests
- With the patient standing with his or her back against a wall, measure the **occiput to wall distance**. The inability to touch the occiput against the wall is abnormal. This measurement may be used to follow the progression of ankylosing spondylitis.
- **Spurling's sign** may be used to identify cervical root impingement. Ask the patient to simultaneously rotate and laterally flex toward the affected side. Reproduction of radicular symptoms suggests cervical root impingement.
- The **compression test** is less specific than Spurling's sign for identifying cervical root impingement. Perform this test with the patient sitting. Exert an axial load by applying downward pressure on the patient's head. Reproduction of radicular pain suggests cervical nerve root impingement.
- **Lhermitte's sign** is nonspecific but should prompt thorough neurologic evaluation. Its presence is associated with conditions like vitamin B_{12} deficiency, multiple sclerosis, and cervical disk disease (nerve impingement) and refers to the presence of electric-like shocks that radiate down the back in response to forward flexion of the neck.

Neurologic Correlates
- A patient with spinal injury, spinal cord injury, or nerve root symptoms should have a complete neurologic examination, including sensory, motor, and reflexes in all limbs.
- Testing specific nerve roots (see Figure 5-4):
  - ▪ C4: Necklace sensory distribution, elevation of scapulae
  - ▪ C5: Anterolateral shoulder sensation, deltoid and biceps weakness, and diminished biceps reflex
  - ▪ C6: Lateral hand (thumb) and forearm sensation, biceps and wrist extensor weakness, and diminished biceps reflex
  - ▪ C7: Index and middle finger and dorsal arm sensation, triceps and digit extensor weakness, and diminished triceps reflex
  - ▪ C8: Small finger and medial arm sensation, hypothenar and hand flexor weakness

PEARL
- **Torticollis** is painful lateral deviation of the neck associated with contralateral SCM muscle tenderness or spasm.

PERFORM AN EXAMINATION OF THE THORACIC SPINE

Patient Positioning
- Cooperative patients with *acute* injuries to the thoracic spine should be examined only in the supine position. "Log rolling" the patient with the help of two or more assistants will allow palpation of the thoracolumbar spine and soft tissues while minimizing further spinal injury.
- Patients without acute traumatic injuries are best examined standing, wearing an examining gown, which opens in the back (to expose the thoracic spinal area).

Inspection

- Inspect the thoracic spine in a resting position, noting the normal slight upper thoracic kyphosis and thoracolumbar lordosis (see Figure 6-2).
- The posterior ribs, shoulder height, scapulae, and iliac crests should be symmetric in upright and flexed positions. Asymmetry may suggest scoliosis (Figure 6-3).

Palpation

- Palpate each spinous process. This may be facilitated by having the patient lean forward, resting his or her elbows on a bed or chair back. Begin palpating at C7-T1, which is typically prominent and easily identified. The L4 process sits on the line joining the iliac crests posteriorly (Figure 6-4). Note any tenderness or step deformities that may indicate spondylolisthesis.
- Palpate the paraspinal muscles for bulk, tenderness, mass, or spasm.
- Place your hands over the scapulae, and ask the patient to bend forward. Note the position of your hands; their height should be symmetric. This technique may detect subtle scoliosis.

Percussion

- Percuss each vertebra with the hypothenar aspect of your closed fist. Deep pain to percussion is nonspecific but may indicate degenerative disease, malignancy, or infection.

Range of Motion

- Inspect the patient's active ROM. With the patient standing, instruct him or her to touch his or her toes (forward flexion). With the patient in flexion, palpate the spinous processes, noting the normal increased interspinous distance. **Finger to floor distance** can be used to measure the extent of flexion. The normal range varies considerably, but this measurement can be used to follow disease progression in ankylosing spondylitis.
- Using your hands to fix the pelvis, ask the patient to bend backward (extension), laterally (lateral flexion), and to rotate from side to side. There is little extension in the thoracic spine itself because of the angulation of the spinous processes.
  - Extension: 30 degrees
  - Lateral flexion: 35 degrees
  - Rotation: 30 degrees

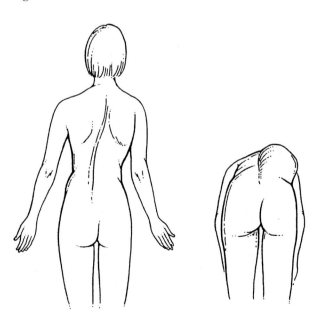

Figure 6-3   Inspecting for scoliosis. (From Swartz M: *Textbook of physical diagnosis: history and examination,* ed 3, Philadelphia, 1998, WB Saunders, p 634, Figure 22-28.)

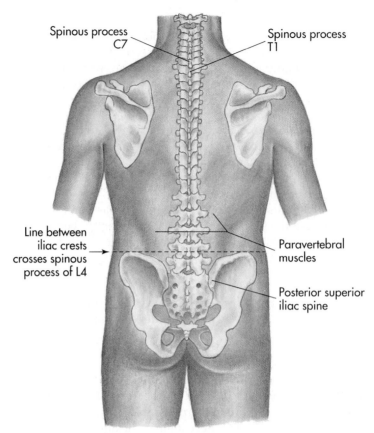

Figure 6-4   Landmarks on the back. (From Seidel HM, Ball JW, Dains JE, Benedict GB: *Mosby's guide to physical examination,* ed 5, St. Louis, 2003, Mosby, p 716, Figure 20-19.)

- Observe for the normal reversal from thoracolumbar lordosis to kyphosis in flexion. Failure to reverse may indicate degenerative disease.

PEARL
- Thoracic disk herniation typically occurs in the mid-lower thoracic spine and presents with radicular pain down the back or along the ribs. A central disk herniation may present with weakness, spasticity below the level of the lesion, or bowel or bladder dysfunction.

PERFORM AN EXAMINATION OF THE LUMBAR SPINE AND SACROILIAC JOINTS

Patient Positioning
- Cooperative patients with *acute* injuries to the thoracic spine should be examined only in the supine position. "Log rolling" the patient with the help of two or more assistants will allow palpation of the thoracolumbar spine and soft tissues while minimizing further spinal injury.
- Patients without acute traumatic injuries are best examined standing, wearing an examining gown, which opens in the back (to expose the lumbosacral spinal area).

Inspection
- Inspect the lumbosacral spine in a resting position, noting the normal lumbar lordotic curve. Note any asymmetry of the iliac crests.

Palpation

- Palpate each spinous process. The L4 process sits on the line joining the iliac crests posteriorly (see Figure 6-4). Note any tenderness or step deformities that may indicate spondylolisthesis. Palpate for tenderness over the posterior superior iliac spine (PSIS) and sacroiliac (SI) joints.
- Palpate the paraspinal muscles for bulk, tenderness, mass, or spasm.

Percussion

- Percuss each vertebra with the hypothenar aspect of your closed fist. Deep pain to percussion is nonspecific but may indicate degenerative disease, malignancy, or infection.

Range of Motion

- Inspect the patient's active ROM. With the patient standing, instruct him or her to touch his or her toes (forward flexion). With the patient in flexion, palpate the spinous processes, noting the normal increased interspinous distance. **Finger to floor distance** can be used to measure the extent of flexion. The normal range varies considerably, but this measurement is useful to follow disease progression in ankylosing spondylitis.
- Using your hands to fix the pelvis, ask the patient to bend backward (extension), laterally (lateral flexion), and rotate from side to side.
  - Extension: 30 degrees
  - Lateral flexion: 35 degrees
  - Rotation: 30 degrees
- Observe for the normal reversal from thoracolumbar lordosis to kyphosis in flexion. Failure to reverse may indicate degenerative disease.

Special Tests

- **SI joint pain** can be reproduced by placing the patient in a supine position with the contralateral hip and knee flexed and the ipsilateral hip hyperextended over the edge of the bed. This maneuver reproduces pain in sacroiliitis.
- Radicular pain from L5 or S1 roots can be reproduced by several techniques that stretch the sciatic nerve roots:
  - **Straight leg raising** is usually performed with the patient supine and legs extended. The symptomatic leg is passively raised off the bed (knee extended). A positive test is indicated by worsened pain in the affected leg at hip flexion <60 to 70 degrees.
  - The **bowstring sign** is elicited by passively raising the patient's symptomatic leg off the bed with the knee in slight flexion until just below the threshold for radicular pain. The bowstring sign is said to be present when pain is then elicited through firm compression of the popliteal fossa (pain radiates from the knee to the back).
  - **Lasègue's sign** is elicited by passively raising the patient's symptomatic leg off the bed with the knee in slight flexion until just below the threshold for radicular pain. Lasègue's sign is said to be present when passive dorsiflexion of the ankle worsens pain.
  - Tests for radicular pain may also be performed in a sitting position and may unveil inconsistencies (Figure 6-5).
  - **Crossed-over** or bilateral leg pain in response to these maneuvers may suggest a central disk herniation or cauda equina involvement.
- **Schober's test** is initiated with the patient in a standing position. Identify the **dimples of Venus** (SI joints), and make a mark on the skin at the midline. Using a measuring tape make a second mark 10 cm above. Ask the patient to bend forward. Remeasure the distance between the two marks (Figure 6-6). It normally measures at least 15 cm. Reduced expansion of the interspinous distance may suggest ankylosing spondylitis.

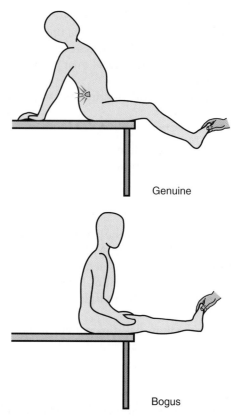

Figure 6-5   Retesting positive straight leg raising in a seated position. (Adapted from Munro JF, Campbell IW, editors: *Macleod's clinical examination,* ed 10, Edinburgh, 2000, Churchill Livingstone, p 271, Figure 8.13 *B, C.*)

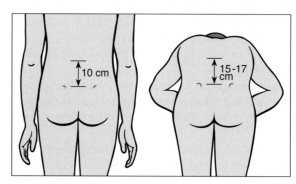

Figure 6-6   Schober's test. (Adapted from Munro JF, Campbell IW, editors: *Macleod's clinical examination,* ed 10, Edinburgh, 2000, Churchill Livingstone, p 269, Figure 8.10.)

PEARLS

- Herniated lumbar disks most commonly occur at L4-L5 and L5-S1 levels. Lateral disk herniation at these levels may produce neurologic findings in the distribution of L5 and S1 nerve roots, respectively.
- Signs of **cauda equina syndrome** include diminished saddle sensation, reduced rectal tone, and urinary retention. Patients with back pain and bowel or bladder symptoms should be examined for sensation in the saddle distribution and rectal tone.
- New onset of atraumatic back pain or tenderness, particularly in patients aged <18 or >60 years, should raise suspicion of serious illness, such as malignancy, pancreatitis, ruptured abdominal aortic aneurysm (AAA), or aortic dissection. A thorough physi-

cal examination searching for thoracic or abdominal causes of referred back pain must be performed.

PERFORM AN EXAMINATION OF THE SHOULDER

Patient Positioning
- The patient should be draped in a manner to allow full exposure of the shoulder and comparison with the other side. An examining gown tied under the arms will leave the shoulders exposed while covering the chest and breasts.

Inspection
- Inspect for **SEADS.**

Palpation
- While palpating the shoulder think of **TEST CA**, and note any asymmetry.
- Palpate the sternoclavicular joint, following the clavicle laterally to the acromioclavicular (AC) joint (Figure 6-7). Palpate the acromion, spine, and body of the scapula. The coracoclavicular joint is situated just medial and inferior to the AC joint. The greater tubercle of the humerus and humeral head are palpated laterally beneath the deltoid muscle. The glenohumeral joint is typically not palpable beneath the overlying musculature.
- Palpate the supraspinatus, infraspinatus, deltoid, and biceps areas for tenderness (Figure 6-8). The tendon of the long head of the biceps is palpable in the groove medial to the greater tuberosity. The subacromial bursa lies deep to the deltoid and just lateral to the acromion. The supraspinatus tendon wraps anteriorly over the glenohumeral joint, inserting on the greater tuberosity.

Range of Motion
- Movement of the shoulder combines motions of the scapula and glenohumeral joint.
- Inspect the patient's active ROM and compare with the contralateral shoulder. Instruct him or her to raise the arms forward (flexion) straight over the head and

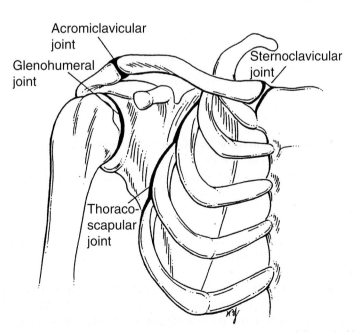

Figure 6-7 Bony anatomy of the shoulder. (From Swartz M: *Textbook of physical diagnosis: history and examination,* ed 4, Philadelphia, 2002, WB Saunders.)

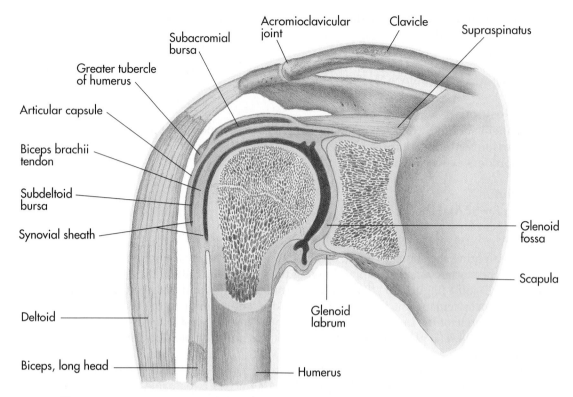

Subacromial bursa

Acromioclavicular joint

Clavicle

Supraspinatus

Greater tubercle of humerus

Articular capsule

Biceps brachii tendon

Subdeltoid bursa

Synovial sheath

Deltoid

Biceps, long head

Glenoid fossa

Scapula

Glenoid labrum

Humerus

Figure 6-8   Glenohumeral and acromioclavicular joints. (From Seidel HM, Ball JW, Dains JE, Benedict GB: *Mosby's guide to physical examination,* ed 5, St. Louis, 2003, Mosby, p 702, Figure 20-6.)

extend them backward (extension). Ask him or her to lift the arms laterally overhead (abduction) and swing them across the chest (adduction). Assess internal and external rotation with the elbows flexed; instruct the patient to put his or her hands behind the head (internal rotation) and behind the back (external rotation).

- Forward flexion: 180 degrees
- Extension: 45 degrees
- Abduction: 180 degrees
- Adduction: 45 degrees
- Internal and external rotation: 90 degrees

• If there is limitation in the active ROM, test the passive ROM by guiding the shoulder through the same motions (flexion, extension, abduction, adduction, internal and external rotation).

Power

• Repeating the motions elicited for ROM, apply an opposing force. Grade the muscle power according to the Oxford Scale.
• Reduced strength, particularly for abduction and external rotation, is common with acute and chronic injuries of the rotator cuff.

Special Tests

• The **drop test** is performed by asking the patient to actively abduct the shoulder 90 degrees. Inability to maintain this position is a positive test and suggests a significant rotator cuff tear.
• The **impingement test** is performed on the patient's right shoulder by fixing the scapula (with your left hand) and flexing the glenohumeral joint (with your right hand) as you stand behind the patient (Figure 6-9). This action impinges the subacromial bursa between greater tuberosity and the acromion. The presence of pain with this maneuver is a positive test and may indicate subacromial bursitis.

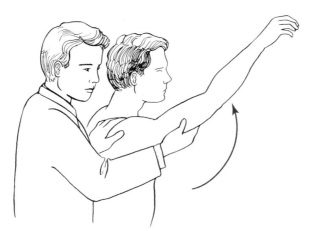

Figure 6-9   Impingement test. (Adapted from Marx JA, Hockberger RS, Walls RM, editors: *Rosen's emergency medicine: concepts and clinical practice,* ed 5, St. Louis, 2002, Mosby, p 601, Figure 46-39.)

PEARL
- A patient with shoulder pain should have an examination of the neck to rule out referred pain. Elicit Spurling's sign, and perform the cervical compression test to detect cervical root impingement or radiculopathy as a source of shoulder pain.

PERFORM AN EXAMINATION OF THE ELBOW

Patient Positioning
- Expose both arms (for comparison purposes) from shoulder to fingers.

Inspection
- Inspect the elbow in its resting position for **SEADS**. The normal carrying angle is 5 to 20 degrees (Figure 6-10).

Palpation
- While palpating the elbow think of **TEST CA**, and note any asymmetry.
- Palpate the olecranon, medial and lateral condyles of the humerus, and the radial head (Figure 6-11). Palpate the forearm and humerus, including the wrist and shoulder joints.
- An elbow effusion will be best palpated in the anatomic triangle formed by the radial head, lateral condyle, and olecranon.
- Palpate the ulnar nerve (between the olecranon and medial epicondyle), the olecranon bursa (normally not palpable), the common extensor insertion at the lateral epicondyle, and the common flexor insertion at the medial epicondyle.

Range of Motion
- Begin by inspecting the patient's active ROM compared with the contralateral elbow. Instruct the patient to bend his or her elbow (flexion) and straighten the elbow (extension). Pronation and supination are assessed with the elbow flexed to 90 degrees and the thumb pointing straight up (neutral position).
  - Flexion: 150 degrees
  - Extension: 0 degrees (mild *symmetrical* hyperextension is within normal limits)
  - Supination: 90 degrees
  - Pronation: 90 degrees
- If there is limitation in the active ROM, test the passive ROM by guiding the elbow through the same motions (flexion, extension, supination, and pronation).

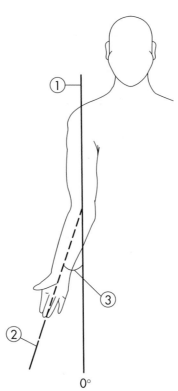

Figure 6-10   Carrying angle (3) is formed by the intersection of lines drawn parallel to the long axis of the humerus (1) and ulna (2). (From Marx JA, Hockberger RS, Walls RM, editors: *Rosen's emergency medicine: concepts and clinical practice,* ed 5, St. Louis, 2002, Mosby, p 558, Figure 45-5.)

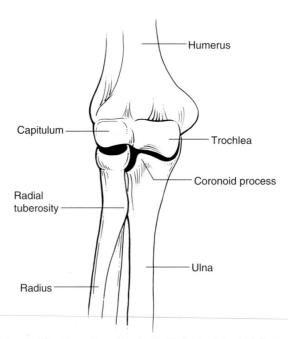

Figure 6-11   Bony anatomy of the elbow. (From Swartz M: *Textbook of physical diagnosis: history and examination,* ed 4, Philadelphia, 2002, WB Saunders, Figure 19-7.)

Power
- Repeating the motions elicited for ROM, apply an opposing force. Grade the muscle power according to the Oxford Scale.

Special Tests
- Look for **tennis elbow** using forced wrist extension. Tenderness over the common extensor insertion at the lateral epicondyle suggests lateral epicondylitis or tennis elbow.
- Similarly look for **golfer's elbow** using forced wrist flexion. Tenderness over the common flexor insertion at the medial epicondyle suggests medial epicondylitis or golfer's elbow.

PEARLS
- In the setting of injury an abnormal or asymmetric carrying angle may indicate a supracondylar fracture.
- Olecranon bursitis, otherwise known as **student's elbow**, is suggested by the presence of point tenderness, swelling, and fluctuance over the olecranon.

PERFORM AN EXAMINATION OF THE WRIST

Patient Positioning
- Expose both arms (for comparison purposes) from elbows to finger tips.

Inspection
- Inspect the dorsal and volar surfaces of the wrist for **SEADS**.

Palpation
- While palpating the wrist think of **TEST CA**, and note any asymmetry.
- Palpate the wrist using both hands with your thumbs positioned dorsally and your index fingers against the volar surface. The wrist joint includes the distal radius and ulna and the carpal bones (Figure 6-12). Identify landmarks, including the radial and ulnar styloid processes and the distal radioulnar articulation.
- The **anatomic snuffbox** is bordered by the abductor pollicis longus/extensor pollicis brevis and extensor pollicis longus. The scaphoid is palpable within the snuffbox (Figure 6-13). The scaphoid tubercle is palpated at the base of the thenar eminence with the wrist in extension.
- **Lister's tubercle** is a bony prominence on the dorsum of the wrist (dorsal tubercle of the radius). The scapholunate joint is just distal to Lister's tubercle and is a common site of ligamentous injury.
- The pisiform is palpated at the base of the hypothenar muscles.
- Palpate the extensor and flexor tendons as they cross the wrist joint (Figure 6-14).
- Palpate the forearm. Palpate the radial and ulnar pulses.

Range of Motion
- Begin by assessing the patient's active ROM and compare with the contralateral wrist, beginning with the wrist in a neutral position, fingers extended.
- Instruct the patient to bend the wrist up and down (flexion and extension) and from side to side (radial and ulnar deviation).
  - Flexion: 90 degrees
  - Extension: 70 degrees
  - Ulnar deviation: 50 degrees
  - Radial deviation: 20 degrees
- If there is limitation of active motion, test the passive ROM by guiding the wrist through the same motions (flexion, extension, ulnar and radial deviation).

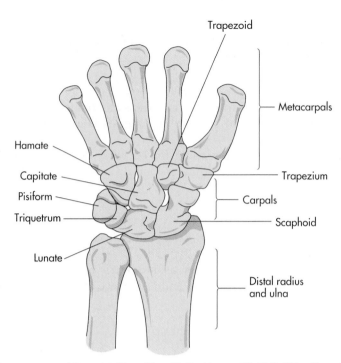

Figure 6-12 Bony anatomy of the wrist. (From Marx JA, Hockberger RS, Walls RM, editors: *Rosen's emergency medicine: concepts and clinical practice,* ed 5, St. Louis, 2002, Mosby, p 535, Figure 44-1.)

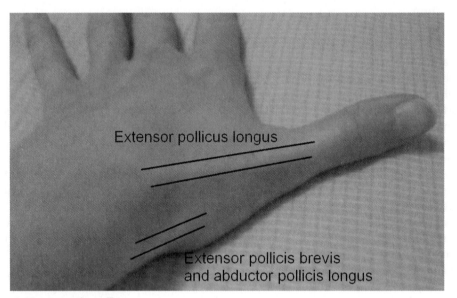

Figure 6-13 Anatomic snuffbox.

Power
- Repeating the motions elicited for ROM, apply an opposing force. Grade the muscle power according to the Oxford Scale.

Special Tests
- **Phalen's test** is performed by asking the patient to hold both wrists in full flexion with the dorsal surfaces pressed together (the opposite of prayer hands) for approximately 60 seconds. Numbness or paresthesias in the distribution of the median nerve suggest CTS.

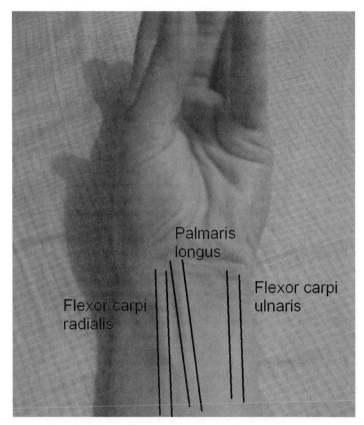

Figure 6-14   Flexor tendons of wrist.

- **Tinel's sign** is tested by percussing the volar aspect of the wrist over the median nerve. Numbness or paresthesias in the distribution of the median nerve suggest CTS.
- **Finkelstein's test** is performed by instructing the patient to place his or her thumb in the palm of the closed fist. Ask the patient to ulnarly deviate the wrist. This test stretches the extensor pollicis brevis and abductor pollicis longus and produces pain in patients with de Quervain's tenosynovitis.

PERFORM AN EXAMINATION OF THE HAND

Patient Positioning
- Expose both arms (for comparison purposes) from elbows to finger tips.

Inspection
- Inspect the dorsal and volar surfaces of the hand for **SEADS** (Figure 6-15).
- Note specifically any pattern of joint inflammation or thickening and any contractures.
- Note any asymmetry or atrophy of the intrinsic muscles of the hand, including the thenar eminence, hypothenar muscles, and interossei.

Palpation
- While palpating the hand think of **TEST CA**, and note any asymmetry.
- Palpate the individual bones of the hands, including the carpals, metacarpals, and phalanges.
- Palpate the MCP joints in slight flexion. Place a thumb on either side of the extensor tendon dorsally with your index fingers supporting the palmar aspect of the joint.

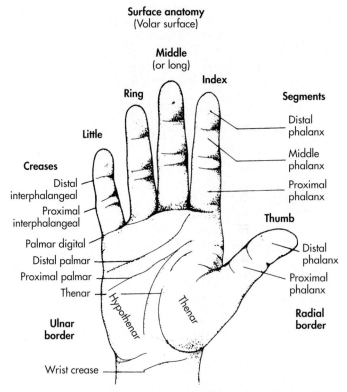

Surface anatomy
(Volar surface)

Figure 6-15   Surface anatomy of the hand. (From Marx JA, Hockberger RS, Walls RM, editors: *Rosen's emergency medicine: concepts and clinical practice,* ed 5, St. Louis, 2002, Mosby, p 494, Figure 43-1.)

- Palpate each interphalangeal (IP) joint using the index finger and thumb of both hands, compressing each joint from lateral and anteroposterior (AP) directions. Check the stability of each joint in all directions (dorsal, volar, radial, and ulnar).

Range of Motion
- Begin by assessing the patient's active ROM and compare with the contralateral hand.
- Instruct the patient to bend the fingers forward at the knuckles (MCP joints) and then stretch them back (flexion and extension). Make a fist (finger flexion). Stretch the fingers apart (abduction), and touch them together again (adduction).
  - MCP joint: 90 degrees flexion, 30 degrees extension
  - PIP joint: 120 degrees flexion, 0 degrees extension
  - DIP joint: 70 degrees flexion, 0 degrees extension
- If there is limitation of active motion or asymmetry, test the passive ROM by gently guiding the wrist through the same planes of movement.

Power
- Repeating the motions elicited for ROM, apply an opposing force. Grade the muscle power according to the Oxford Scale.
  - Lumbricals: Flexion of the MCP joint with IP joints in extension
  - Flexor digitorum superficialis: Flexion of the PIP joint with immobilization of the MCP joint
  - Flexor digitorum profundus: Flexion of the DIP joint with immobilization of the PIP joint
  - Dorsal interossei (digit abduction) and volar interossei (digit adduction)
  - Thenar eminence: Opposition of thumb and small finger (the hypothenar muscles also play a role), elevation of the thumb from the palm against resistance

■ Adductor pollicis: Test by asking the patient to grip a sheet of paper between the thumb and index metacarpal.

PEARLS

- Symmetrical involvement of the MCP and PIP joints suggests rheumatoid arthritis (RA). Digits tend to swell in a fusiform fashion.
- Degenerative osteoarthritis affects the PIP and DIP joints but rarely affects the MCP joints. **Heberden nodes** occur at the DIP joints, and **Bouchard nodes** occur at the PIP joints.
- Atrophy of the intrinsic hand muscles may occur as a result of joint disease and disuse or secondary to specific nerve dysfunction (e.g., advanced CTS is characterized by atrophy of the thenar eminence supplied by the median nerve).

PERFORM AN EXAMINATION OF THE HIP

Patient Positioning

- Inspection should be performed with the patient in a standing position.
- Palpation is best done with the patient supine.

Inspection

- Inspect the hips anteriorly and posteriorly with the patient in a standing position, noting any **SEADS**.
- Observe the stance, posture, and gait.
- Note any asymmetry in the height of the iliac crests or the gluteal folds (see Figure 6-4).

Palpation

- While palpating the hip and pelvis think of **TEST CA**, and note any asymmetry.
- Palpate the anterior superior iliac spine (ASIS), femurs, and greater trochanters (Figure 6-16). Exerting pressure on both sides of the pelvis simultaneously, test its stability.

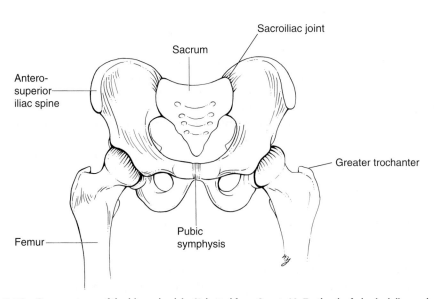

Figure 6-16   Bony anatomy of the hip and pelvis. (Adapted from Swartz M: *Textbook of physical diagnosis: history and examination,* ed 4, Philadelphia, 2002, WB Saunders, Figure 19-13.)

Range of Motion

- Begin by inspecting the patient's active ROM compared with the contralateral hip. From a supine position, instruct the patient to lift his or her straightened leg from the examining table (hip flexion). Lower the leg, and swing it outward (abduction) and then medially (adduction). Flex the knee, and rotate it outward, placing the lateral aspect of the foot on the contralateral knee (external rotation), and then rotate it inward (internal rotation). With the patient standing extend the leg backward without arching the back (extension).
  - Flexion: 90 to 120 degrees
  - Extension: Up to 30 degrees
  - Abduction: Up to 45 degrees
  - Adduction: Up to 30 degrees
  - External rotation: 45 degrees
  - Internal rotation: 40 degrees
- If there is limitation in the active ROM, test the passive ROM by guiding the hip through the same motions (flexion, extension, abduction, adduction, external and internal rotation).

Power

- Repeating flexion, extension, abduction, and adduction, apply an opposing force. Grade the muscle power according to the Oxford Scale.

Special Tests

- Perform the **Trendelenburg test** to detect weak hip abductors. Standing behind the patient, ask him or her to stand on one leg and then on the other. Note any change in the level of the iliac crests or gluteal folds during this maneuver. If the iliac crest drops toward the non–weight-bearing side, it indicates weakness of the hip abductors in the weight-bearing limb.
- Measure **true leg length** from the ASIS to the medial malleolus (measuring tape crosses the knee medially). Discrepancy within 1 cm is acceptable.

PERFORM AN EXAMINATION OF THE KNEE

Patient Positioning

- Expose both knees (for comparison purposes) from groin to ankles.

Inspection

- Inspect the knee in flexed and extended positions for **SEADS**.
- Effusions are best observed by inspecting the suprapatellar region. The anteromedial depression may be obliterated if there is a large effusion.
- Observe the stance, posture, and gait.
- **Genu varum** is considered to be present when there is >2.5 cm of space between the knees with the medial malleoli together (bow-legged).
- **Genu valgum** is considered to be present when there is >2.5 cm of space between the medial malleoli when the knees are together (knock-knees).

Palpation

- While palpating the knee think of **TEST CA**, and note any asymmetry.
- Palpate the patella, tibial tuberosity, tibial condyles, and femoral epicondyles (Figure 6-17).
- The normal knee is cooler than its surrounding tissue. Palpate for temperature with the dorsum of your hand, using the mid-thigh and shin for comparison. To determine symmetry compare with the contralateral knee.

In extension: posterior view   In flexion: anterior view

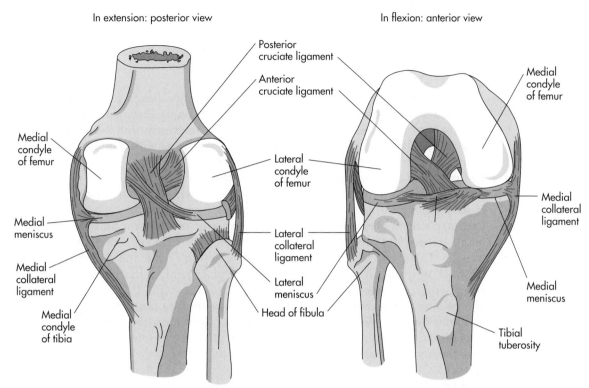

Figure 6-17 Bony and ligamentous anatomy of the knee. (Adapted from Marx JA, Hockberger RS, Walls RM, editors: *Rosen's emergency medicine: concepts and clinical practice,* ed 5, St. Louis, 2002, Mosby, p 675, Figure 50-1.)

- Examining for effusions:
  - Immobilize the patella with the thumb and index finger (suprapatellar). Use the free hand to milk the medial aspect of the knee (upward strokes). Using a downward stroke on the lateral aspect of the knee, fluid is displaced and may be visible as a bulge medially, known as the **bulge sign**.
  - A large effusion can be assessed by immobilizing the knee and **balloting** the patella against the femur while maintaining suprapatellar compression with the immobilizing hand.
- The quadriceps angle, or **Q angle**, is measured with the knee extended. The angle is formed by intersecting lines drawn from the tibial tubercle to the ASIS and from the center of the patella to the ASIS. Normal is <10 to 15 degrees. An increased Q angle predisposes to dislocation of the patella.

Range of Motion
- Begin by inspecting the patient's active ROM compared with the contralateral knee. Instruct the patient to bend his or her knee (flexion) and straighten it (extension).
  - Flexion: Up to 130 degrees
  - Extension: 0 degrees (mild *symmetrical* hyperextension is within normal limits)
- If there is limitation in the active ROM, test the passive ROM by guiding the knee through the same motions (flexion, extension).

Power
- Repeating the motions elicited for ROM, apply an opposing force. Grade the muscle power according to the Oxford Scale.

Special Tests

- Ligaments, a fibrocartilaginous capsule, and the surrounding muscles stabilize the knee. Test the stability of the knee using the following maneuvers with the patient in the supine position. These tests should be performed on both knees to compare symmetry.
  - The **anterior drawer test** is performed with the knee flexed to 90 degrees and anchored on the examining table (the examiner sits on it). Placing the fingers in the popliteal fossa and the thumbs over the joint line anteriorly, pull the tibia forward. A "positive" test occurs when a palpable step develops with anterior force, indicating an anterior cruciate ligament (ACL) tear.
  - The **posterior drawer test** is performed in the same position as above. Apply a backward force on the tibia. A positive test occurs when the tibia displaces >5mm posteriorly, indicating a torn posterior cruciate ligament (PCL).
  - **Lachman's test** is more sensitive than the anterior drawer test for detecting ACL injury but requires an intact PCL. The test is performed with the patient's knee flexed at 15 degrees. The left hand stabilizes the thigh while the right hand grasps the tibia and pulls it anteriorly. Anterior displacement of the tibia >5mm (compared with contralateral knee) indicates injury to the ACL.
  - The **collateral ligament stress test** is performed in two positions: knee extended and knee flexed to 30 degrees. Using one arm to support the leg, the other hand rests on the knee to apply a varus or valgus stress. Joint line opening (compared with the normal knee) on valgus stress indicates injury to the medial collateral ligament (MCL), whereas opening on varus stress indicates lateral collateral ligament (LCL) damage. Instability with the knee fully extended indicates a complete injury, whereas instability at 30 degrees may indicate more limited injury.
- **McMurray's test** is performed with the patient supine. Place your left hand on the patient's knee, ensuring you are able to feel the joint line. Using your right hand to grasp the foot, flex and extend the knee while simultaneously internally and externally rotating it. External rotation tests the medial meniscus, and internal rotation tests the lateral meniscus. Palpable clicking in the joint line or pain constitutes a positive test.

PEARLS

- Swelling over the patella itself is more often caused by prepatellar bursitis than effusion.
- A unilateral, swollen, erythematous knee is almost always pathologic.

SAMPLE OSCE SCENARIOS

> INSTRUCTIONS TO CANDIDATE: A 33-year-old administrative assistant complains of tingling and pain in her right hand that wakes her up from sleep at night. Perform a focused physical examination.

DD$_X$ Carpal Tunnel Syndrome (VITAMINS C)
- **T**raumatic: Chronic repetitive use syndrome
- **A**utoimmune/**A**llergic: RA
- **M**etabolic: Diabetes mellitus (DM), hypothyroidism, acromegaly, gout, and obesity
- **I**diopathic
- **C**ongenital/genetic: Congenitally narrowed carpal tunnel
- Pregnancy

Patient Positioning
- Expose both arms (for comparison purposes) from elbows to finger tips.

Inspection
- Inspect the dorsal and volar surfaces of the hand for **SEADS**.
- Note any asymmetry or atrophy of the intrinsic muscles of the hand, including the thenar eminence, hypothenar muscles, and interossei.
- Thenar atrophy is observed as a concavity of the eminence best noted when inspected tangentially.

Palpation
- While palpating the hand think of **TEST CA**, and note any asymmetry.
- Palpate the individual bones of the hands, including the carpals, metacarpals, and phalanges. Palpate the MCP and IP joints.

Range of Motion
- Begin by assessing the patient's active ROM and compare with the contralateral hand.
- Instruct the patient to bend the fingers forward at the knuckles (MCP joints), and then stretch them back (flexion and extension). Make a fist (finger flexion). Stretch the fingers apart (abduction), and touch them together again (adduction).
- Ask the patient to oppose the thumb and small finger (opposition), point the thumb up as if hitchhiking (extension), and point it across the palm (flexion). Also abduct and adduct the thumb.
- If there is limitation of active motion or asymmetry, test the passive ROM by gently guiding the wrist through the same planes of movement.

Power
- The **thumb abduction test** detects weakness of the abductor pollicis brevis, which is innervated solely by the median nerve. Ask the patient to raise his or her thumb perpendicular to the palm against resistance. Weakness is characteristic of median nerve neuropathy or CTS.
- Repeating the motions elicited for ROM, apply an opposing force. Grade the muscle power according to the Oxford Scale.

Special Tests
- Test two-point discrimination and vibration sense (low frequency tuning fork). Decreased pain sensation in the distribution of the median nerve (thumb, index finger, and radial half of ring finger) compared with the small finger suggests CTS. Mapping sensation may delineate any nerve root involvement.

- Test the brachioradialis (C5-C6), biceps (C5-C6), and triceps (C7) reflexes to delineate any nerve root involvement.
- **Phalen's test** is performed by asking the patient to hold both wrists in full flexion with the dorsal surfaces pressed together (the opposite of prayer hands) for approximately 60 seconds. Numbness or paresthesias in the distribution of the median nerve suggest CTS.
- **Tinel's sign** is tested by percussing the volar aspect of the wrist over the median nerve. Numbness or paresthesias in the distribution of the median nerve suggest CTS.
- The **flick test** is performed by asking the patient what maneuver he or she performs when experiencing symptoms. If the patient demonstrates a flicking motion of the hands, the test is said to be positive.

PEARLS
- **Carpal tunnel syndrome** is a compression neuropathy whereby the median nerve (C5-T1) is compressed within the carpal tunnel.
- It is often considered to be an overuse syndrome from gross or repetitive microtrauma, such as when typing with improper ergonomic wrist position.
- Common systemic causes decrease the volume of the carpal tunnel by increasing the size of the tendons from tissue infiltration or myxomatous enlargement. These etiologies include pregnancy, diabetes, hypothyroidism, acromegaly, gout, and obesity. RA is a common inflammatory cause of CTS.

INSTRUCTIONS TO CANDIDATE: A 29-year-old male with a known diagnosis of ankylosing spondylitis presents to your office for a recheck. Perform an appropriate physical examination.

Definition
- **Ankylosing spondylitis** is a seronegative spondyloarthropathy. Like all chronic inflammatory disorders, it is systemic with some organs affected to a greater extent than others. The physical manifestations are divided into articular and extraarticular categories:
  - Articular involvement: Axial skeleton, peripheral joints, and enthesitis
  - Extraarticular involvement: Ocular, cardiac, respiratory, renal, and neurologic (in decreasing order of incidence)

Inspection
- Inspect the back. Note any spinal deformity such as loss of lumbar lordosis and pronounced thoracic kyphosis. Look at the patient's gait, stance, and posture.
- Inspect for peripheral joint involvement (hips, shoulders, and knees).

Palpation
- **SI joint pain** can be reproduced by placing the patient in a supine position with the contralateral hip and knee flexed and the ipsilateral hip hyperextended over the edge of the bed. This maneuver reproduces pain in sacroiliitis.
- **Enthesitis** is tenderness over tendinous insertions, found commonly at the chest wall, Achilles tendon, plantar fascia near the heel, tibial tuberosity, patella, and iliac crests.

Tests Requiring Active/Passive Range of Motion
- The spine shows a progressively more limited ROM.
- **"FABERE"** maneuvers at the hip joint (Flexion, **AB**duction, **E**xternal **R**otation, and **E**xtension) stress the SI joint and elicit pain.

- Lumbar spine: Flexion is the most affected movement, although extension, axial rotation, and lateral bending are also affected.
  - **Schober's test** is initiated with the patient in a standing position. Identify the **dimples of Venus** (SI joints), and make a mark on the skin at the midline. Using a measuring tape make a second mark 10 cm above. Ask the patient to bend forward. Remeasure the distance between the two marks (see Figure 6-6). It normally measures at least 15 cm. Reduced expansion suggests ankylosing spondylitis.
- Cervical spine: Decreased ROM with lateral flexion, forward flexion, hyperextension, and rotation. Depending on the patient's position of function, they may develop a stoop forward. With the patient standing with his or her back against a wall, measure the **occiput to wall distance.** The inability to touch the occiput against the wall is abnormal. This measurement may be used to follow disease progression.
- Chest expansion: The chest normally expands 5 cm from expiration to maximal inspiration. This should be measured at the fourth intercostal space in men and immediately below the breasts in women.

Extraarticular Manifestations

- Ocular: The most common extraarticular manifestation of ankylosing spondylitis is acute anterior uveitis/iridocyclitis. It is accompanied by photophobia and increased lacrimation.
- Cardiovascular system (CVS): Aortic regurgitation (AR; see pp 15-16) is the most common cardiac manifestation. Atrioventricular (AV) conduction abnormalities, ascending aortitis, and pericarditis can also occur but may be undetectable clinically.
- Respiratory (Resp): Progressive fibrosis of the upper lobes rarely occurs and is usually a late finding. It usually presents with cough and rarely with hemoptysis.

> INSTRUCTIONS TO CANDIDATE: A 62-year-old male complains of "terrible" knee pain. Take a detailed history, exploring possible etiologies.

DD$_X$ VITAMINS C

- **V**ascular: Vasculitis
- **I**nfectious: Septic arthritis
- **T**raumatic: Hemarthrosis
- **A**utoimmune/**A**llergic: RA, systemic lupus erythematosus (SLE), scleroderma, ankylosing spondylitis, reactive arthritis, rheumatic fever, and sarcoidosis
- **M**etabolic: Gout, pseudogout
- **I**diopathic/**I**atrogenic: Osteoarthritis
- **N**eoplastic: Metastasis, primary tumor of bone or cartilage, and paraneoplastic syndrome

History

- **Ch**aracter: What does the pain feel like? Do you have any stiffness?
- **L**ocation: Where is the pain (in which knee and in what part of the knee)? Do you have pain in any other joints (distal versus proximal, monoarticular versus polyarticular)?
- **O**nset: How did this start (sudden versus gradual)? Does it start in the morning, day, or evening? Does it take >30 minutes after waking for the joints to "loosen up" (morning stiffness)?
- **R**adiation: Does the pain move anywhere? Down your leg or up your leg?
- **I**ntensity: How severe is the pain on a scale of 1 to 10, with 1 being mild pain and 10 being the worst pain? How does it affect your ADLs?

- **Duration:** How long does the pain last (constant versus intermittent, acute versus chronic)?
- **Events associated:**
  - Redness, swelling, deformity, or muscle atrophy?
  - Limitation of movement, weakness
  - Trauma (recent or past), anticoagulants/bleeding diathesis (hemarthrosis)
  - Diarrhea, stomatitis
  - Skin changes (rashes, nodules, psoriasis, tophi, shiny skin)
  - Conjunctivitis, oral ulcers, STI, or enthesopathy (reactive arthritis)
  - Raynaud's phenomenon
  - Constitutional symptoms: Fever, chills, night sweats, weight loss, anorexia, and asthenia
  - Recent medication changes
- **Frequency:** Has this ever happened to you before? How often does it happen?
- **Palliative factors:** What makes it better, if anything?
  - Activity versus rest? Activity exacerbates osteoarthritis, whereas rest worsens inflammatory arthritides.
  - Antiinflammatory drugs?
- **Provocative factors:** What makes it worse, if anything?
  - Activity versus rest?
  - Weight bearing (osteoarthritis)?
  - Stair climbing (patellofemoral arthritis)?
- **PMH:** Arthritis, inflammatory bowel disease (IBD), bleeding diathesis, lung disease, renal disease, psoriasis, STI, HIV, or connective tissue disease
- **PSH:** Trauma, previous joint surgery, or arthroscopy
- **MEDS:** NSAID, ASA, steroids, warfarin, or allopurinol
- **SH:** EtOH, recreational drugs, IV drug use, smoking, recent travel, multiple sexual partners, and unprotected sex
- **FH:** Arthritis, connective tissue disease, or IBD

INSTRUCTIONS TO CANDIDATE: An 85-year-old female presents after a "broken arm" with concerns about osteoporosis. Take a detailed history, focusing on risk factors.

Definition

- **Osteoporosis** is a disorder characterized by markedly decreased bone density or bone mass leading to an increased risk of developing a fracture from elevated bone fragility (Figure 6-18).
- A **fragility fracture** is most commonly considered to be one of the hip, vertebra, or distal forearm. The following factors increase the risk of frailty fractures:
  - Poor overall health
  - Nursing home patients, especially those with dementia
  - Bed-bound or immobilized patients
  - Poor eyesight
  - Poor balance
  - Falls

Risk Factors

- Primary osteoporosis is almost always diagnosed clinically and can be confirmed with a bone densitometry. A complete assessment of the patient's risk factors is essential when taking the history.
  - Age: Postmenopausal
  - Female sex
  - Estrogen status: Decreased production or any postpubertal deficiency

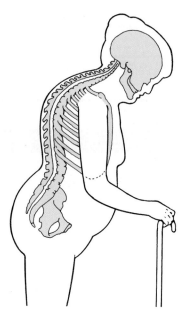

Figure 6-18   Posture of osteoporosis: dowager hump. (From Seidel HM, Ball JW, Dains JE, Benedict GB: *Mosby's guide to physical examination,* ed 5, St. Louis, 2003, Mosby, p 764, Figure 20-77.)

- ■ Low peak bone mass: Malnutrition, genetic (multifactorial)
- ■ Race: White, East Asian
- ■ FH: Osteoporosis or a fragility fracture in a first-degree relative
- ■ History of a fragility fracture as an adult
- ■ Lifestyle: Smoking, alcoholism
- ■ Diet: Inadequate calcium and/or vitamin D intake
- ■ Physical activity: Sedentary
- ■ Body habitus: Low body weight with the highest risk in thin females
- • Secondary causes of osteoporosis may be approached with a "review of systems" assessment, focusing on kidney, liver, endocrine, gastrointestinal, and malignant etiologies.
  - ■ Renal disease: Chronic renal failure impairs metabolism of vitamin D (renal osteodystrophy).
  - ■ Liver disease: Chronic liver disease impairs metabolism of vitamin D.
  - ■ Endocrine: Hyperparathyroidism, hyperthyroidism, Cushing's syndrome (endogenous or exogenous corticosteroid intake), hypogonadism, and acromegaly
  - ■ Gastrointestinal: Malabsorption states (e.g., IBD, celiac disease, pancreatic insufficiency), bowel resection, and long-term total parenteral nutrition (TPN)
  - ■ Malignancy: Multiple myeloma, leukemia, lymphoma, and solid tumors (breast, thyroid, lung, colorectal cancer)
- • Medications: Corticosteroids, anticonvulsants, aluminium-containing antacids, and immunosuppressants (e.g., methotrexate [MTX] and cyclosporine)

SAMPLE CHECKLISTS

> INSTRUCTIONS TO CANDIDATE: Perform an examination of the cervical spine. Describe your actions.

Key Points	Satisfactorily Carried out
Introduces self to the patient	❏
Determines how the patient wishes to be addressed	❏
Explains nature of the examination to the patient	❏
Examines the patient in a logical fashion	❏
Inspection	
• Posterior	❏
• Lateral	❏
• Curvature: Note normal lordotic curvature with patient supine or with occiput to wall	❏
Notes any	
• **S**welling	❏
• **E**rythema, **e**cchymosis	❏
• **A**trophy	❏
• **D**eformity	❏
• **S**kin changes	❏
Palpation	
• Patient positioning: Sitting	❏
• Cervical spinous processes	❏
• SCM, trapezius muscles	❏
• Paraspinal muscles	❏
Notes any	
• **T**enderness	❏
• **E**ffusion	❏
• **S**welling	❏
• **T**emperature	❏
• **C**repitus	❏
• **A**trophy	❏
Tests active ROM	
• Flexion	❏
• Extension	❏
• Rotation	❏
• Lateral flexion	❏
Tests passive ROM	
• Flexion	❏
• Extension	❏
• Rotation	❏
• Lateral flexion	❏
Tests power	
• Flexion	❏
• Extension	❏
• Rotation	❏
• Lateral flexion	❏
Measures occiput to wall distance	❏
Drapes the patient appropriately	❏
Makes appropriate closing remarks	❏

INSTRUCTIONS TO CANDIDATE: Perform an examination of the lumbar spine. Describe your actions.

Key Points	Satisfactorily Carried out
Introduces self to the patient	❑
Determines how the patient wishes to be addressed	❑
Explains nature of the examination to the patient	❑
Examines the patient in a logical fashion	❑
Inspection	
• Gait	❑
• Notes normal lordotic curve	❑
• Notes presence of any kyphosis or scoliosis	❑
Notes any	
• **S**welling	❑
• **E**rythema, **e**cchymosis	❑
• **A**trophy	❑
• **D**eformity	❑
• **S**kin changes	❑
Palpation	
• Patient positioning: Sitting or standing	❑
• Lumbar spinous processes	❑
• Paraspinal muscles	❑
Notes any	
• **T**enderness	❑
• **E**ffusion	❑
• **S**welling	❑
• **T**emperature	❑
• **C**repitus	❑
• **A**trophy	❑
Tests ROM	
• Finger to floor distance	❑
• Schober's test	❑
• Extension	❑
• Lateral flexion	❑
• Rotation	❑
Special tests	
• Straight leg raising	❑
• Bowstring sign	❑
• Lasègue's sign	❑
Drapes the patient appropriately	❑
Makes appropriate closing remarks	❑

> INSTRUCTIONS TO CANDIDATE: Perform an examination of the right shoulder. Describe your actions.

Key Points	Satisfactorily Carried out
Introduces self to the patient	❏
Determines how the patient wishes to be addressed	❏
Explains nature of the examination to the patient	❏
Examines the patient in a logical fashion	❏
Inspection	
• Anterior	❏
• Posterior	❏
• Compares with contralateral shoulder (asymmetry)	❏
Notes any	
• **S**welling	❏
• **E**rythema, **e**cchymosis	❏
• **A**trophy	❏
• **D**eformity	❏
• **S**kin changes	❏
Palpation	
• Sternoclavicular joint	❏
• Acromioclavicular joint	❏
• Coracoclavicular joint	❏
• Greater tuberosity of humerus	❏
• Scapula	❏
• Supraspinatus, infraspinatus, deltoid, and biceps tendons	❏
Notes any	
• **T**enderness	❏
• **E**ffusion	❏
• **S**welling	❏
• **T**emperature	❏
• **C**repitus	❏
• **A**trophy	❏
Tests active ROM	
• Flexion	❏
• Extension	❏
• Abduction	❏
• Adduction	❏
• Internal rotation	❏
• External rotation	❏
Tests for passive ROM	
• Flexion	❏
• Extension	❏
• Abduction	❏
• Adduction	❏
• Internal rotation	❏
• External rotation	❏

Key Points	Satisfactorily Carried out
Tests power	
• Flexion	❏
• Extension	❏
• Abduction	❏
• Adduction	❏
• Internal rotation	❏
• External rotation	❏
Special tests	
• Impingement test	❏
• Drop test	❏
Bonus	
• Recognizes neck as source of referred pain (Spurling's sign, compression test)	❏
Drapes the patient appropriately	❏
Makes appropriate closing remarks	❏

INSTRUCTIONS TO CANDIDATE: Perform an examination of the left elbow. Describe your actions.

Key Points	Satisfactorily Carried out
Introduces self to the patient	❏
Determines how the patient wishes to be addressed	❏
Explains nature of the examination to the patient	❏
Examines the patient in a logical fashion	❏
Inspection	
• Carrying angle	❏
• Compares with contralateral elbow (asymmetry)	❏
Notes any	
• **S**welling	❏
• **E**rythema, **e**cchymosis	❏
• **A**trophy	❏
• **D**eformity	❏
• **S**kin changes	❏
Palpation	
• Olecranon	❏
• Medial and lateral humeral condyles	❏
• Radial head	❏
• Medial epicondyle	❏
• Lateral epicondyle	❏
• Effusion (anatomic triangle formed by radial head, lateral condyle, and olecranon)	❏
Notes any	
• **T**enderness	❏
• **E**ffusion	❏

Key Points	Satisfactorily Carried out
• **S**welling	❏
• **T**emperature	❏
• **C**repitus	❏
• **A**trophy	❏
Tests active ROM	
• Flexion	❏
• Extension	❏
• Supination	❏
• Pronation	❏
Tests passive ROM	
• Flexion	❏
• Extension	❏
• Supination	❏
• Pronation	❏
Tests power	
• Flexion	❏
• Extension	❏
• Supination	❏
• Pronation	❏
Special tests	
• Tennis elbow (forced wrist extension, lateral epicondyle tenderness)	❏
• Golfer's elbow (forced wrist flexion, medial epicondyle tenderness)	❏
Drapes the patient appropriately	❏
Makes appropriate closing remarks	❏

INSTRUCTIONS TO CANDIDATE: Perform an examination of the right hand and wrist. Describe your actions.

Key Points	Satisfactorily Carried out
Introduces self to the patient	❏
Determines how the patient wishes to be addressed	❏
Explains nature of the examination to the patient	❏
Examines the patient in a logical fashion	❏
Inspection	
• Volar	❏
• Dorsal	❏
• Thenar eminence	❏
• Compares with contralateral wrist/hand (asymmetry)	❏
Notes any	
• **S**welling	❏
• **E**rythema, **e**cchymosis	❏
• **A**trophy	❏

Key Points	Satisfactorily Carried out
• **D**eformity (e.g., swan neck deformity)	❏
• **S**kin changes	❏
Palpation	
• Radioulnar groove	❏
• Radiocarpal groove	❏
• MCP joints	❏
• PIP joints	❏
• DIP joints	❏
• IP joints (thumbs)	❏
Notes any	
• **T**enderness	❏
• **E**ffusion	❏
• **S**welling	❏
• **T**emperature	❏
• **C**repitus	❏
• **A**trophy	❏
Tests active ROM	
• Wrist flexion/extension	❏
• Wrist ulnar/radial deviation	❏
• Flexion/extension of MCP joints	❏
• Flexor digitorum superficialis/profundus	❏
• Finger abduction/adduction	❏
• Finger opposition	❏
• Thumb abduction/adduction	❏
Tests passive ROM	
• Wrist flexion/extension	❏
• Wrist ulnar/radial deviation	❏
• Flexion/extension of MCP joints	❏
• Flexion/extension of PIP and DIP joints	❏
• Finger abduction/adduction	❏
• Finger opposition	❏
• Thumb abduction/adduction	❏
Tests power	
• Wrist flexion/extension	❏
• Wrist ulnar/radial deviation	❏
• Flexion/extension of MCP joints	❏
• Flexor digitorum superficialis/profundus	❏
• Finger abduction/adduction	❏
• Finger opposition	❏
• Thumb abduction/adduction	❏
Special tests	
• Tinel's sign	❏
• Phalen's test	❏
Drapes the patient appropriately	❏
Makes appropriate closing remarks	❏

INSTRUCTIONS TO CANDIDATE: Perform an examination of the left knee. Describe your actions.

Key Points	Satisfactorily Carried out
Introduces self to the patient	❏
Determines how the patient wishes to be addressed	❏
Explains nature of the examination to the patient	❏
Examines the patient in a logical fashion	❏
Inspection • Compares with contralateral knee (asymmetry)	❏
Notes any • **S**welling (suprapatellar convexity versus concavity) • **E**rythema, **e**cchymosis • **A**trophy • **D**eformity (e.g., genu valgum, genu varum) • **S**kin changes	❏ ❏ ❏ ❏ ❏
Palpation • Patella • Tibial tuberosity • Tibial condyles • Femoral epicondyles	❏ ❏ ❏ ❏
Notes any • **T**enderness • **E**ffusion: Patellar tap, bulge sign • **S**welling • **T**emperature • **C**repitus: Throughout the ROM • **A**trophy	❏ ❏ ❏ ❏ ❏ ❏
Tests active ROM • Flexion • Extension	❏ ❏
Tests passive ROM • Flexion • Extension	❏ ❏
Tests power • Flexion • Extension	❏ ❏
Tests stability • Collateral ligament stress test • Anterior drawer test or Lachman's test • Posterior drawer test	❏ ❏ ❏
McMurray's test	❏
Determines Q angle	❏
Drapes the patient appropriately	❏
Makes appropriate closing remarks	❏

INSTRUCTIONS TO CANDIDATE: Perform an examination of the left ankle and foot. Describe your actions.

Key Points	Satisfactorily Carried out
Introduces self to the patient	❏
Determines how the patient wishes to be addressed	❏
Explains nature of the examination to the patient	❏
Examines the patient in a logical fashion	❏
Inspection	
• Inspects while weight bearing and while sitting	❏
• Compares with contralateral ankle/foot (asymmetry)	❏
Notes any	
• **S**welling	❏
• **E**rythema, **e**cchymosis	❏
• **A**trophy	❏
• **D**eformity (e.g., pes planus, pes cavus)	❏
• **S**kin changes	❏
Palpation	
• Medial malleolus	❏
• Lateral malleolus	❏
• Talus (anterior)	❏
• Calcaneus	❏
• Achilles tendon	❏
• MTP joints	❏
• Toes	❏
Notes any	
• **T**enderness	❏
• **E**ffusion	❏
• **S**welling	❏
• **T**emperature	❏
• **C**repitus	❏
• **A**trophy	❏
Tests active ROM	
• Dorsiflexion	❏
• Plantar flexion	❏
• Inversion	❏
• Eversion	❏
• Flexion of great toe	❏
• Extension of great toe	❏
Tests passive ROM	
• Dorsiflexion	❏
• Plantar flexion	❏
• Inversion	❏
• Eversion	❏
• Abduction/adduction of ankle	❏
• Flexion of great toe	❏
• Extension of great toe	❏
Tests stability	
• Anterior drawer test	❏
• Inversion stress test	❏
• External rotation test	❏
Drapes the patient appropriately	❏
Makes appropriate closing remarks	❏

INSTRUCTIONS TO CANDIDATE: Perform a focused physical examination of the hand in this patient with a history of rheumatoid arthritis. Describe your actions and expected findings (Figures 6-19 and 6-20).

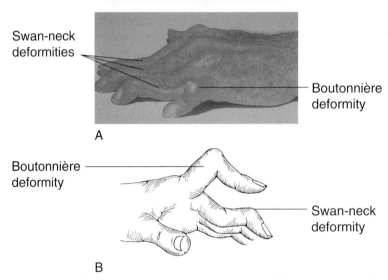

Figure 6-19   Swan-neck and boutonnière deformities in rheumatoid arthritis. (From Wison SF, Giddens JF: *Health assessment for nursing practice*, ed 2, St. Louis, 2001, Mosby, p 658, Figure 24-31.)

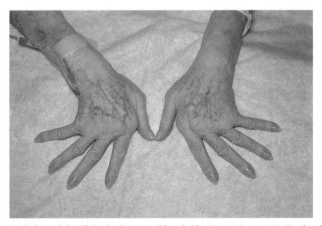

Figure 6-20   Ulnar deviation of the digits in rheumatoid arthritis. (From Swartz M: *Textbook of physical diagnosis: history and examination,* ed 4, Philadelphia, 1998, WB Saunders, Figure 19-56.)

Key Points	Satisfactorily Carried out
Introduces self to the patient	❑
Determines how the patient wishes to be addressed	❑
Explains nature of the examination to the patient	❑
Examines the patient in a logical fashion	❑
Inspection • Compares with contralateral hand (asymmetry)	❑

Key Points	Satisfactorily Carried out
Notes any	
• **S**welling (fusiform)	❏
• **E**rythema, **e**cchymosis	❏
• **A**trophy	❏
• **D**eformity	❏
• **S**kin changes (rheumatoid nodules)	❏
Identifies ulnar drift of digits	❏
Identifies subluxations	❏
Identifies "typical" rheumatoid deformities	
• Swan neck	❏
• Boutonnière	❏
Palpation	
• Nodules	❏
• Tendons	❏
• MCP joints	❏
• PIP joints	❏
• DIP joints	❏
• IP joints (thumbs)	❏
Notes any	
• **T**enderness	❏
• **E**ffusion	❏
• **S**welling	❏
• **T**emperature	❏
• **C**repitus	❏
• **A**trophy	❏
Tests active ROM	
• Flexion/extension of MCP joints	❏
• Flexor digitorum superficialis/profundus	❏
• Finger abduction/adduction	❏
• Finger opposition	❏
• Thumb abduction/adduction	❏
Tests passive ROM	
• Flexion/extension of MCP joints	❏
• Flexion/extension of PIP and DIP joints	❏
• Finger abduction/adduction	❏
• Finger opposition	❏
• Thumb abduction/adduction	❏
Tests power	
• Grip strength	❏
• Flexion/extension of MCP joints	❏
• Flexor digitorum superficialis/profundus	❏
• Finger abduction/adduction	❏
• Finger opposition	❏
• Thumb abduction/adduction	❏
Drapes the patient appropriately	❏
Makes appropriate closing remarks	❏

> INSTRUCTIONS TO CANDIDATE: Examine this patient with a suspected right L4-L5 or L5-S1 disk protrusion causing root compression.

Key Points	Satisfactorily Carried out
Introduces self to the patient	❑
Determines how the patient wishes to be addressed	❑
Explains nature of the examination to the patient	❑
Examines the patient in a logical fashion	❑
Inspection	
• Gait	❑
• Looks for loss of normal lordotic curvature (spasm)	❑
• Notes presence of any kyphosis or scoliosis	❑
• Notes any fasciculations in the lower limb	❑
Notes any	
• **S**welling	❑
• **E**rythema, **e**cchymosis	❑
• **A**trophy (lower limbs, especially right leg)	❑
• **D**eformity	❑
• **S**kin changes	❑
Palpation	
• Patient positioning: Sitting or standing	❑
• Lumbar spinous processes	❑
• SI joints	❑
• Paraspinal muscles	❑
Notes any	
• **T**enderness	❑
• **E**ffusion	❑
• **S**welling	❑
• **T**emperature	❑
• **C**repitus	❑
• **A**trophy	❑
Tests ROM	
• Finger to floor distance	❑
• Schober's test	❑
• Extension	❑
• Lateral flexion	❑
• Rotation	❑
Muscle strength	
• Plantar flexion (walking on toes)	❑
• Dorsiflexion (walking on heels)	❑
• Flexion of great toe	❑
• Extension of great toe	❑
• Knee flexion	❑
Tests muscle tone (notes any clonus)	❑
Special tests	
• Straight leg raising	❑
• Bowstring sign	❑
• Lasègue's sign	❑

Key Points	Satisfactorily Carried out
Deep tendon reflexes	
• Knee (compares with contralateral knee)	❏
• Ankle (compares with contralateral ankle)	❏
• Plantar (compares with contralateral foot)	❏
Sensation	
• L4 dermatome	❏
• L5 dermatome	❏
• S1 dermatome	❏
• Perineal (saddle region)	❏
Rectal examination for tone	❏
Drapes the patient appropriately	❏
Makes appropriate closing remarks	❏

CHAPTER 7

Dermatology

OBJECTIVES

ANATOMY

CARDINAL SIGNS AND SYMPTOMS

ESSENTIAL CLINICAL COMPETENCIES
APPROACH TO SKIN EXAMINATION

SAMPLE OSCE SCENARIOS

- A 23-year-old female presents with a history of facial acne unresponsive to over-the-counter products. Obtain an appropriate history, and perform a focused physical examination, identifying morphology and type of acne.
- A 28-year-old male presents with large linear blisters on the lower extremities that are weeping and crusting, having returned from a camping trip approximately 5 days ago. Perform a focused history and physical examination.
- An 18-year-old male presents with a flare of his lifelong eczema that he attributes to increased school stressors. He has been more pruritic with "juicy, sometimes oozing bumps." He has tried numerous creams and ointments in the past for his skin but tells you that no prescription has ever worked and is therefore using an "all natural" cream. Obtain an appropriate history. What relevant information will help you determine the factors responsible for this recent flare?
- A 23-year-old male presents with acute onset of multiple scaly droplike plaques on the trunk after a sore throat. He had a similar episode 2 years ago and uses a topical corticosteroid for chronic psoriasis on the elbows and knees. Obtain an appropriate history. What type of psoriasis is this, and what other papulosquamous diseases should be considered?
- A 34-year-old female nurse presents with a 1-week history of raised, markedly pruritic wheals in the skin. This has occurred daily and leaves no residual skin changes. Obtain an appropriate history. What information will be helpful to sort out the nature of these plaques?
- A 62-year-old male presents with a persistent ankle ulcer after accidentally hitting it on a chair 4 weeks ago. Obtain an appropriate history. What information do you need to determine the type of ulcer he has?
- A 35-year-old female presents with a 1-week history of painful nodules, swelling, and "bruising" localized to the shins with no ulceration. Obtain an appropriate history. What history is important in delineating cause and associated illness for this eruption?
- A 65-year-old female presents with a new-onset, widespread, symmetrical red itchy eruption of 3 days' duration. She is well, other than hypothyroidism for which she takes thyroxin. After a recent upper respiratory illness she was prescribed an oral amino penicillin antibiotic, which she stopped taking 1 week ago. Obtain an appropriate history. What information is required to sort out the nature of this eruption?
- A 65-year-old male presents with a bump on his face of 6 months' duration that bleeds when he shaves. He has applied a topical antibiotic, but the lesion has never healed. He sunburns easily and worked outside in construction for many years, never wearing sunscreen. Obtain an appropriate history. What background information do you need to determine the most likely causes for this lesion?

Continued

• A 63-year-old male presents with a changing pigmented lesion on his back. He estimates its duration to be 1 year or more, and his wife had noticed it getting larger and darker. Obtain an appropriate history. What important information do you need to assess this patient?

SAMPLE CHECKLIST
❑ This 25-year-old male with psoriasis is referred to your clinic for follow-up evaluation. Perform a focused physical examination, and describe your findings.

OBJECTIVES

*The successful student should be able to take a **focused** dermatologic **history** and formulate a differential diagnosis for:*
• Acne
• Blistering disorders
• Dermatitis
• Psoriasis
• Urticaria
• Leg ulcers
• Erythema nodosum
• Exanthems
• Non-melanoma skin cancer
• Pigmented lesions

Formulating a differential diagnosis for unknown skin disease is facilitated by identification of a primary lesion (e.g., scaly papules and plaques characterize psoriasis, pityriasis versicolor, and lichen planus), and students should familiarize themselves with these terms.

*A complete dermatologic **examination** will include:*
• All hair-bearing and non–hair-bearing cutaneous surfaces
• Hair
• Mucous membranes
• Nails

ANATOMY

• The skin functions primarily as a barrier. It protects the delicate internal environment against physical trauma, ultraviolet damage, and potentially infectious agents. Secondary functions include temperature regulation, sensation, vitamin D synthesis, body odor, and aesthetic appearance.
• Skin consists of the following elements (Figure 7-1):
  ▪ Epidermis
  ▪ Dermis
  ▪ Appendageal structures
  ▪ Subcutaneous fat
• The epidermis is an avascular structure composed of keratinocytes, cells that are constantly undergoing differentiation and migration to produce a dead layer of cells termed the stratum corneum. The end result is an effective protective barrier as outlined previously.
• The dermis is a vascular structure that also contains nerves and cutaneous appendages, meaning eccrine and apocrine sweat glands, hair follicles, and sebaceous glands.
• The dermis is anchored to the epidermis by interlocking rete pegs (epidermal origin) to dermal papillae. The basement membrane zone (BMZ) represents the interface

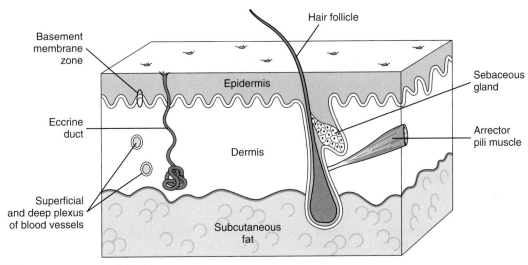

Figure 7-1   Anatomy of the skin.

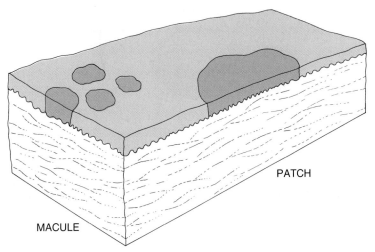

Figure 7-2   Nonpalpable primary skin lesions. (From Swartz M: *Textbook of physical diagnosis: history and examination*, ed 4, Philadelphia, 2002, WB Saunders, p 135, Figure 7-17.)

between these two structures, and through a series of interactions it effectively cements the two surfaces together. Disruption of the BMZ leads to a number of blistering disorders, depending on the origin of separation within the BMZ. The dermis also houses blood vessels (responsible for the erythema seen in many skin conditions) and nerves that provide touch, temperature, and pain sensation.
• The underlying layer of fat provides insulation and functions also to cushion from blunt trauma.

CARDINAL SIGNS AND SYMPTOMS

Nonpalpable Primary Skin Lesions (Figure 7-2)
• A **macule** is a circumscribed nonpalpable area of skin discoloration <0.5 cm.
• A **patch** is a circumscribed nonpalpable area of skin discoloration >0.5 cm.

Palpable Primary Skin Lesions (Figure 7-3)
• A **papule** is a solid elevated lesion <0.5 cm.
• A **plaque** is an elevated lesion >0.5 cm without significant depth.

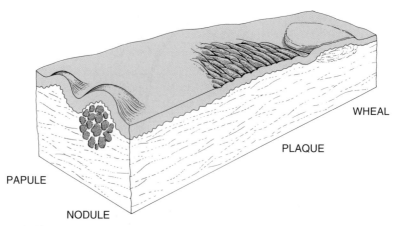

Figure 7-3   Palpable primary skin lesions. (Adapted from Swartz M: *Textbook of physical diagnosis: history and examination*, ed 4, Philadelphia, 2002, WB Saunders, p 136, Figure 7-18.)

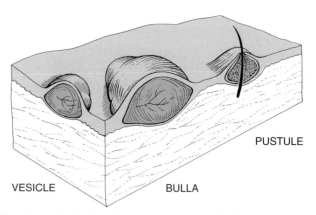

Figure 7-4   Fluid-filled primary skin lesions. (From Swartz M: *Textbook of physical diagnosis: history and examination*, ed 4, Philadelphia, 2002, WB Saunders, p 136, Figure 7-19.)

- A **nodule** is a solid lesion in the skin >0.5 cm with considerable depth by palpation.
- A **wheal** is an elevated white papule or plaque secondary to dermal edema that resolves within hours, leaving no cutaneous abnormality.

Fluid-Filled Primary Skin Lesions (Figure 7-4)
- A **vesicle** is a circumscribed fluid-filled lesion <0.5 cm.
- A **bulla** is a circumscribed fluid-filled lesion >0.5 cm.
- A **pustule** is a circumscribed lesion filled with pus.

Secondary Skin Lesions (Figure 7-5)
- An **erosion** represents focal, partial thickness loss of epidermis.
- An **ulcer** represents focal, complete thickness loss of epidermis.
- A **fissure** is a linear crack or cleavage in the skin.
- **Excoriations** are a superficial loss of epidermis, often linear, created by scratching.
- **Atrophy** in dermatology refers to loss of size as a result of thinning of part of the epidermis or dermis.
- A **scale** is an abnormal accumulation or shedding of flakes of skin (representing stratum corneum).
- **Crusts** are dried deposits of serum, blood, or pus on the skin.
- **Purpura** is any area of extravasation of blood into skin.
- **Petechiae** are palpable or nonpalpable extravasations of blood into skin involving an area of <0.5 cm.

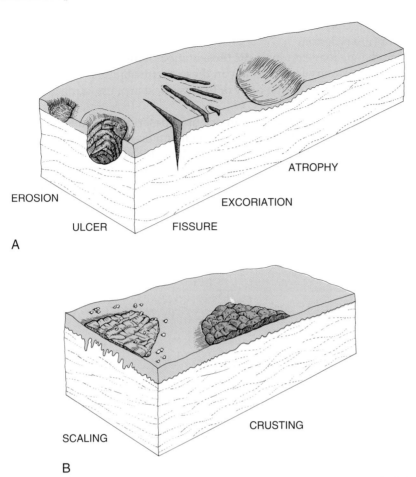

Figure 7-5 **A,** Secondary skin lesions below the skin plane. (Adapted from Swartz M: *Textbook of physical diagnosis: history and examination,* ed 4, Philadelphia, 2002, WB Saunders, p 138, Figure 7-21.) **B,** Secondary skin lesions above the skin plane. (From Swartz M: *Textbook of physical diagnosis: history and examination,* ed 4, Philadelphia, 2002, WB Saunders, p 138, Figure 7-22.)

- **Ecchymosis** is extravasation of blood into skin involving an area >2 cm.
- A **scar** is an area of induration or depression in the skin secondary to healing. It may be normal, hypertrophic, or keloidal in nature.

Arrangement
- Groups of lesions can be described according to certain patterns.
- These include grouped, linear, serpiginous, arcuate, nummular, annular, and reticular.
- Individual lesions may also be described as nummular or annular, such as in a nummular plaque of eczema.

ESSENTIAL CLINICAL COMPETENCIES

Approach to Skin Examination
A complete dermatologic examination includes inspection of:

- All hair-bearing and non–hair-bearing cutaneous surfaces
- Hair
- Mucous membranes
- Nails

- In describing a cutaneous eruption (avoid the term "rash") you should attempt to identify a primary lesion.
- Secondary change may dominate the presentation of the primary eruption, and a diligent search for primary lesions is key in these circumstances.
- It is helpful to comment on the color of the lesion, sharpness, surface contour, shape, and texture.
- Arrangement and distribution are important in describing a skin eruption.
- As in other areas of clinical examination when you do not recognize something in the skin, adopt the **VITAMINS C** approach; it will enable you to expand your list of possibilities for a problem and ensure you do not forget relevant historical questions.
- Using the correct terms enables you to communicate more effectively with colleagues and ultimately benefits your patient.

SAMPLE OSCE SCENARIOS

INSTRUCTIONS TO CANDIDATE: A 23-year-old female presents with a history of facial acne unresponsive to over-the-counter products. Obtain an appropriate history, and perform a focused physical examination, identifying morphology and type of acne.

DD$_X$ VITAMINS C

- **V**ascular: Think of rosacea (Figures 7-6 and 7-7)
- **I**nfectious: Bacterial folliculitis
- **T**raumatic: Acne excoriée (Figure 7-8)
- **A**utoimmune/**A**llergic
- **M**etabolic: Steroid acne (from either oral or topical steroids; Figure 7-9)
- **I**diopathic/**I**atrogenic: Perioral dermatitis (iatrogenic steroid use; Figure 7-10)
- **C**ongenital/genetic: Adenoma sebaceum in tuberous sclerosis
- Acne vulgaris (Figure 7-11)

History

- **Ch**aracter: What is the nature of the acneiform eruption?
  - Are primary lesions of acne vulgaris present (i.e., comedones [open and closed], papules, pustules, and nodules)?
  - Is the acne noninflammatory (comedonal), inflammatory (papules, pustules, nodules), or mixed? Rosacea lacks comedones.
  - Is there scarring, and is it linear? Scarring may occur with acne vulgaris. Isolated linear scarring suggests acne excoriée.
  - Are lesions the same size and shape (monomorphic), or are there different morphologies? Monomorphic lesions are more often seen in perioral dermatitis and steroid acne.
  - Are there associated telangiectasias and flushing or erythema on the nose and cheeks (suggestive of rosacea)?

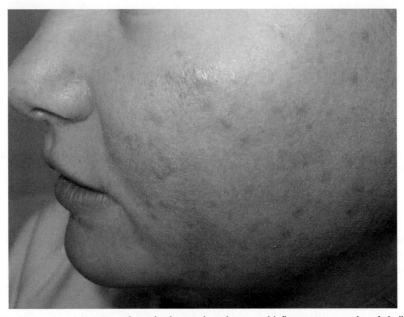

Figure 7-6 Acne rosacea. Note prominent background erythema and inflammatory papules of similar size and shape in the absence of comedones. Note subtle telangiectasias (small threadlike blood vessels) account for the erythema but are not clearly visible in this image. (Used with permission of Dr. Peter Green.)

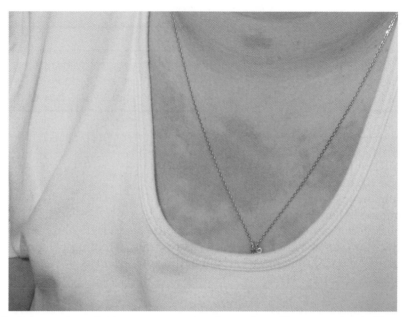

Figure 7-7 Note prominent flushing response on chest in a patient with rosacea. (Used with permission of Dr. Peter Green.)

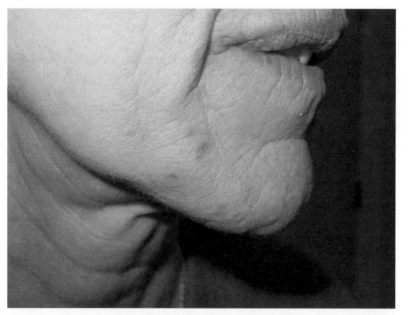

Figure 7-8 Acne excoriée. Patient presented with "acne unresponsive to treatment." Note absence of any primary acne excoriée; only excoriations are present. (Used with permission of Dr. Peter Green.)

- Location: Where do the lesions predominate?
  - Sebaceous gland–rich areas such as cheeks, forehead, upper chest, and back?
  - Perioral distribution, sparing cheeks, and forehead (perioral dermatitis)?
  - Papules and pustules confined to nose, cheeks, forehead, and chin, sparing peri-ocular skin, with significant background erythema and telangiectasia (acne rosacea)?
  - Are the lesions unilateral (suggestive of bacterial folliculitis)?
- Onset: Gradual progression of acne or acute onset over days? Sudden onset suggests bacterial folliculitis.

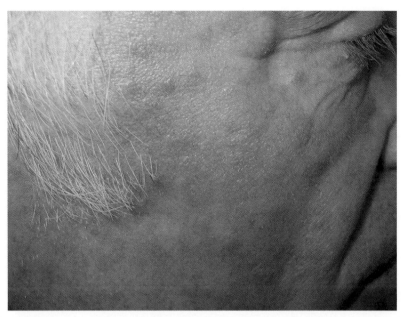

Figure 7-9 Steroid acne. An acneiform eruption confined to cheeks and temples where moderate potency topical steroids had been applied over a number of years. Again note the presence of telangiectasias and absence of comedones. Rosacea could have a similar appearance; thus the history was instrumental in making the appropriate diagnosis. (Used with permission of Dr. Peter Green.)

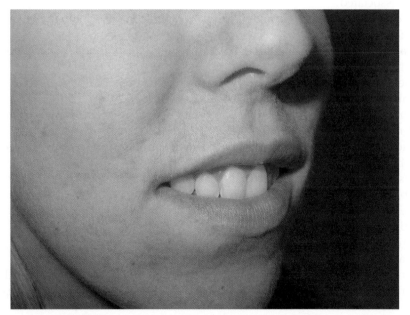

Figure 7-10 Perioral dermatitis: A subtle collection of monomorphic red papules in a perioral distribution. (Used with permission of Dr. Peter Green.)

- Intensity: Must be measured by the physician's assessment and the patient's perception of severity.
  - Inflammatory (papules and pustules) versus noninflammatory (comedones)
  - Extent of cutaneous involvement
  - Presence of scarring
  - Presence of nodules
  - Psychologic impact on patient

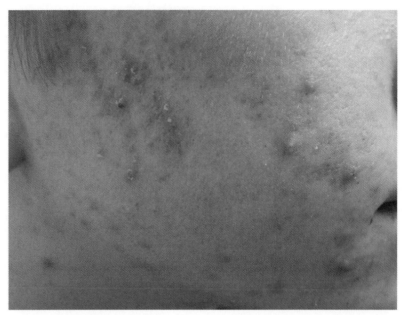

Figure 7-11   Acne vulgaris. Note simultaneous presence of closed comedones (blackheads), open comedones (whiteheads), papules, pustules, small nodules, and subtle early scarring. This patient was treated successfully with oral isotretinoin. (Used with permission of Dr. Peter Green.)

- **Duration:** How long has the acne been present in its current state?
- **Events associated:**
    - Polycystic ovarian syndrome (PCOS): Irregular menses, hirsutism, acanthosis nigricans
    - Rosacea: Flushing with EtOH, hot beverages, spicy foods, social stressors, or weather
    - Acne excoriée or acne vulgaris with secondary excoriations: Does the patient manipulate (squeezing, picking, excoriating) the acne?
    - Adenoma sebaceum in tuberous sclerosis: History of seizures, white patches (ash leaf macules), digital fibromas, tooth pits, cutaneous collagenomas
    - Topical moisturizer application? Excessive, chronic application causes perioral dermatitis.
    - Does the patient use excessive makeup to cover the acne? Makeup may worsen the problem.
- **Frequency:** Is the acne of recent onset or a recurrent issue?
- **Palliative factors:** What treatments, if any, have worked?
    - Isotretinoin
    - Tetracycline
- **Provocative factors:** Have you noted worsening with any previous topical therapy (prescription or over-the-counter [OTC])? Does the patient believe that stress or diet causes the acne?
- **Past medical history (PMH):** PCOS, irregular menses
- **Medication (MEDS; including OTC medications):** Previous isotretinoin use, oral steroids, oral contraceptive pill (OCP), antidepressants (may suggest acne excoriée or a relative contraindication for isotretinoin)
- **Social history (SH):** Occupation, sexual activity (pregnancy is contraindicated while on isotretinoin or tetracyclines), and use of EtOH and tobacco
- **Family history (FH):** Severe or scarring acne, rosacea

INSTRUCTIONS TO CANDIDATE: A 28-year-old male presents with large linear blisters on the lower extremities that are weeping and crusting, having returned from a camping trip approximately 5 days ago. Perform a focused history and physical examination.

DD$_X$ VITAMINS C
- **Vascular:** Vasculitis
- **Infectious:** Bacterial infection (bullous erysipelas or cellulitis), viral infection (herpes simplex, herpes zoster; Figures 7-12 and 7-13)
- **Traumatic:** Burn
- **Autoimmune/Allergic:** Autoimmune blistering disorders (bullous pemphigoid, pemphigus vulgaris; Figure 7-14), acute allergic contact dermatitis (poison ivy, oak, or sumac; Figure 7-15)

History
- **Character:** Are the primary lesions vesicles (<0.5 to 1.0 cm) or bullae (>0.5 to 1.0 cm)?
  - Are they grouped into small grapelike clusters (herpes simplex) or along a dermatome (herpes zoster)?
  - Are they arranged in a linear fashion (allergic contact dermatitis)?
  - Do the blisters rupture easily (pemphigus), or are they more tense (bullous pemphigoid)?
- **Location:**
  - Are the blisters more generalized (pemphigus, bullous pemphigoid) or localized?
  - Unilateral? Bilateral (NOT cellulitis, or bullous erysipelas)?
  - Do they involve the lip, lumbar spine, or other isolated area of skin (herpes simplex)?
  - Do they involve a truncal or head and neck dermatome (herpes zoster)?
  - Are they isolated to the lower extremity (allergic contact dermatitis to poison ivy, bullous erysipelas, cellulitis)?
- **Onset:** Gradual onset or acute?
- **Radiation:** Linear or dermatomal?

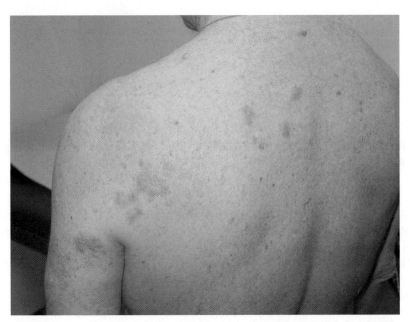

Figure 7-12 Dermatomal pattern of herpes zoster on trunk; note clusters of vesicles. (Used with permission of Dr. Peter Green.)

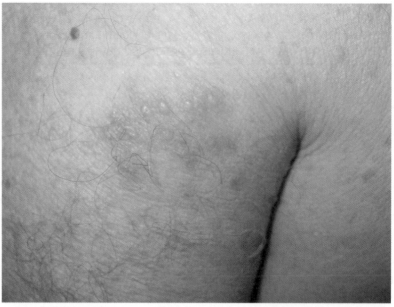

Figure 7-13   Close-up of herpes zoster demonstrating vesicles on an erythematous base. (Used with permission of Dr. Peter Green.)

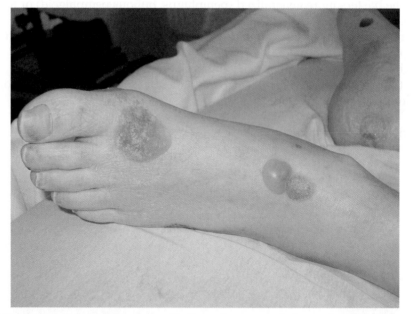

Figure 7-14   Tense bullae adjacent to ruptured bullae on lower extremity in a male with bullous pemphigoid. (Used with permission of Dr. Peter Green.)

- Intensity: What is the extent of cutaneous surface involved? More extensive blisters are not likely to be herpes simplex (exception: eczema herpeticum; i.e., generalized herpes simplex infection).
- Duration: Do blisters rupture quickly or remain tense (implies superficial versus deeper process)?
- Events associated:
  - Mucosal membrane blisters (pemphigus, rarely bullous pemphigoid)?
  - Associated itch (allergic contact dermatitis, early phase of bullous pemphigoid)?

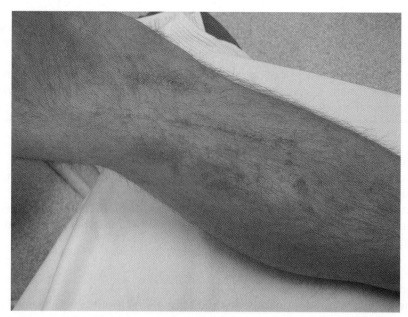

Figure 7-15 Linear vesicles on an urticarial, erythematous base of poison ivy allergic contact dermatitis. (Used with permission of Dr. Peter Green.)

- ■ Fever, chills, nausea, vomiting, and painful limb (bullous erysipelas, cellulitis, secondary infection with widespread blisters)?
- ■ Preceding pain or burning sensation (herpes zoster)
- **Frequency:** Recurrent localized blistering in the same area (herpes simplex)?
- **Palliative factors:** Is there anything that makes it better? If so, what?
- **Provocative factors:**
  - ■ Recent exposure to shrubbery, wooded areas (poison ivy, oak, or sumac)?
  - ■ Any new recent contacts (e.g., topical moisturizer, itch creams with "caine" suffix, or nickel; allergic contact dermatitis)?
  - ■ Recent burn or trauma?

Physical Examination
- **Vitals:** Heart rate (HR), blood pressure (BP), and temperature: Fever is associated with bacterial infection but not primary blistering disorders unless significant secondary infection is present
- **General:** Looks well but uncomfortable because of itch versus looks unwell because of extensive blistering or infection
- **Skin:** Examine all hair-bearing and non–hair-bearing cutaneous surfaces, hair, mucous membranes, and nails.

PEARLS
- Localized linear unilateral lower extremity bullae and vesicles in a well individual most likely are caused by allergic contact dermatitis (e.g., poison ivy, oak, or sumac).
- A pattern on the lower extremity of circumferential or extensive painful erythema with associated bullae and systemic symptoms is compatible with bullous erysipelas (sharply circumscribed erythema) or cellulitis (poorly circumscribed erythema).
- Zoster would be unusual on a lower extremity.
- Autoimmune blistering disorders would not generally affect a young person and would not be localized to the lower extremity.

INSTRUCTIONS TO CANDIDATE: An 18-year-old male presents with a flare of his lifelong eczema that he attributes to increased school stressors. He has been more pruritic with "juicy, sometimes oozing bumps." He has tried numerous creams and ointments in the past for his skin but tells you that no prescription has ever worked and is therefore using an "all natural" cream. Obtain an appropriate history. What relevant information will help you determine the factors responsible for this recent flare?

DD$_X$ VITAMINS C

- **Infectious:** Atopic dermatitis with secondary *Staphylococcus aureus* infection, eczema herpeticum (widespread herpes simplex 1)
- **Autoimmune/Allergic:** Atopic dermatitis with episodic flare (Figure 7-16), secondary allergic contact dermatitis to preservative or medicated ingredient in natural remedy
- **Idiopathic/Iatrogenic:** Drug reaction

History

- **Character:**
  - Is the dermatitis predominantly dry and scaly with chronically thickened skin?
  - Is there oozing and crusting (suggests secondary bacterial infection with *S. aureus*)?
  - Are small, deep, intensely itchy vesicles present within the eczema (vesicular nature suggests more acute flare of chronic atopic dermatitis or allergic contact dermatitis)?
  - Is pruritus a prominent feature?
  - Are weeping, umbilicated vesicles present in a generalized or widespread distribution (eczema herpeticum)?
- **Location:** Predominantly flexor surfaces (antecubital and popliteal fossae more common areas of eczema)? Are new areas flaring?
- **Onset:** Has this flared up quickly or been progressive?
- **Radiation:** Is the eczema localized, or is there generalized involvement? Has the eczema spread beyond its usual areas of involvement?

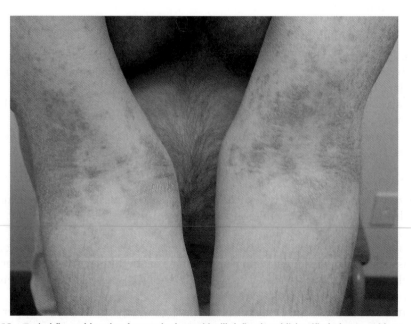

Figure 7-16   Typical flexural location for atopic dermatitis; ill-defined, red lichenified plaques with no vesicles or evidence of secondary infection. (Used with permission of Dr. Peter Green.)

- **Intensity:** To what degree has the eczema impacted the patient's life? Is the itch bad enough to interfere with normal daily activities or interrupt sleep? Has the itch been severe enough to trigger excoriations or secondary infection?
- **Duration:** How long has this particular flare lasted?
- **Events associated:** Fever or chills (suggest serious secondary infection or widespread involvement)?
- **Frequency:** How often does the eczema flare and under what circumstances?
- **Palliative factors:** How has the patient been managing the eczema?
  - How often does the patient apply topical moisturizers or medicated ointment (important to determine compliance)?
  - How much of the medication has the patient used (make sure to look at the jar or tube to see how much is gone)?
  - Does the patient prefer creams (slightly less effective but cosmetically more elegant) or ointments (consistency of petroleum jelly)?
  - How often does the patient bathe or shower (daily optimizes moisture in the skin)?
- **Provocative factors:**
  - Dust? Pets? Wool? Foods (egg, milk, peanut)?
  - Occupational factors (hand washing, exposure to irritants, potential allergens [e.g., rubber gloves])?
  - Stress (may flare but not the primary cause of eczema)?
  - Has the patient started any new topical products with potential allergens (fragrance, formaldehyde releasers, lanolin, parabens)?
  - Does the patient's medicated cream "burn" the skin on contact (usually because of preservatives and not an allergic response but it often causes patients to stop therapy)?
- **PMH:** Has the patient ever been admitted to the hospital for eczema or required oral antibiotics to manage secondary infection? Associated asthma, rhinitis?
- **MEDS:** Current prescription for topical therapy? Recent oral antibiotics? Previous oral corticosteroids?
- **Allergies:** Known medication allergies or documented allergies by prick testing
- **FH:** Atopic dermatitis

INSTRUCTIONS TO CANDIDATE: A 23-year-old male presents with acute onset of multiple scaly droplike plaques on the trunk after a sore throat. He had a similar episode 2 years ago and uses a topical corticosteroid for chronic psoriasis on the elbows and knees. Obtain an appropriate history. What type of psoriasis is this, and what other papulosquamous diseases should be considered?

DD$_X$ VITAMINS C
- **Infectious:** Secondary syphilis (Figure 7-17), tinea corporis (Figure 7-18), pityriasis versicolor and pityriasis rosea (presumed viral) (Figure 7-19)
- **Autoimmune/Allergic:** Psoriasis (Figure 7-20), allergic contact dermatitis
- **Idiopathic/Iatrogenic:** Drug reaction
- **Neoplastic:** Cutaneous T-cell lymphoma (usually large plaques, chronic)

History
- **Character:**
  - Are the plaques beefy red with thicker, adherent silvery scale?
  - Are the plaques droplike (i.e., 1 to 2 cm; guttate psoriasis)?
  - Is the eruption symmetrical or asymmetrical (tinea corporis)?
  - Are the plaques pink with a collar of fine scale, and is there a larger herald patch that preceded the smaller plaques (pityriasis rosea)?

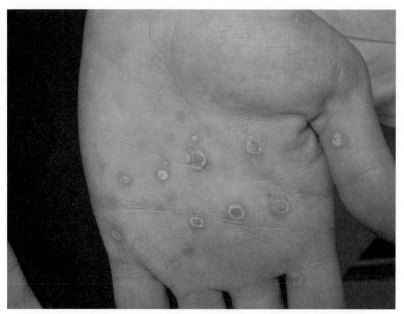

Figure 7-17 Secondary syphilis involving palm. (Used with permission of Dr. Peter Green.)

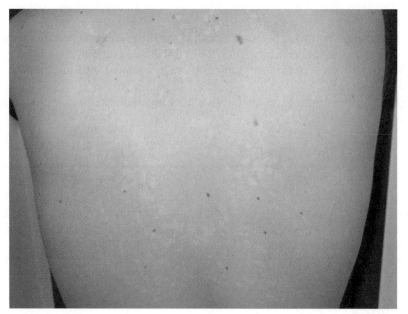

Figure 7-18 Tinea versicolor with predominance of hypopigmentation and subtle scale. (Used with permission of Dr. Peter Green.)

- Are there copper-colored (yellowish) or "ham"-colored (reddish brown) scaly plaques on palms or soles? Lymphadenopathy? Oral ulceration (secondary syphilis)?
- Are there subtle scaly plaques with associated hypopigmentation (pityriasis versicolor)?
- Location:
  - Truncal and proximal extremities (guttate psoriasis and pityriasis versicolor)?
  - Above with palmar involvement (secondary syphilis)?
  - Upper back and chest (pityriasis versicolor)?
  - Concurrent nail changes (plaque psoriasis, tinea corporis)?

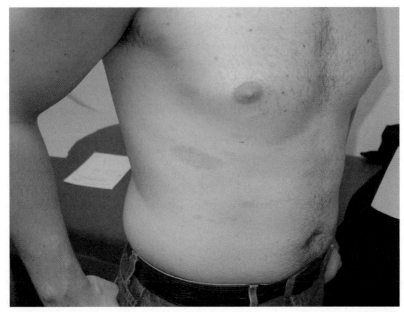

Figure 7-19   Herald patch of pityriasis rosea; note adjacent smaller, oval, and scaly plaques. (Used with permission of Dr. Peter Green.)

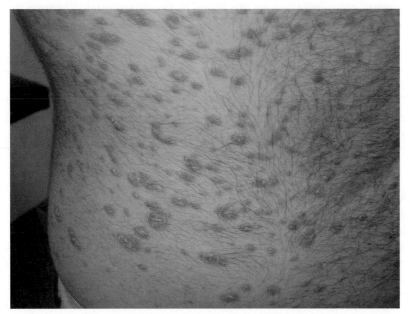

Figure 7-20   Guttate psoriasis on trunk following streptococcal pharyngitis. (Used with permission of Dr. Peter Green.)

- **O**nset: Acute presentation (guttate psoriasis, pityriasis rosea, secondary syphilis) versus chronic (tinea corporis, pityriasis versicolor)?
- **R**adiation: "Christmas tree" pattern of scaly plaques on back (pityriasis rosea)
- **I**ntensity: Extent of eruption, intensity of pruritus
  - Guttate psoriasis: Pruritus varies.
  - Syphilis: Usually minimal itch
  - Pityriasis rosea: Itch varies, mild to marked.
  - Pityriasis versicolor: Asymptomatic to minimal itch
- **D**uration: Weeks or months? Guttate psoriasis and pityriasis rosea last approximately 6 to 8 weeks, even without treatment. Secondary syphilis lasts approximately 4 to 12 weeks.

- Events associated:
  - Strep throat (precedes guttate psoriasis)?
  - Viral pharyngitis may precede pityriasis versicolor.
  - Tinea unguium in toenails/fingernails as source for tinea corporis?
  - Previous genital ulceration? Fever, flulike symptoms, myalgia, stiff neck, and lymphadenopathy (secondary syphilis)?
- Frequency: Previous similar episode (guttate psoriasis)? Note: Pityriasis rosea rarely recurs.
- Palliative factors: Any treatment to date?
- Provocative factors: Is there anything that makes it worse? If so, what?
- PMH: Psoriasis (guttate flares may occur in isolation or with associated chronic plaque psoriasis), HIV (associated risk for syphilis)
- MEDS: Oral antibiotic for pharyngitis often falsely implicated as allergic reaction in guttate psoriasis
- SH: Risk factors for secondary syphilis?

PEARLS

- Secondary syphilis is a papulosquamous eruption that can have considerable variation in clinical appearance with macules, papules, and plaques. Identification of risk factors, involvement of palms and soles, presence of lymphadenopathy, oral ulcers, and systemic symptoms will be helpful to make the diagnosis.
- Pityriasis lichenoides, small plaque parapsoriasis, and pityriasis rubra pilaris are more unusual papulosquamous eruptions in the differential diagnosis and are not covered here.

INSTRUCTIONS TO CANDIDATE: A 34-year-old female nurse presents with a 1-week history of raised, markedly pruritic wheals in the skin. This has occurred daily and leaves no residual skin changes. Obtain an appropriate history. What information will be helpful to sort out the nature of these plaques?

DD$_X$ VITAMINS C

- Vascular: Urticarial vasculitis
- Infectious: Cellulitis (will not migrate like urticaria)
- Traumatic: Physical urticaria: Pressure, vibration, cold, solar, and aquagenic
- Autoimmune/Allergic: Acute urticaria, angioedema (hereditary or acquired), type 1 allergic reaction, and serum sickness or serum sickness–like reaction
- Idiopathic/Iatrogenic: Drug reaction

History

- Character:
  - Are the plaques migratory (moving to different parts of skin)? Do they disappear, leaving no residual skin changes? Are they edematous and intensely pruritic? Are they large plaques or smaller papules (urticaria)?
  - Is there marked subcutaneous or more extensive swelling (angioedema)?
  - Is there residual purpura (suggests urticarial vasculitis)?
- Location: Are they confined to skin? Is there airway involvement (angioedema or type 1 allergic reaction)?
- Onset: Acute or chronic (6 weeks for urticaria)?
- Radiation: Are the lesions regional or generalized?
- Intensity: How severe are the hives?
- Duration: Do individual lesions last <24 hours (urticaria or angioedema)? Do they last longer (urticarial vasculitis)?

- Events associated:
  - Is there throat swelling or tightness (angioedema, type 1 allergic reaction)?
  - Is there marked swelling (angioedema)?
  - Joint paint (serum sickness or serum sickness–like reaction)?
- Frequency: Are there repeated episodes of angioedema (hereditary or acquired angioedema)? How often do the hives occur?
- Palliative factors: Has anything been tried for the hives? Antihistamines?
- Provocative factors:
  - Are there physical triggers for the hives (e.g., pressure, vibration, cold, sweating, water)?
  - Any food triggers (e.g., egg, seafood, strawberries)?
  - Any exposure to latex products (possible type 1 latex allergy)?
  - Recent infectious symptoms?
- **PMH:** Any previous episodes of anaphylaxis? Any history of lupus (urticarial vasculitis)? Other illness? Hepatitis? Thyroid disease (rarely implicated in urticaria)? Lymphoma (acquired angioedema)?
- **MEDS (including OTC medications):** Any new medications? Recent nonsteroidal antiinflammatory drugs (NSAIDs; trigger for urticaria)?
- **Allergies:** Known medication allergies or documented allergies by prick testing. Does the patient carry an EpiPen?
- **FH:** Hereditary angioedema

INSTRUCTIONS TO CANDIDATE: A 62-year-old male presents with a persistent ankle ulcer after accidentally hitting it on a chair 4 weeks ago. Obtain an appropriate history. What information do you need to determine the type of ulcer he has?

DD$_X$ VITAMINS C
- **V**ascular: Venous stasis ulcer (Figure 7-21), arterial ulcer, and vasculitis
- **I**nfectious: Cellulitis
- **T**raumatic: Traumatic ulcer
- **A**utoimmune/**A**llergic: Connective tissue disease–related vasculitis
- **M**etabolic: Diabetic ulceration, necrobiosis lipoidica
- **I**diopathic/**I**atrogenic
- **N**eoplastic: Squamous cell carcinoma, basal cell carcinoma, and lymphoma
- **S**ubstance abuse and **P**sychiatric: Artifactual ulcers (often linear or bizarre geographic shapes)

History
- **C**haracter:
  - Does the ulcer have ill-defined, shaggy borders? Is there moderate discomfort? Is there associated edema? Are there associated areas of venous stasis (hyperpigmentation, fibrosis, dermatitis, venous varicosities [venous stasis ulcer])?
  - Is the ulcer punched out with well-defined borders? Is the ulcer markedly painful? Dependent rubor? Is there a lack of edema (arterial ulcers)?
  - Are the ulcers surrounded by callus and painless (diabetic ulcer)?
- **L**ocation:
  - Medial malleolus or calf (stasis ulcer)?
  - Distal extremity (i.e., toes or foot: arterial ulcer)?
  - Pressure points (i.e., ball of foot, heel, or toe: diabetic ulcer)?
- **O**nset: How did it start (sudden versus gradual)?
- **R**adiation: Isolated or multiple ulcers? What is the extent of venous stasis changes?
- **I**ntensity: Severity of symptoms and size of ulcers
- **D**uration: How long has this been going on (longstanding versus recent ulceration)?

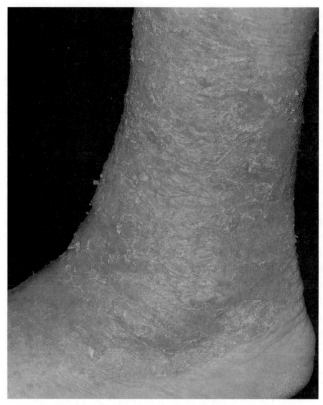

Figure 7-21   Venous stasis ulcer. (From Habif TP: *A color guide to diagnosis and therapy: clinical dermatology*, ed 3, St. Louis, 1996, Mosby, p 75, Figure 3-57.)

- Events associated:
  - Is there a history of chronic edema or venous varicosities?
  - Any recent infectious signs or symptoms of associated cellulitis?
  - Any recent trauma?
  - History of peripheral vascular disease with claudication?
  - Diabetic neuropathy?
- Frequency: Any previous leg ulcers?
- Palliative factors: Does dependent position (e.g., hanging leg over bed) make the ulcer LESS painful (arterial ulcer) or MORE painful (venous ulcer)?
- Provocative factors: Pressure induced? Trauma induced? Local infection? Edema?
- **PMH:** Diabetes? Associated neuropathy? Peripheral vascular disease? Chronic lymphedema?
- **MEDS:** Recent antibiotics to manage infection
- **SH:** Smoking, EtOH, and recreational drugs

PEARLS
- Ill-defined ulcers on ankle(s) with shaggy borders, in background of pitting edema, erythema, and hyperpigmentation with preserved peripheral pulses represent **venous stasis ulceration**.
- Punched-out ulcers on distal extremity(ies) (e.g., toe, lateral surface of fifth metatarsal) with no edema, reduced or absent peripheral pulses, and dependent rubor with risk factors for peripheral vascular disease are **arterial ulcers.**
- Painless and/or calloused ulcer or hematoma on weight-bearing surfaces (e.g., plantar toes, metatarsal heads, heels) in a diabetic patient with known neuropathy is a **diabetic or neuropathic ulcer**.
- Rule out unilateral ill-defined painful erythema with fever, chills, or malaise, which suggests concurrent cellulitis.

- Note that some patients may have combined risk factors for ulceration (e.g., arterial and venous disease).

INSTRUCTIONS TO CANDIDATE: A 35-year-old female presents with a 1-week history of painful nodules, swelling, and "bruising" localized to the shins with no ulceration. Obtain an appropriate history. What history is important in delineating cause and associated illness for this eruption?

DD$_X$ VITAMINS C
- **V**ascular: Vasculitis, thrombophlebitis
- **I**nfectious: Cellulitis, tuberculosis
- **T**rauma
- **A**utoimmune/**A**llergic: Systemic lupus erythematosus (SLE)–associated panniculitis
- **M**etabolic: Pancreatic panniculitis, necrobiosis lipoidica
- **I**diopathic/**I**atrogenic: Fixed drug eruption
- **N**eoplastic: Lymphoma
- **C**ongenital/genetic: α_1-Antitrypsin deficiency panniculitis
- Erythema nodosum (Figure 7-22)
- Panniculitis of other cause

History
- Character:
  - Are there discrete nodules that are red and tender? Are they palpable? Is there associated bruising?
  - Is ulceration present? Erythema nodosum does not ulcerate. Ulceration is more associated with vasculitis.
  - Is there significant diffuse or circumferential unilateral erythema (cellulitis)?
  - Is there a localized painful nodule with adjacent venous varicosities (superficial thrombophlebitis)?
  - Is there surrounding purpura (palpable or nonpalpable) or livedo reticularis (netlike bluish discoloration) suggestive of vasculitis?

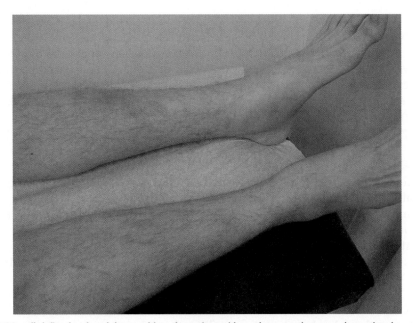

Figure 7-22   Ill-defined red nodules on shins of a patient with erythema nodosum and associated asymptomatic pulmonary sarcoid. (Used with permission of Dr. Peter Green.)

- **L**ocation: Are the nodules on the shins only? Are extensor surfaces of upper extremities involved (sometimes with erythema nodosum)?
- **O**nset: Are the nodules of recent onset?
- **R**adiation: Are both legs involved symmetrically, or is it unilateral (less likely erythema nodosum, may be cellulitis)?
- **I**ntensity: How painful are the nodules? Do they interfere with walking?
- **D**uration: How long have the nodules been present (erythema nodosum lasts approximately 2 to 4 weeks)? If there is only bruising at the site of previous nodules, it may represent resolving erythema nodosum.
- **E**vents associated:
  - Was there preceding sore throat (streptococcal pharyngitis may be a trigger for erythema nodosum)?
  - Arthralgias (may accompany erythema nodosum)?
  - Is the patient systemically unwell (cellulitis, lymphoma, pancreatic disease, lupus, vasculitis)?
  - Is there a history or pulmonary symptoms of sarcoidosis (erythema nodosum associated with mild pulmonary sarcoid: Löfgren's syndrome, which is most often asymptomatic)?
  - Any travel to areas with endemic histoplasmosis, coccidioidomycosis (infectious trigger for erythema nodosum)?
  - Fever/chills (infectious causes; low-grade fever may be seen with erythema nodosum)?
- **F**requency: Previous similar episodes (erythema nodosum may be recurrent)?
- **P**alliative factors: Does elevating legs reduce discomfort (erythema nodosum)?
- **P**rovocative factors: Is there anything that makes it worse? If so, what?
- **PMH:** Inflammatory bowel disease (IBD; associated with erythema nodosum), sarcoidosis, SLE (lupus panniculitis), pancreatic disease (pancreatic panniculitis), and pregnancy (trigger for erythema nodosum)
- **MEDS:** Recent OCP or sulfa ingestion (trigger for erythema nodosum)

PEARL
- Erythema nodosum is the most common cause of panniculitis (inflammation of subcutaneous fat). However, a deep elliptical biopsy may be necessary to determine the exact cause.

INSTRUCTIONS TO CANDIDATE: A 65-year-old female presents with a new-onset, widespread, symmetrical red itchy eruption of 3 days' duration. She is well, other than hypothyroidism for which she takes thyroxin. After a recent upper respiratory illness she was prescribed an oral amino penicillin antibiotic, which she stopped taking 1 week ago. Obtain an appropriate history. What information is required to sort out the nature of this eruption?

DD$_X$ VITAMINS C
- **I**nfectious: Viral eruption, toxin-mediated exanthem (e.g., scarlet fever, staphylococcal scalded skin syndrome [SSSS], toxic shock syndrome [TSS])
- **A**utoimmune/**A**llergic: Allergic contact dermatitis, erythema multiforme (Stevens-Johnson's syndrome)
- **I**diopathic/**I**atrogenic: Drug eruption (Figure 7-23)
- NOTE: The words "exanthem" and "eruption" may be used interchangeably here.

History
- **C**haracter:
  - Is there urticarial (edematous or raised) erythema?
  - Is it partially or completely blanchable (early drug eruptions usually completely blanch with pressure; contact dermatitis does not)?

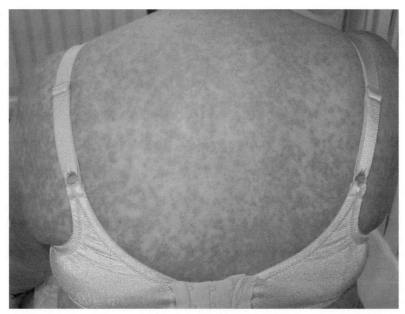

Figure 7-23   Drug exanthem following ingestion of amoxicillin. (Used with permission of Dr. Peter Green.)

- Is it macular and confluent (drug exanthem)?
- Is there a palpable or "sandpaper" quality (scarlet fever)?
- Is there blistering or peeling of the skin (Stevens-Johnson's syndrome, SSSS)?
- Is there an eczema-like quality with scale and vesicles (allergic contact dermatitis)?
- Target lesions (i.e., central dusky necrosis with surrounding erythema and edema [Stevens-Johnson's syndrome])?
- Location:
  - Generalized (all skin affected) or truncal and extremities? Isolated regional involvement (e.g., extremities only) is unlikely to be a drug eruption.
  - Mucosal membrane involvement (blistering, crusting) of Stevens-Johnson's syndrome? Peeling of palms and soles (follows scarlet fever, TSS)?
  - Drug and viral eruptions often spare palms.
- Onset: Sudden onset? BEFORE or AFTER new medications or infectious symptoms?
- Radiation:
  - Symmetrical, bilateral involvement with confluence of erythema over large areas but most often truncal and proximal extremities, later spreading to distal extremities (drug or viral exanthem)
  - Predominant involvement in folds (neck, axilla, groin) with erythema and peeling seen in SSSS? Regional involvement (e.g., neck, chest, face) with eczema-like eruption (allergic contact dermatitis)?
- Intensity: Is the eruption *itchy* (drug, viral, allergic contact dermatitis) or *painful* (Stevens-Johnson's syndrome, SSSS).
- Duration: Drug or viral eruptions generally last approximately 2 weeks; allergic contact dermatitis will continue with reexposure to antigen. Toxin-mediated disease will evolve through stages over time.
- Events associated:
  - Upper respiratory or gastrointestinal (GI) symptoms (viral eruption OR drug taken for same)?
  - Patient systemically unwell (Stevens-Johnson's syndrome or toxin-mediated illness)?
  - Fever, hemodynamic instability, and visceral involvement (TSS)?
  - Recent pharyngitis, systemic symptoms, and strawberry tongue (scarlet fever)?
- Frequency: Any previous reactions to drugs?
- Palliative factors: Has there been application of any OTC or prescription topical therapy (some may cause allergic contact dermatitis)?

- **Provocative factors**: Is there anything that makes it worse? If so, what? Does firm stroking of affected skin lead to spread of blistering (positive Nikolsky's sign) as seen in SSSS?
- **PMH**: Previous drug hypersensitivity or medication-induced life-threatening skin eruptions
- **MEDS (including OTC medications)**: Detailed account of ALL medications

PEARLS

- Onset of drug eruption with medication is delayed and may occur from 1 to 2 weeks after primary exposure; patients may neglect to mention ingestion of medication that they are no longer taking, erroneously assuming that it could not be causing the eruption.
- A drug eruption will evolve and spread during 2 weeks, regardless of intervention (including discontinuation of implicated medication), and patients must be reassured that the eruption is not "getting worse." However, new development of blisters may indicate development of more serious drug reaction (i.e., Stevens-Johnson's syndrome).
- In the absence of a history implicating a specific medication, drug eruptions and viral eruptions are often clinical and histologically indistinguishable.

> INSTRUCTIONS TO CANDIDATE: A 65-year-old male presents with a bump on his face of 6 months' duration that bleeds when he shaves. He has applied a topical antibiotic, but the lesion has never healed. He sunburns easily and worked outside in construction for many years, never wearing sunscreen. Obtain an appropriate history. What background information do you need to determine the most likely causes for this lesion?

DD$_X$ VITAMINS C

- **Vascular**: Rosacea
- **Infectious**: Folliculitis
- **Traumatic**
- **Neoplastic**: Basal cell carcinoma (BCC; Figure 7-24), squamous cell carcinoma (SCC), or other tumor (e.g., keratoacanthoma, atypical fibroxanthoma)
- **Congenital/genetic**: Nevus
- Seborrheic keratosis (Figure 7-25)
- Actinic keratosis
- Irritated nevus
- Sebaceous gland hyperplasia (Figure 7-26)

History

- **Character**:
  - Is the lesion a papule, ulcer (BCC, SCC), or scaly plaque (actinic keratosis, seborrheic keratosis)?
  - Is there a shiny, pearly quality with associated telangiectasia (BCC)?
  - Does the lesion bleed easily (BCC, SCC)?
  - Does the lesion have a warty, brown, stuck-on appearance (seborrheic keratosis)?
  - Is the lesion flat, rough, and scaly with ill-defined borders (actinic keratosis)?
  - Is there a flesh-colored papule with associated inflammation of surrounding skin (suggestive of irritated nevus)?
  - Are there multiple soft, yellow, umbilicated (indented) papules (sebaceous hyperplasia)?
- Location: Sun-exposed skin
- **Onset**: New (i.e., weeks to months favors BCC, SCC) or longstanding (i.e., years favors noncancerous cause such as seborrheic keratosis, irritated nevus, sebaceous hyperplasia)?

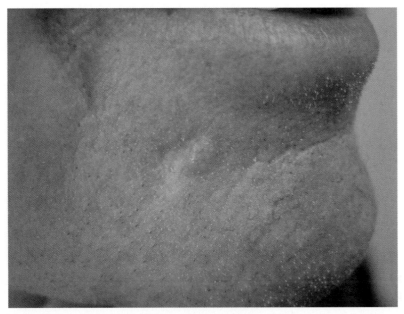

Figure 7-24   Basal cell carcinoma of the chin. (Used with permission of Dr. Peter Green.)

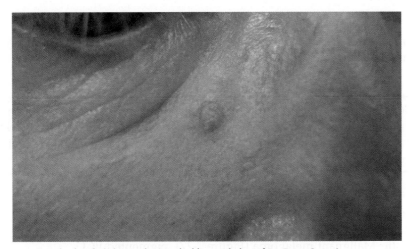

Figure 7-25   Irritated seborrheic keratosis. (Used with permission of Dr. Peter Green.)

- **R**adiation: What is the size of the lesion? Are there multiple lesions (more suggestive of a benign process: seborrheic keratosis, sebaceous hyperplasia, and actinic keratosis)?
- **I**ntensity: Is the lesion painful (may not help differentiate causes)?
- **D**uration: New-onset lesions more likely to be cancerous.
- **E**vents associated:
  - Tendency to sunburn easily?
  - History of significant sun exposure or blistering sunburns?
- **F**requency: Any previous similar problems? How was it managed?
- **P**alliative factors: Any treatments attempted to date (e.g., antibiotics, liquid nitrogen, excision)?
- **P**rovocative factors: Does trauma induce bleeding (suggestive of BCC, SCC but may also occur with others)?
- **PMH**: Previous skin malignancy, immunosuppression (SCC more common than BCC in this setting; may be multiple; also may have multiple actinic keratosis)

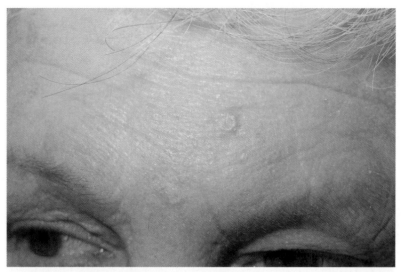

Figure 7-26 Sebaceous gland hyperplasia of the forehead; a soft yellow papule with central umbilication. (Used with permission of Dr. Peter Green.)

- **MEDS**: acetylsalicylic acid (ASA; may enhance bleeding tendency), immunosuppressants

PEARL
- Although actinic keratoses are considered precancerous, they may be present for years and not develop into cancer.

> INSTRUCTIONS TO CANDIDATE: A 63-year-old male presents with a changing pigmented lesion on his back. He estimates its duration to be 1 year or more, and his wife had noticed it getting larger and darker. Obtain an appropriate history. What important information do you need to assess this patient?

DD$_X$ VITAMINS C
- **Vascular**: Pyogenic granuloma, thrombosed or irritated hemangioma
- **Neoplastic**: Malignant melanoma (Figure 7-27), pigmented BCC
- **Congenital/genetic**: Irritated congenital or compound nevus
- **Dysplastic nevus** (Figure 7-28)
- **Seborrheic keratosis** (Figure 7-29)

History
- **Character**:
  - Is the lesion pigmented? What is the predominant color (black, brown, pink, gray), or are there multiple colors?
  - Is the lesion asymmetrical? Is there an irregular border?
  - Is the lesion >0.5 cm?
  - Is there ulceration?
  - Are there other pigmented lesions present, and if so, do they look irregular or dysplastic?
- **Location**: Sun-exposed or non–sun-exposed skin? Location of other pigmented lesions? Do not neglect scalp, palm, sole, nail, and mucosal surface assessment.
- **Onset**: Is the lesion of new onset? Has there been recent change in size, shape, or color?
- **Radiation**: Measure size of the lesion in broadest diameter in millimeters.

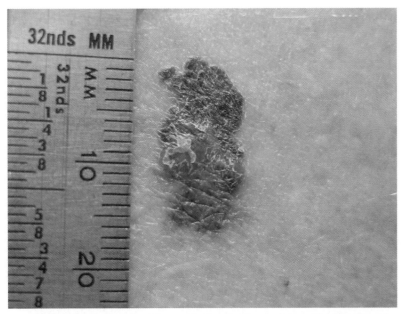

Figure 7-27   Malignant melanoma of the right scapula. (Used with permission of Dr. Peter Green.)

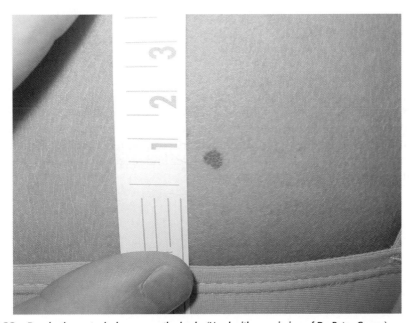

Figure 7-28   Dysplastic or atypical nevus on the back. (Used with permission of Dr. Peter Green.)

- Intensity: Any pain or itch associated with the lesion?
- Duration: How long has the lesion been present? If there has been change in the lesion, how long has the original lesion been present?
- Events associated:
  - Any bleeding of the lesion?
  - Any ulceration?
  - Any lymph node involvement noted by the patient or other symptoms of metastases?
  - Multiple nevi, typical or atypical (increased risk of melanoma)?
  - Any history of excess sun exposure or blistering sunburns?
  - Does the patient burn easily in the sun? Blond or red hair color?
- Frequency: Have you had any other lesions like this? If so, when? How many?

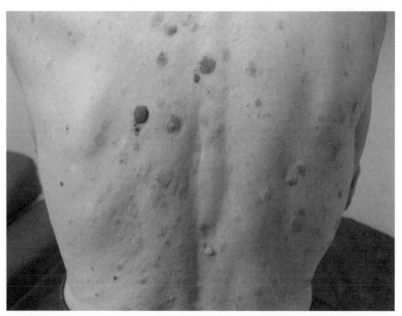

Figure 7-29   Multiple seborrheic keratosis on the back. (Used with permission of Dr. Peter Green.)

- **PMH**: Previous skin biopsies for pigmented lesions, previous malignancy, or immunosuppression
- **FH**: Multiple atypical nevi, melanoma

PEARL
- Patients with an abnormal or changing mole must undergo a complete examination of their skin, including palms, soles, scalp, genital skin, and mucosal surfaces. Patient modesty must be respected; however, failure to perform a complete examination may result in missed lesions with significant adverse consequences for the patient. Lymph node examination and examination of the liver and spleen should also take place in patients with suspected melanoma.

SAMPLE CHECKLIST

INSTRUCTIONS TO CANDIDATE: This 25-year-old male with psoriasis is referred to your clinic for follow-up evaluation. Perform a focused physical examination, and describe your findings.

Key Points	Satisfactorily Completed
Introduces self to the patient	❏
Determines how the patient wishes to be addressed	❏
Explains nature of the examination to the patient	❏
Drapes the patient properly during the examination, and ensures patient comfort	❏
Examines the patient in a logical fashion	❏
Inspection	
• Examines the entire skin surface, including palms and soles, scalp, anogenital area, and nails	❏
• Notes any excoriations	❏
• Nails: Pitting, onycholysis, and oil drop sign	❏
• Scalp: Predominates along hair line with silvery scales	❏
• Köebner's phenomenon (inspection only: linear or traumatized areas involved)	❏
• Sausage digits	❏
Palpation	
• Raised plaques versus erythema only (treated psoriasis)	❏
• Auspitz sign (should be described only and not performed)	❏
• Examines large joints (hips, lumbosacral area) for range of motion (ROM), tenderness	❏
• Examines large tendinous insertions for swelling and tenderness	❏
• Examines hands for ROM, swelling, and tenderness (sausage digits)	❏
Description of findings	
• Describes location and amount of skin involvement	❏
• Notes predominant extensor and scalp involvement (guttate psoriasis involves the trunk and proximal extremities)	❏
• Salmon-pink or beefy red plaques with overlying silvery scales	❏
• Plaques are well demarcated from surrounding normal skin	❏
• Presence of widespread pustules or erythroderma (both medical emergencies)	❏
• Notes scalp and nail findings	❏
• Notes associated arthritic features	❏
Makes appropriate closing remarks	❏

CHAPTER 8

Hematology

OBJECTIVES

ANATOMY

ESSENTIAL CLINICAL COMPETENCIES

EXAMINE THE LYMPH NODES OF THE HEAD AND NECK. DESCRIBE YOUR FINDINGS.

SAMPLE OSCE SCENARIOS

- A 36-year-old male presents with recent onset of easy bruising and nosebleeds. Take a detailed history, exploring possible etiologies.
- A 19-year-old student visits the university health clinic for the first time. On routine history, he notes that he has "some kind of bleeding problem." Take a detailed history, exploring possible etiologies.
- A 27-year-old male presents to his family physician complaining of weight loss and night sweats. Take a detailed history of his symptoms, exploring possible etiologies.
- You are doing a rotation in hematology and are asked to see a 22-year-old male referred with a tentative diagnosis of lymphoma. Examine the patient, and describe your findings.
- A 55-year-old female presents to the emergency department feeling generally unwell. She has a low-grade fever (temperature 38°C). Her complete blood count shows hemoglobin 95 g/L, white blood cells 100×10^9/L, and platelets 40×10^9/L. Take a detailed history, exploring possible etiologies, and perform a focused physical examination.
- A 60-year-old female presents to the emergency department complaining of fatigue and weakness. She visited her family doctor 3 days ago with the same complaint, and he ordered some "tests." The astute triage nurse checks for recent laboratory investigations and brings you the results of her complete blood count: hemoglobin 68 g/L, white blood cells 8.6×10^9/L, and platelets 115×10^9/L. The mean corpuscular volume is 66 fL. Take a detailed history, exploring possible etiologies, and perform a focused physical examination.
- A 47-year-old female presents to the emergency department with a swollen and painful right calf. Take a detailed history, focusing on risk factors for thromboembolic disease, and perform a focused physical examination.
- The previous patient has a Doppler ultrasound of the right leg, confirming a below-knee deep venous thrombosis. She is discharged with appropriate treatment and follow-up evaluation. She returns to the emergency department the next day with shortness of breath and chest discomfort. Take an appropriate history, and perform a focused physical examination.

SAMPLE CHECKLIST

❑ Examine the lymph nodes of the head and neck. Describe your findings.

OBJECTIVES

*The successful student should be able to take a **focused history** of the hematologic system, including:*
- Enlarged nodes: Location, duration, number, and tenderness
  - Fever, redness, warmth, streaking
- Constitutional symptoms: Fever, chills, night sweats, weight loss, anorexia, and asthenia
- Anemia
- Bleeding: Easy bruising, epistaxis, hematuria, postoperative, and so on
- Blood type, previous transfusions
- History of infection

*The hematologic **examination** will include:*
LYMPH NODES

Inspection
- Size
- Number
- Presence of redness

Palpation
- Describe characteristics of enlarged nodes and location.
  - Consistency: Rubbery, hard, fluctuant, and matted
  - Size
  - Tenderness
  - Mobility
  - Warmth
- Spleen
- Liver

SYSTEMIC MANIFESTATIONS OF HEMATOLOGIC DISEASE

- Petechiae (thrombocytopenia)
- Gum hypertrophy (infiltrative process, leukemia)
- Bruises, joint effusions (hemarthrosis)
- Jaundice (hemolysis)
- Angular cheilosis, glossitis, stomatitis, and koilonychia (anemia)
- Peripheral sensory neuropathy, impaired proprioception (B_{12} deficiency)
- Thromboembolic disease

ANATOMY

- Blood cells originate from bone marrow. Active marrow in normal adults is confined to ends of long bones, pelvis, ribs, and vertebral bodies. In some situations other regions of bone marrow are recruited. There are three types of blood cells: erythrocytes (red blood cells [RBCs]), leukocytes (white blood cells [WBCs]), and platelets (Plts).
- The lymphatic vasculature drains lymph from bodily tissues and returns it to the venous circulation (at the formation of the brachiocephalic veins). Lymph is filtered through lymph nodes, which are able to detect and remove debris and respond to antigens. Lymph nodes are oval or bean shaped, vary in size, and may not be palpable (Figure 8-1). Inguinal lymph nodes are relatively large (often 1 to 2 cm in an adult). The central nervous system contains no lymphatics.
- Axillary lymph (lateral, medial, infraclavicular, supraclavicular, pectoral) nodes drain most of the arm and breast (Figure 8-2). The ulnar surface of the forearm and

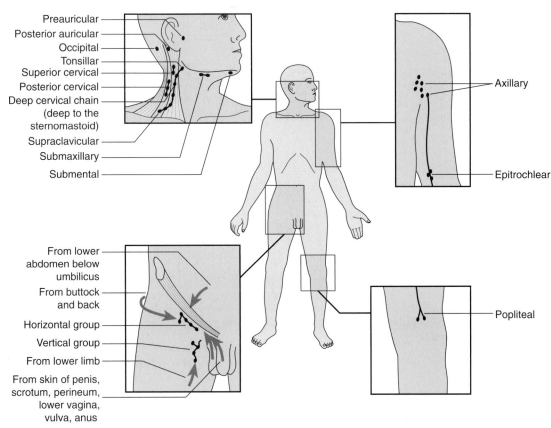

Figure 8-1 Distribution of palpable lymph nodes. (From Munro JF, Campbell IW, editors: *Macleod's clinical examination,* ed 10, Edinburgh, 2000, Churchill Livingstone, p 59, Figure 2.42.)

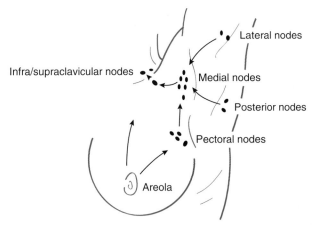

Figure 8-2 Axillary lymph nodes.

hand drain first to the epitrochlear nodes, which are proximal to the medical epicondyle.

• Only the superficial system of lymphatics is palpable in the lower limb (Figure 8-3). The superficial inguinal nodes are composed of two groups: horizontal and vertical (see Figure 8-1). The horizontal group lies below the inguinal ligament and drains the superficial portions of the lower abdomen and buttock, external genitalia (not the testes), anal area, and lower third of the vagina. The vertical group clusters

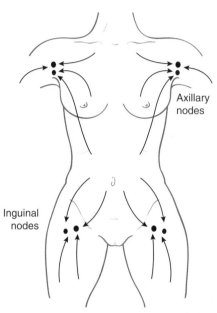

Figure 8-3   Superficial routes of lymphatic drainage. (Used with permission of Dr. Tom Scott, Memorial University of Newfoundland.)

near the great saphenous vein and drains the portion of the leg drained by the small saphenous vein.

PEARLS
- Whenever a node is enlarged or tender, look for a source such as infection in the area that it drains.
- Whenever a malignant or inflammatory lesion is observed, look for involvement of the regional lymph nodes to which it drains.

ESSENTIAL CLINICAL COMPETENCIES

EXAMINE THE LYMPH NODES OF THE HEAD AND NECK. DESCRIBE YOUR FINDINGS

DD$_X$ Lymphadenopathy (VITAMINS C)
- **I**nfection
- **A**utoimmune/Allergic: Collagen vascular disease, infiltration with sarcoid/amyloid, and serum sickness
- **M**etabolic: Drug hypersensitivity
- **N**eoplastic: Lymphoma, leukemia, and metastatic disease

Patient Positioning
- Seat the patient in a chair and stand behind him or her. Flex the neck slightly.

Palpation
- Palpate using the pads of the fingers in a rotatory motion (moving the skin over the underlying tissues). You may examine both sides of the head and neck simultaneously.
- Palpate the following nodes (see Figure 8-1):
    - Occipital: Base of skull posteriorly
    - Postauricular: Superficial to mastoid process

- Preauricular: Anterior to ear
- Tonsillar: Angle of mandible
- Submandibular: Midway between the angle and the tip of the mandible
- Submental: Midline behind tip of mandible (helpful to palpate with one hand while bracing the top of the head with the other hand)
- Anterior cervical: Along the anterior border of the sternocleidomastoid (SCM) muscle
- Superficial cervical: Superficial to SCM muscle
- Posterior cervical: Along anterior edge of trapezius muscle
- Deep cervical: Deep to SCM muscle and often inaccessible (hook thumb and fingers around SCM, and roll the muscle between the fingers)
- Supraclavicular: Deep in the angle between clavicle and SCM muscle
- Infraclavicular: Inferior to the clavicle

You may appreciate the following mnemonic:
"**P**rofessors **T**each **S**lick **M**ed **S**tudents to **C**orrectly **D**efine **N**e**W** **L**umps"

- **P**ulsatility
- **T**enderness: Tenderness on palpation versus constant pain
- **S**hape
- **M**obility: Fixed versus mobile
- **S**ize: Estimated measurement in centimeters
- **C**onsistency: Hard versus soft, firm versus rubbery; compressible, fluctuant
- **D**efinition: Well-defined or irregular margins
- **N**umber: Solitary versus multiple, and **N**odularity: Lumpy versus smooth
- **W**armth
- **L**ocation

PEARLS

- The supraclavicular, submandibular, and submental nodes drain the mouth, throat, and part of the face.
- Enlargement of a supraclavicular node, especially on the left (Virchow's node), suggests possible metastasis from a thoracic or abdominal malignancy.
- The submandibular nodes are smaller and smoother than the underlying submandibular salivary gland.
- Tender nodes suggest inflammation; hard or fixed nodes suggest malignancy.

SAMPLE OSCE SCENARIOS

> INSTRUCTIONS TO CANDIDATE: A 36-year-old male presents with recent onset of easy bruising and nosebleeds. Take a detailed history, exploring possible etiologies.

DD_X VITAMINS C
- **Infectious:** Hypersplenism (e.g., mononucleosis), hemolytic uremic syndrome (HUS)
- **Autoimmune/Allergic:** Idiopathic thrombocytopenic purpura (ITP), thrombotic thrombocytopenic purpura (TTP), Henoch-Schönlein purpura, and Wegener's granulomatosis
- **Metabolic:** Disseminated intravascular coagulation (DIC), vitamin K deficiency (malabsorption syndromes, malnutrition), and Cushing's syndrome (endogenous/exogenous)
- **Idiopathic/Iatrogenic:** Hypersplenism caused by portal hypertension
- **Neoplastic:** Leukemia, lymphoma

History
- **Character:** Describe the bleeding. Are bruises unexplained or associated with injury?
- **Location:** Where is the blood coming from? Where are the bruises?
  - Petechiae
  - Ecchymosis
  - Joint bleed/swelling (hemarthrosis)
  - Mucous membranes (epistaxis, gingival bleeding associated with tooth brushing)
  - Hemoptysis
  - Hematuria
  - Melena, hematochezia, or hematemesis
  - Menorrhagia: Presence of clots, number of pads/tampons needed per day
- **Onset:** When did the bleeding start (hereditary versus acquired)?
- **Radiation:** Any other bleeding (bleeding from another location)?
- **Intensity:** How severe is the bleeding (quantify)? Has it gotten worse?
- **Duration:** How long has the bleeding been going on?
- Events associated:
  - Left upper quadrant (LUQ) pain (splenomegaly), lymphadenopathy
  - Henoch-Schönlein purpura: Recent upper respiratory tract infection (URTI), purpuric skin rash, abdominal pain, polyarthralgias
  - Vitamin K deficiency: Malabsorption (steatorrhea, weight loss)
  - Cushing's syndrome (endogenous/exogenous): Moon facies, truncal obesity, striae
  - TTP: Jaundice, fever, neurologic findings, and renal disease
  - Wegener's granulomatosis: Epistaxis, sinusitis, hematuria, constitutional symptoms, skin lesions
  - Constitutional symptoms: Fever, chills, night sweats, weight loss, anorexia, and asthenia (leukemia, lymphoma)
  - Anemia: Pallor, weakness, fatigue, palpitations
- **Frequency:** How often does the bleeding happen (intermittent versus constant)?
- **Palliative factors:** Is there anything that makes it better? If so, what?
- **Provocative factors:** Is there anything that makes it worse? If so, what?
- **Past medical history (PMH):** Liver disease, renal disease, collagen vascular disease, hemophilia, von Willebrand's disease, HIV, or blood transfusions
- **Past surgical history (PSH):** History of hemorrhage associated with surgery
- **Medications (MEDS):** Nonsteroidal antiinflammatory drugs (NSAIDs), acetylsalicylic acid (ASA), warfarin, steroids, antibiotics, or chemotherapy
- **Social history (SH):** EtOH, smoking
- **Family history (FH):** Bleeding diathesis (hemophilia, von Willebrand's disease), collagen vascular disease

INSTRUCTIONS TO CANDIDATE: A 19-year-old student visits the university health clinic for the first time. On routine history, he notes that he has "some kind of bleeding problem." Take a detailed history, exploring possible etiologies.

Pathophysiology

- Three processes act to achieve hemostasis: vasoconstriction, formation of a platelet plug, and the coagulation cascade. The manifestations of disease vary according to the pathophysiology (Table 8-1).

History

- **Character:** Do you bleed or bruise easily? Are bruises unexplained or associated with injury?
- **Location:** Where do you note bruises/bleeding (if at all)?
  - Petechiae
  - Mucous membranes (epistaxis, gingival bleeding associated with tooth brushing)
  - Bleeding scratches
  - Joint bleeding/swelling (hemarthrosis)
  - Ecchymosis: Torso, points of trauma (e.g., knee, shin, or elbow)
  - Hemoptysis
  - Hematuria
  - Melena, hematemesis, or hematochezia
- **Onset:** Onset of bleeding relative to injury (delayed versus immediate)?
- **Radiation:** Any other bleeding (bleeding from another location)?
- **Intensity:** How severe is your bleeding problem? How large are the bruises (if any)?
  - Is it getting better, worse, or staying the same? Does it limit your activities?
  - Have you ever required a blood transfusion?
- **Duration:** How old were you when this became a problem (hereditary versus acquired)?
- **Events associated:**
  - Hemorrhages: Tooth extraction, surgery, cutting of umbilical cord, and venipuncture sites
  - LUQ pain (splenomegaly), lymphadenopathy
  - Headache: Intracerebral hemorrhage
  - Visual changes: Retinal hemorrhages
  - Henoch-Schönlein purpura: Recent URTI, purpuric skin rash, abdominal pain, polyarthralgias
  - Anemia: Pallor, weakness, fatigue, palpitations

Table 8-1   Characteristics of Bleeding Disorders

Characteristic	Vascular and Platelet Disorders	Coagulation Disorders
Onset of bleeding	Immediate prolonged bleeding	Delayed bleeding after injury
Petechiae	Characteristic	Rare
Large hematomas	Rare	Characteristic
Superficial ecchymosis	Common (small and multiple)	Common (large and solitary)
Hemarthrosis	Rare	Characteristic
Bleeding from superficial cuts and scratches	Persistent, often profuse	Minimal
Sex	Relatively more common in ♀	Most patients with hemophilia are ♂
Family history	Rarely positive	Commonly positive

- Constitutional symptoms: Fever, chills, night sweats, weight loss, anorexia, and asthenia (leukemia, lymphoma)
  - Diet: Vitamin K, C, B_{12} deficiency, iron deficiency, or folate deficiency?
- **Frequency**: How often does the bleeding happen (intermittent versus constant)?
- **Palliative factors**: Is there anything that makes it better? If so, what? Have you responded well to treatments in the past?
- **Provocative factors**: Is there anything that makes it worse? If so, what?
- **PMH/PSH**: Liver disease, renal disease, collagen vascular disease, malabsorption, HIV status, infectious hepatitis, or blood transfusions
- **MEDS**: Steroids, ASA, anticoagulation therapy, chemotherapy, or radiation
- **SH**: Smoking, EtOH, street drugs, diet, travel, and sexual practices
- **FH**: Bleeding diathesis (hemophilia, von Willebrand's disease), collagen vascular disease, infant deaths, or infectious hepatitis

---

INSTRUCTIONS TO CANDIDATE: A 27-year-old male presents to his family physician complaining of weight loss and night sweats. Take a detailed history of his symptoms, exploring possible etiologies.

DD$_X$ VITAMINS C

- **Infectious**: Tuberculosis (TB), HIV
- **Autoimmune/Allergic**: Collagen vascular disease
- **Neoplastic**: Lymphoma (Hodgkin's and non-Hodgkin's [NHL] types), leukemia, and other malignancy

History

- **Character**: Describe how you are feeling.
- **Onset**: When did you first notice the weight loss? When did you first notice the night sweats?
- **Radiation**: Any history of exposure to radiation (therapeutic, occupational)?
- **Intensity**: How much weight have you lost? How severe are the night sweats? Do you soak your pajamas? Your sheets?
- **Duration**: Over what period of time has this weight loss occurred?
- **Events associated**:
  - Other constitutional symptoms: Fever, chills, anorexia, pruritus, and asthenia
  - Lymphadenopathy: "Gland" enlargement (neck, armpit, or groin), cough/shortness of breath (SOB; mediastinal enlargement), EtOH-induced pain (rare)
  - Pel-Ebstein fever: Fever alternating with periods of 15 to 28 days of normal/low temperature
  - Anemia (caused by bone marrow infiltrate, hypersplenism): Pallor, weakness, fatigue
  - Pain caused by bony infiltration or nerve root compression
  - Easy bruising, infections (pancytopenia)
  - Leg edema caused by lymphatic obstruction in the pelvis or groin
  - Early satiety and nausea/vomiting (N/V) caused by compression of the stomach by enlarged spleen
  - Horner's syndrome caused by cervical sympathetic chain compression
  - Hoarseness caused by recurrent laryngeal nerve compression
  - TB: History of exposure to TB, fever, cough, SOB, hemoptysis
  - HIV: Multiple sexual partners, IV drug use, blood transfusions, diarrhea, opportunistic infection
- **Frequency**: How often do the night sweats happen (intermittent versus every night)?
- **Palliative factors**: Is there anything that makes it better? If so, what?
- **Provocative factors**: Is there anything that makes it worse? If so, what?

- **PMH/PSH:** Malignancy, past surgeries, organ transplant, or HIV
- **MEDS:** Immunosuppressants, hypersensitivity to allopurinol/phenytoin may cause lymphadenopathy
- **FH:** Lymphoma, familial malignancies

INSTRUCTIONS TO CANDIDATE: You are doing a rotation in hematology and are asked to see a 22-year-old male referred with a tentative diagnosis of lymphoma. Examine the patient, and describe your findings.

Physical Examination
- **Vitals:** Heart rate (HR), respiratory rate (RR), blood pressure (BP), and temperature (may find low-grade fever)
- **General:** Cachexia, diaphoresis
- **Skin:** Jaundice, pallor (lips, buccal mucosa, conjunctiva, palmar creases), petechiae, ecchymosis
- **Lymphatic system:** Examine lymph nodes in head and neck, axilla, and groin (note size, shape, mobility, consistency, tenderness, warmth, and number of enlarged nodes). Enlarged lymph nodes are rubbery and discrete and later become matted with disease progression.
- **Respiratory (Resp):** Note any signs of infection, pleural effusion, or tracheobronchial compression.
- **Cardiovascular system (CVS):** Look for signs of severe anemia (hyperdynamic precordium, bounding pulses, and aortic flow murmur). Also look for signs of superior vena cava (SVC) syndrome (congestion and edema of the face and neck caused by compression of the SVC).
- **Abdomen:** Examine the liver and spleen (looking for organomegaly). Significantly enlarged paraaortic nodes may be palpable as a deep central mass.
- Note any signs and sources of infection.

PEARL
- Two problems commonly associated with NHL and rarely associated with Hodgkin's lymphoma are SVC syndrome and renal failure (caused by ureteral compression from large pelvic lymph nodes).

INSTRUCTIONS TO CANDIDATE: A 55-year-old female presents to the emergency department feeling generally unwell. She has a low-grade fever (temperature 38°C). Her complete blood count (CBC) shows hemoglobin 95 g/L, white blood cells 100×10^9/L, and platelets 40×10^9/L. Take a detailed history, exploring possible etiologies, and perform a focused physical examination.

DD$_X$ VITAMINS C
- **I**diopathic/**I**atrogenic: Myeloproliferative disorders
- **N**eoplastic: Acute leukemia

History
- **Character:** How are you feeling? Constitutional symptoms (fever, chills, night sweats, weight loss, anorexia, and asthenia)?
- **Onset:** How did this start?
- **Radiation:** Any history of radiation exposure (therapeutic, occupational)?
- **Intensity:** Has it gotten worse (ask about symptom progression)?
- **Duration:** How long have you been feeling unwell?

- Events associated:
  - Infection: Fever, productive cough (pneumonia), dysuria/urinary frequency (urinary tract infection [UTI]), or diarrhea
  - Anemia: Fatigue, weakness, SOB on exertion (SOBOE), chest pain (CP), palpitations
  - Thrombocytopenia: Easy bruising, petechiae, bleeding from mucosal surfaces
  - Early satiety and N/V caused by compression of stomach by hepatosplenomegaly
  - SOB caused by pleural effusion or mediastinal enlargement
  - Infiltration of normal tissues by leukemic cells: Bone pain, cord compression, gum hypertrophy, proptosis, testicular enlargement, hepatosplenomegaly, lymphadenopathy, polyarthritis, SOB, pancytopenia
- Frequency: Has this ever happened to you before?
- Palliative/Provocative factors: Does anything make you feel better or worse? If so, what?
- **PMH/PSH:** Malignancy
- **MEDS, Allergies, SH**
- **FH:** Hematologic malignancy

Physical Examination
- **Vitals:** HR, RR, BP, and temperature
- **General:** Cachexia, diaphoresis
- **Skin:** Pallor (lips, buccal mucosa, conjunctiva, palmar creases), petechiae
- **Head, eyes, ears, nose, and throat (HEENT):** Gum hypertrophy, proptosis, or mucosal bleeding
- **Lymphatic system:** Examine lymph nodes in head and neck, axilla, and groin (note size, shape, mobility, consistency, tenderness, warmth, and number of enlarged nodes).
- **Resp:** Note any signs of infection, pleural effusion, or tracheobronchial compression.
- **CVS:** Look for signs of anemia (hyperdynamic precordium, bounding pulses, and aortic flow murmur).
- **Abdomen:** Examine the liver and spleen (look for organomegaly).

PEARL
- Look for signs and sources of infection. Although the patient has a profound leukocytosis (100×10^9/L), these cells are likely not functioning adequately, leaving the patient vulnerable to infection.

INSTRUCTIONS TO CANDIDATE: A 60-year-old female presents to the emergency department complaining of fatigue and weakness. She visited her family doctor 3 days ago with the same complaint, and he ordered some "tests." The astute triage nurse checks for recent laboratory investigations and brings you the results of her CBC: hemoglobin 68 g/L, white blood cells 8.6×10^9/L, and platelets 115×10^9/L. The mean corpuscular volume is 66 fL. Take a detailed history, exploring possible etiologies, and perform a focused physical examination.

Definition
- **Anemia** results from decreased production of RBCs, increased destruction or loss of RBCs, or sequestration of RBCs. Anemias are commonly classified using the mean corpuscular volume (Table 8-2). Microcytic hypochromic anemia is characterized by the presence of small, pale RBCs on blood smear. Iron deficiency is the most common cause, and the most common etiology is blood loss.
- This patient has a marked microcytic anemia (Table 8-3).

Table 8-2 Classification of Anemia

Microcytic (MCV <80 fL)	Normocytic (MCV 80–95 fL)	Macrocytic (MCV >95 fL)
Iron deficiency	Acute blood loss	B_{12} deficiency
Thalassemia	Hemolysis	Folate deficiency
Sideroblastic anemia	Hypoproduction of RBCs	Alcohol
	Anemia of chronic disease	

MCV, Mean corpuscular volume.

Table 8-3 Differentiating Microcytic Anemia

Type of Anemia	Serum Iron	Ferritin	Total Iron Binding Capacity (TIBC)
Iron deficiency anemia	↓	↓	↑
Thalassemia	↑	↑	↓
Congenital sideroblastic anemia	↑	↑	↓

History
- **Character:** How are you feeling? Tell me about your weakness and fatigue.
- **Location:** Look for sources of possible blood loss:
  - Gastrointestinal (GI) blood loss: Melena, hematochezia, or hematemesis
  - Mucous membranes (epistaxis, gingival bleeding associated with tooth brushing)
  - Hemoptysis
  - Hematuria
  - Menorrhagia: Presence of clots, number of pads/tampons needed per day
  - Trauma
- **Onset:** How did this start?
- **Intensity:** Has it gotten worse (ask about symptom progression)?
- **Duration:** How long have you been feeling unwell?
- **Events associated:**
  - Pica: Craving for dirt, paint, or ice
  - Brittle nails, smooth tongue, angular cheilosis
  - Plummer-Vinson syndrome (associated pharyngeal web): Dysphagia
  - Dyspnea, palpitations, or chest pain on exertion
  - Malnutrition: Iron, vitamin C
  - Constitutional symptoms: Fever, chills, night sweats, weight loss, anorexia, and asthenia (malignancy)
- **Frequency:** Has this ever happened to you before?
- **Palliative factors:** Does anything make you feel better? If so, what?
- **Provocative factors:** Does anything make you feel worse? If so, what?
  - Exertional symptoms?
- **PMH/PSH:** Anemia, bleeding diathesis, malignancy, cardiovascular disease, liver/renal disease, or blood transfusions
- **MEDS:** NSAIDs, ASA, iron supplements, or anticoagulants
- **SH:** EtOH, smoking
- **FH:** Thalassemia, familial malignancy (e.g., colon cancer), or bleeding diathesis

Physical Examination
- **Vitals:** HR, RR, BP, and temperature
- **General:** Cachexia, jaundice

- **Skin:** Pallor (lips, buccal mucosa, conjunctiva, palmar creases), koilonychia (brittle, ridged, or spoon nails)
- **HEENT:** Glossitis, angular cheilosis, frontal bossing, or abnormal facies
- **Lymphatic system:** Examine lymph nodes in the head and neck, axilla, and groin (note size, shape, mobility, consistency, tenderness, warmth, and number of enlarged nodes).
- **CVS:** Look for signs of cardiac compromise: Displaced apical impulse (cardiac dilatation), hyperdynamic precordium, bounding pulses, and aortic flow murmur.
- **Abdomen:** Examine the liver and spleen (look for organomegaly). Note any masses. Perform a digital rectal examination (DRE).

INSTRUCTIONS TO CANDIDATE: A 47-year-old female presents to the emergency department with a swollen and painful right calf. Take a detailed history, focusing on risk factors for thromboembolic disease, and perform a focused physical examination.

DD$_X$ VITAMINS C
- **Vascular:** Deep venous thrombosis (DVT), thrombophlebitis, and arterial insufficiency
- **Infectious:** Cellulitis
- **Traumatic:** Traumatic injury, ruptured Baker's cyst
- **Idiopathic/Iatrogenic:** Neuropathy, referred pain

History
- **Character:** Describe the pain in your leg.
- **Location:** What part of your leg is swollen? What part of your leg is painful?
- **Onset:** How did the leg pain start (sudden versus gradual)?
- **Radiation:** Does the pain move anywhere? Into your foot? Or up your leg?
- **Intensity:** How severe is your pain right now, on a scale of 1 to 10 with 1 being mild and 10 being the worst? Has your pain gotten worse?
- **Duration:** How long has your leg been painful? Swollen?
- **Events associated:**
  - Clinical diagnosis of DVT is unreliable.
  - Fever, localized redness and swelling, and heat may be consistent with infection.
  - Trauma
  - Back pain: Neuropathy
  - Knee effusion, sudden onset of pain and swelling, popliteal mass: Rupture of Baker's cyst
  - Red, tender cord in calf: Superficial thrombophlebitis
- **Frequency:** Has this ever happened to you before? If so, how often does it happen? When did you last have leg pain and swelling?
- **Palliative factors:** Is there anything that makes your leg pain better? If so, what?
- **Provocative factors:** Is there anything that makes your leg pain worse? If so, what?
  - Calf pain that occurs with activity and resolves with rest is called claudication (arterial insufficiency).
- **PMH/PSH:** Thromboembolic disease, blood dyscrasias, polycythemia, recent surgery, pregnancy, diabetes mellitus (DM), or obesity
- **MEDS:** Estrogens, anticoagulants (noncompliance or addition of a new medication may alter efficacy)
- **FH:** Thromboembolic disease, antithrombin III deficiency, protein C and/or S deficiency, or factor V Leiden

Risk Factors for Thromboembolic Disease
- **Virchow's triad:** Endothelial injury, hypercoagulability, and stasis
- **Injury:** Vascular catheter insertion, injection of irritating substances, trauma, and surgery (especially abdominal, pelvic, and orthopedic procedures)

- Hypercoagulability: Malignancy, polycythemia, estrogen administration, thrombophlebitis, dehydration, nephrotic syndrome, inflammatory bowel disease (IBD), infusion of prothrombin complex concentrates, factor V Leiden mutation, antithrombin III deficiency, protein C and/or S deficiency, lupus anticoagulant, and antiphospholipid syndrome
- Stasis: Myocardial infarction (MI), heart failure, pregnancy (inferior vena cava [IVC] compression), and prolonged immobility (e.g., long trips in car/plane)
- Other: Smoking, age >60 years, history of thromboembolic disease, obesity, and DM

Physical Examination
- **Vitals:** HR and rhythm, RR, BP, and temperature
- **General:** Gait, patient position on stretcher or chair
- **Skin:** Peripheral edema, skin color, skin temperature over feet and legs (using back of fingers), skin quality (atrophic changes, ulcers), capillary refill
- **Resp:** Auscultation (breath sounds, adventitious sounds, pleural friction rub)
- **CVS:** Auscultation, pulses (dorsalis pedis, posterior tibial, popliteal, femoral), and "6 Ps" of arterial occlusion:
  - Pain
  - Pulselessness
  - Pallor
  - Polar (cool temperature)
  - Paresthesia
  - Paralysis
- **Musculoskeletal (MSK):** Note any signs of trauma or varicose veins (dilated and tortuous veins)
  - Swelling: Measure circumference of the thigh and leg 10 cm below the tibial tuberosity. A difference of >3 cm is considered significant.
  - Look for knee effusion. Palpate popliteal fossa for protrusion cyst of the knee known as Baker's cyst.

PEARLS
- **Homans's sign:** Flex the patient's knee. Forcefully and abruptly dorsiflex the ankle. This produces pain in *some* patients with DVT but may also be positive with intervertebral disk herniation and other conditions. Some believe that performing this examination may dislodge the clot and precipitate pulmonary embolism (PE).
- **Lisker sign:** Percuss the surface of the tibia, medial to the crest. Bone tenderness (Lisker sign) is present in some patients with DVT. This sign should not be positive in patients with disk herniation.

INSTRUCTIONS TO CANDIDATE: The previous patient has a Doppler ultrasound of the right leg, confirming a below-knee DVT. She is discharged with appropriate treatment and follow-up evaluation. She returns to the emergency department the next day with shortness of breath and chest discomfort. Take an appropriate history, and perform a focused physical examination.

DD$_X$
- PE until proven otherwise.

Definition
- PE obstructs flow in the pulmonary arterial circulation and commonly arises from thrombi in deep leg or pelvic veins (less commonly from the arm or right side of the heart). If the PE is not fatal, the clot will lyse, and symptoms will resolve (unless infarction occurs). Pulmonary infarction is rare because the lung has a dual blood

supply (pulmonary and bronchial circulation). Symptoms of embolization occur abruptly; infarction develops over hours. Massive PE may present as cardiac arrest or shock.

- **First evaluate** Airway, Breathing, and Circulation. It may be necessary to perform an immediate intervention, such as supplemental O_2, IV access, or intubation.
  - Is the patient able to talk? Swallow? Cough?
  - Are both lungs ventilated? Is the patient oxygenating (mentation, pulse oximetry)?
  - Abnormal vitals? Peripheral circulation (pulses, capillary refill)?
  - If no immediate interventions are required, proceed to take the history, and perform the physical examination.

History
- **Character:** Describe the nature of your breathing difficulty.
- **Location:** Where were you when you became SOB?
- **Onset:** How did the SOB start (sudden versus gradual)? What were you doing when you became SOB?
- **Intensity:** How severe is your SOB right now, on a scale of 1 to 10 with 1 being mild and 10 being the worst? Has your SOB gotten worse?
- **Duration:** How long have you been SOB?
- **Events associated:**
  - PE triad (rare): Sudden SOB, hemoptysis, and pleuritic CP
  - Fever, palpitations, or syncope
  - Pulmonary infarction: Hemoptysis, pleuritic CP, fever, consolidation, pleural effusion, pleural friction rub
- **Frequency:** Has this ever happened to you before? If so, how often does it happen? When was the last time you became SOB?
- **Palliative factors:** Is there anything that makes your SOB better? If so, what?
- **Provocative factors:** Is there anything that makes your SOB worse? If so, what?
- **PMH/PSH:** Thromboembolic disease, ischemic heart disease (IHD), asthma, or pericardial disease
- **MEDS:** Anticoagulants

Physical Examination
- **Vitals:** HR and rhythm (sinus tachycardia is common), RR (depth, effort, and pattern), BP, and temperature
- **General:** Respiratory distress, unilateral splinting of chest (pleuritic chest pain)
- **Skin:** Peripheral edema, cyanosis, clubbing, capillary refill
- **HEENT:** Central cyanosis, tracheal position
- **Resp:** Chest expansion (symmetry), tactile fremitus, percussion, and auscultation (breath sounds, adventitious sounds, pleural friction rub)
- **CVS:** Signs of cor pulmonale (increased jugular venous pressure, positive hepato-jugular reflux, and right ventricular heave), peripheral pulses, palpate apical impulse, and auscultate, looking for loud P_2, S_3, or murmurs
- **Neurologic (Neuro):** Mental status (adequate brain oxygenation)

SAMPLE CHECKLIST

INSTRUCTIONS TO CANDIDATE: Examine the lymph nodes of the head and neck. Describe your findings.

Key Points	Satisfactorily Completed
Introduces self to the patient	❏
Determines how the patient wishes to be addressed	❏
Explains nature of the examination to the patient	❏
Examines the patient in a logical fashion	❏
Inspection	
• Symmetry	❏
• Visible masses	❏
Nodes	
• Occipital	❏
• Postauricular	❏
• Preauricular	❏
• Tonsillar	❏
• Submandibular	❏
• Submental	❏
• Anterior cervical	❏
• Posterior cervical	❏
• Supraclavicular	❏
• Infraclavicular	❏
Description	
• Location and number	❏
• Size and shape	❏
• Mobility	❏
• Consistency	❏
• Tenderness	❏
• Warmth	❏
Drapes the patient appropriately	❏
Makes appropriate closing remarks	❏

CHAPTER 9

Endocrinology

OBJECTIVES

ANATOMY OF THE THYROID GLAND

ESSENTIAL CLINICAL COMPETENCIES
PERFORM AN EXAMINATION OF THE THYROID GLAND

SAMPLE OSCE SCENARIOS
- A 25-year-old female presents to her family doctor with "milk" leaking from her breasts intermittently during the past month. Perform a focused history and physical examination.
- A 36-year-old female presents to her family physician complaining of heat intolerance and weight loss despite increased appetite. Her thyroid-stimulating hormone is 0.07 mU/L. Perform a focused history and physical examination.
- A 49-year-old female presents to the emergency department with facial swelling and weakness. When asked about past medical problems, she admits that she used to have "low thyroid." She stopped taking her medications several months ago when her drug plan expired. Perform a focused history and physical examination.
- A 37-year-old female presents with complaint of increased hair growth on her body. Take a detailed history, exploring possible etiologies.
- A 53-year-old female is referred with central obesity and "stretch marks" on her abdomen and torso. Perform a focused history and physical examination.
- A 38-year-old male with type 1 diabetes mellitus presents to his family doctor for routine evaluation. Perform a focused history and funduscopy on this patient. Describe your findings.
- A 62-year-old male presents for surgical consultation. He has a "lump" in his neck anteriorly. Take a detailed history, focusing on risk factors for malignancy.

SAMPLE CHECKLISTS
- ❏ Perform a physical examination of the thyroid gland.
- ❏ A 28-year-old female is referred for assessment of Addison's disease. Perform a focused physical examination and describe your findings.
- ❏ A 32-year-old male with acromegaly presents to his endocrinologist for follow-up evaluation. Examine the head, neck, and skin for clinical signs associated with this condition. Describe your findings.

OBJECTIVES

*The successful student should be able to take a **focused history** of the endocrine system, including:*
- Galactorrhea
- Gynecomastia
- Amenorrhea
- Hirsutism
- Polyuria, polydipsia
- Cold or heat intolerance
- Neck swelling, goiter
- Increased prominence of the eyes, puffiness in preorbital area

- Changes in skin and hair
- Constipation, diarrhea
- Weight loss, weight gain
- Loss of libido, impotence
- Osteoporosis
- Diabetes mellitus (DM)

*The endocrine **examination** will include:*

Inspection
- Skin: Hirsutism, dry/oily skin, sallow skin, striae, and foot ulcers
- Face: Facial edema, moon facies, coarse facial features, prognathism, exophthalmos, and Queen Anne's eyebrows
- Body habitus: Central obesity, supraclavicular fat pad, "buffalo hump," and large hands and feet
- Neck: Static and on swallowing

Palpation
- Thyroid: Static and on swallowing
- Isthmus and lobe margins using a bimanual technique
  - Size and symmetry
  - Consistency
  - Nodularity
  - Tenderness

Auscultation
- Thyroid for bruits (hyperdynamic circulation)

ANATOMY OF THE THYROID GLAND

- In terms of embryology the **thyroid** develops from the floor of the pharynx. The primitive thyroid gland migrates caudally to rest anterior to the trachea. If migration fails to stop anterior to the second or third tracheal ring, the thyroid may become partially or wholly substernal. If the migratory tract fails to obliterate, a thyroglossal cyst may develop.
- The normal thyroid gland is located inferior to the cricoid cartilage, anterior and lateral to the trachea (Figure 9-1). The two lateral lobes are connected by an **isthmus,**

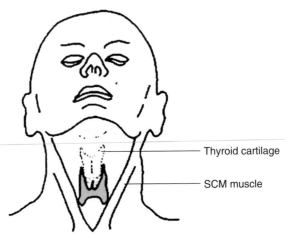

Figure 9-1   Surface anatomy of the thyroid. (Used with permission of Dr. Tom Scott, Memorial University of Newfoundland.)

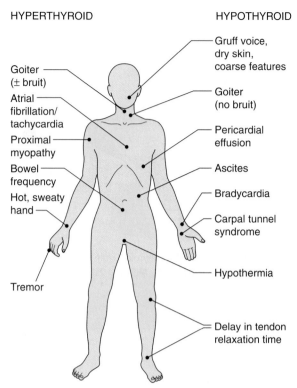

HYPERTHYROID   HYPOTHYROID

Goiter
(± bruit)

Atrial
fibrillation/
tachycardia

Proximal
myopathy

Bowel
frequency

Hot, sweaty
hand

Tremor

Gruff voice,
dry skin,
coarse features

Goiter
(no bruit)

Pericardial
effusion

Ascites

Bradycardia

Carpal tunnel
syndrome

Hypothermia

Delay in tendon
relaxation time

Figure 9-2   Features of hyperthyroidism and hypothyroidism. (From Munro JF, Campbell IW, editors: *Macleod's clinical examination,* ed 10, Edinburgh, 2000, Churchill Livingstone, p 63, Figure 2.47.)

which extends across the trachea anterior to the second tracheal ring. The thyroid gland is often not palpable (the isthmus may be palpable).

- The thyroid is firmly embedded in the pretracheal fascia. Therefore it ascends with swallowing. This movement helps distinguish the thyroid from other masses in the neck.
- The recurrent laryngeal nerve lies deep to the medial aspect of the thyroid and may be damaged during thyroid surgery or in invasive malignant disease, causing hoarseness.
- The thyroid hormone produced by the thyroid gland influences cellular metabolism (Figure 9-2).

ESSENTIAL CLINICAL COMPETENCIES

PERFORM AN EXAMINATION OF THE THYROID GLAND

Inspection
- Ask the patient to extend the neck slightly. Use tangential lighting to inspect the region below the cricoid cartilage for the thyroid gland. Ask the patient to take a sip of water, slightly extend the neck, and swallow. Watch for movement of the thyroid, noting contour and symmetry. Normally the thyroid gland, thyroid cartilage, and cricoid cartilage rise with swallowing.

Palpation
- **Posterior approach**: Palpation is most precisely done from behind the patient. Slightly extend the patient's neck. Overextending will interfere with palpation (taut muscles). Palpate the lateral lobes of the thyroid (Figure 9-3). The isthmus is more often palpable than the lateral lobes. Ask the patient to sip and swallow as necessary.

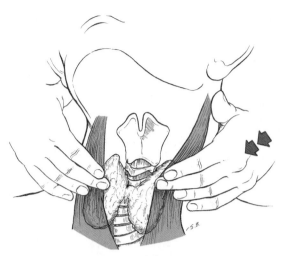

Figure 9-3 Posterior approach to examination of the thyroid. (From Barkauskas VH, Baumann LC, Darling-Fisher CS: *Health and physical assessment*, ed 3, St. Louis, 2002, Mosby, p 238, Figure 11-16[1].)

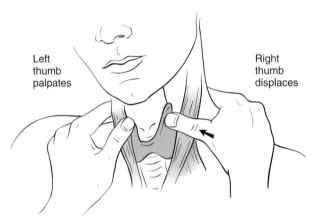

Figure 9-4 Anterior approach to examination of the thyroid. (From Jarvis CJ: *Physical examination and health assessment*, ed 2, Philadelphia, 1996, WB Saunders, p 284, Figure 11-15.)

Feel for any glandular tissue rising under your finger pads. Note size, shape, consistency, nodularity, and tenderness of the gland. The physical characteristics of the thyroid gland are NOT a reflection of its function.

- **Anterior approach**: Sit in front of the patient. To palpate the right lobe, slightly flex the neck, and turn the chin toward the right side. Displace the left lobe with your right hand, and palpate the right lobe with your left hand (Figure 9-4). Ask the patient to swallow, and feel the tissue rising under your fingers.

Auscultation

- If the thyroid gland is enlarged, auscultate over the lateral lobes with the bell of your stethoscope to detect a bruit (hyperdynamic circulation).

SAMPLE OSCE SCENARIOS

> INSTRUCTIONS TO CANDIDATE: A 25-year-old female presents to her family doctor with "milk" leaking from her breasts intermittently during the past month. Perform a focused history and physical examination.

Definition
- **Galactorrhea** is the abnormal presence of lactation, specifically lactation that is persistent and takes place outside the context of breast-feeding or during the peripartum period.

DD$_X$ VITAMINS C
- Metabolic: Drugs, breast-feeding, acromegaly, and hypothyroidism
- Idiopathic/Iatrogenic: Liver failure
- Neoplastic: Prolactinoma
- Pregnancy, pseudocyesis (false pregnancy)

History
- **Ch**aracter: What is the discharge like? Describe the color, odor, and consistency of the discharge.
- **L**ocation: From where does the discharge come? Areola? Other location? From one or both breasts?
- **O**nset: How did this come about (sudden versus gradual)?
- **I**ntensity: Quantify the amount of daily discharge. Does it leak through your clothes? Is it getting better, worse, or staying the same? Does it limit your activities?
- **D**uration: How long has this been going on (acute versus chronic)?
- **E**vents associated:
  - Any rashes or ulcers on the breasts? Any redness or pain?
  - Have you found any lumps on breast self-examination?
  - Last menstrual period (LMP)? Amenorrhea? Pregnant? Postpartum?
  - Decreased libido?
  - Headache? Visual disturbance (bitemporal hemianopsia)?
  - Constitutional symptoms: Fever, chills, night sweats, weight loss, anorexia, and asthenia
- **F**requency: Has this ever happened to you before? If so, when? Does it happen every day (intermittent versus constant)?
- **P**alliative factors: Is there anything that makes it better? If so, what?
- **P**rovocative factors: Is there anything that makes it worse? If so, what?
  - Breast stimulation?
- **Past medical history (PMH)/past surgical history (PSH):** Breast/thoracic surgery, breast cancer, endocrine disease, pregnancy, or pseudocyesis
- **Medications (MEDS):** Hormones, antipsychotics, antidepressants, or methyldopa
- **Social history (SH):** Smoking, EtOH, street drugs, and sexual practices
- **Family history (FH):** Breast cancer, endocrine disease

Physical Examination
- **Vitals:** Heart rate (HR), respiratory rate (RR), blood pressure (BP), and temperature
- **General:** Body habitus, distribution of body hair
- **Skin:** Skin quality (dry/oily), hyperpigmentation
- **Lymphatic system:** Examine lymph nodes in the head, neck, and axilla. Note size, shape, mobility, consistency, tenderness, warmth, and number of enlarged nodes.
- **Respiratory (Resp):** Chest expansion (symmetry), auscultation (breath sounds, adventitious sounds)

- **Cardiovascular system (CVS):** Palpate peripheral pulses. Note pulse volume, contour, and rhythm. Auscultate the heart, looking for extra heart sounds or flow murmurs associated with hyperdynamic circulation.
- **Abdomen:** Inspect the abdomen. Auscultate for bowel sounds. Percuss lightly in all four quadrants. Perform light and deep palpation, and identify any masses or areas of tenderness. Check for rebound tenderness. Examine the liver and spleen. Perform a digital rectal examination (DRE).
- **Neurologic (Neuro):** Perform a cranial nerve (CN) examination with attention to CNs II, III, IV, and VI. A macroadenoma of the pituitary may cause bitemporal hemianopsia as a result of compression of the optic chiasm. Perform a funduscopic examination, and note any papilledema.
- **Gynecologic (Gyne):** Perform a thorough examination of the breasts. Note any discharge, skin changes, masses, or tenderness.

INSTRUCTIONS TO CANDIDATE: A 36-year-old female presents to her family physician complaining of heat intolerance and weight loss despite increased appetite. Her thyroid-stimulating hormone is 0.07 mU/L. Perform a focused history and physical examination.

Definition

- **Hyperthyroidism** is an abnormality in thyroid regulation that results in a high level of thyroid hormone and low levels of thyroid stimulating hormone (TSH). This typically manifests as a hypermetabolic state. Beware of hyperthyroidism in elderly patients, in whom it may present with an "apathetic" picture rather than a hypermetabolic state. **Thyroid storm** is a *life-threatening emergency* of profound thyrotoxicosis. It is characterized by fever, weakness, cardiovascular collapse, and shock. A number of precipitants have been identified, including infection, trauma, and surgery.

DD$_X$ VITAMINS C

- **Autoimmune/Allergic:** Subacute thyroiditis, Hashimoto's thyroiditis, and Graves' disease (diffuse toxic goiter)
- **Metabolic:** Exogenous thyroid hormone, excessive iodine ingestion
- **Idiopathic/Iatrogenic:** Plummer's disease (nodular toxic goiter)

History

- **Ch**aracter: Describe how you are feeling.
- **O**nset: How has this come about (sudden versus gradual)? When did you first notice the weight loss? Increased appetite? Heat intolerance?
- **R**adiation: Any previous radiation to the neck or known radiation exposure (occupational, therapeutic)?
- **I**ntensity: How much weight have you lost? Do your clothes still fit you? How severe is the heat intolerance? Do you get sweaty? Does it soak your clothes? How often do you eat? Are your symptoms getting better, worse, or staying the same?
- **D**uration: Over what period of time have these symptoms occurred (acute versus chronic)?
- **E**vents associated:
  - Any change in bowel habit? Diarrhea?
  - Palpitations? Irritability? Difficulty sleeping?
  - Any tremor or shakes? Muscle weakness (e.g., difficulty standing from a sitting position)?
  - Any change in your menstrual periods (e.g., decreased duration and frequency)? LMP? Are you pregnant?

- Any swelling in your legs (pretibial myxedema)? Itching? Any eye changes (e.g., bulging)?
  - Any changes in vision? Diplopia (infiltration of eye muscles in Graves' disease may lead to diplopia)?
  - Constitutional symptoms: Fever, chills, night sweats, anorexia, and asthenia
- **Frequency:** How often do you notice these symptoms (intermittent versus constant)?
- **Palliative factors:** Is there anything that makes it better? If so, what?
- **Provocative factors:** Is there anything that makes it worse? If so, what?
- **PMH/PSH:** Thyroid disease, radiation, or malignancy (thyroid, multiple endocrine neoplasia [MEN])
- **MEDS:** Sources of exogenous thyroid such as propylthiouracil (PTU) and thyroxine
- **SH:** Smoking, EtOH, street drugs, and diet (excessive iodine)
- **FH:** Thyroid disease, MEN

Physical Examination

- **Vitals:** HR and rhythm, RR, BP, and temperature
  - Tachycardia or atrial fibrillation may be present. Note a widened pulse pressure or fever.
- **General:** Body habitus, diaphoresis, anxiety
- **Skin:** Nonpitting edema (lower limb), clubbing, excoriations
- **Head, eyes, ears, nose, and throat (HEENT):** Inspect the eyes, noting any eye protrusion, lid retraction, or lid lag. Exophthalmos is unique to Graves' disease. Inspect and palpate the thyroid gland. Note the size, shape, consistency, nodularity, and any tenderness. Auscultate over the lateral lobes with the bell to detect a bruit (hyperdynamic circulation).
- **Resp:** Chest expansion (symmetry), auscultation (breath sounds, adventitious sounds)
- **CVS:** Palpate peripheral pulses. Note pulse volume, contour, and rhythm. Auscultate the heart, looking for extra heart sounds or flow murmurs associated with hyperdynamic circulation.
- **Abdomen:** Inspect the abdomen. Auscultate for bowel sounds (may be increased sounds in hyperthyroidism). Percuss lightly in all four quadrants. Perform light and deep palpation, and identify any masses or areas of tenderness. Check for rebound tenderness. Examine the liver and spleen. Perform a DRE.
- **Neuro:** Inspect for tremor. Examine the reflexes (may have hyperreflexia). Test muscle strength, especially proximal muscles (e.g., ask the patient to stand from a seated position). Examine the extraocular eye movements. Perform a funduscopic examination, and note any papilledema.

INSTRUCTIONS TO CANDIDATE: A 49-year-old female presents to the emergency department with facial swelling and weakness. When asked about past medical problems, she admits that she used to have "low thyroid." She stopped taking her medications several months ago when her drug plan expired. Perform a focused history and physical examination.

Definition

- **Hypothyroidism** is an abnormality in thyroid regulation that results in a low level of thyroid hormone and high levels of TSH. This typically manifests as a hypometabolic state. Tissues may be infiltrated by mucopolysaccharides. **Myxedema coma** is a *life-threatening complication* of hypothyroidism. It is characterized by hypothermia, coma, and respiratory depression. A number of precipitants have been identified, including infection, trauma, and exposure to cold.

DD~X~ VITAMINS C

- **Traumatic:** Radioactive thyroid ablation, thyroidectomy
- **Autoimmune/Allergic:** Hashimoto's thyroiditis
- **Metabolic:** Hypopituitarism
- **Idiopathic/Iatrogenic:** Idiopathic atrophy of the thyroid

History

- **Character:** Describe your facial swelling. What do you mean by weakness? Do you mean weakness of your muscles or fatigue or something else?
- **Location:** Where have you noticed the swelling? Around your eyes? Your whole face? Where is the weakness? Arms? Legs?
- **Onset:** How did this come about (sudden versus gradual)? When did you first notice the swelling? Weakness?
- **Radiation:** Any previous radiation to the neck or known radiation exposure (occupational, therapeutic)?
- **Intensity:** How swollen is your face compared with normal? How weak are you? Are you able to get around? Does it limit your activities? Is it getting better, worse, or staying the same?
- **Duration:** Over what period of time have these symptoms occurred (acute versus chronic)?
- **Events associated:**
  - Any change in bowel habit? Constipation? Weight gain? Decreased appetite?
  - Have you noticed any sleepiness? Slowed thought or speech? Difficulty with memory?
  - Any fatigue? Muscle cramps? Cold intolerance?
  - Any changes in your skin or hair, such as dryness or hair loss?
  - Any change in your menstrual periods (e.g., increased duration, frequency)? LMP? Are you pregnant?
  - Any hand numbness or weakness (carpal tunnel syndrome [CTS])?
- **Frequency:** How often do you notice these symptoms (intermittent versus constant)?
- **Palliative factors:** Is there anything that makes it better? If so, what?
- **Provocative factors:** Is there anything that makes it worse? If so, what?
- **PMH/PSH:** Thyroid disease, radiation, thyroidectomy, DM, Addison's disease, or pernicious anemia
- **MEDS:** Amiodarone, lithium
- **SH:** Smoking, EtOH, and street drugs
- **FH:** Thyroid disease

Physical Examination

- **Vitals:** HR and rhythm, RR, BP, and temperature
  - Bradycardia may be present. Note a narrowed pulse pressure or low temperature.
- **General:** Body habitus, dulled facial expression
- **Skin:** Dry, coarse skin, yellow-red pigmentation on palms and soles (carotenemia), brittle nails
- **HEENT:** Inspect the hair. It may be coarse and brittle. Note loss of the lateral third of the eyebrows (Queen Anne's eyebrows). Inspect the face, noting edema around the eyes and macroglossia. Inspect and palpate the thyroid gland. Note the size, shape, consistency, nodularity, and any tenderness. Auscultate over the lateral lobes with the bell to detect a bruit (hyperdynamic circulation).
- **Resp:** Chest expansion (symmetry), percussion, and auscultation (breath sounds, adventitious sounds). Note signs consistent with pleural effusion.
- **CVS:** Palpate peripheral pulses. Note pulse volume, contour, and rhythm. Auscultate the heart, looking for extra heart sounds or murmurs. Muffled heart sounds and an elevated jugular venous pressure (JVP) may suggest pericardial effusion.
- **Abdomen:** Inspect the abdomen. Auscultate for bowel sounds (may be decreased sounds in hypothyroidism). Percuss lightly in all four quadrants. Perform light and

deep palpation, and identify any masses or areas of tenderness. Check for rebound tenderness. Examine the liver and spleen. Perform a DRE.

- **Neuro:** Inspect for tremor. Examine the reflexes. Note a slow return phase of deep tendon reflexes (DTRs). Test muscle strength, and examine for CTS.

> INSTRUCTIONS TO CANDIDATE: A 37-year-old female presents with complaint of increased hair growth on her body. Take a detailed history, exploring possible etiologies (Figure 9-5).

Definition

- **Hypertrichosis** or hirsutism is excessive hair growth in androgenic-dependent hair patterns secondary to increased androgenic activity.

DD$_X$ VITAMINS C

- **Metabolic:** Cushing's syndrome, androgen-secreting ovarian tumors, polycystic ovarian syndrome (PCOS), congenital adrenal hyperplasia (CAH), acromegaly, and drugs
- **Idiopathic/Iatrogenic:** Obesity
- **Congenital/genetic:** Familial (especially in families of Mediterranean origin)

History

- **ID:** Ethnic origin
- **Character:** What does the hair look like (coarse versus fine, pigmented versus light)?
- **Location:** Where is the hair growth (face, upper arms, chest, upper abdomen, back, inner thighs, buttocks)?
- **Onset:** When did it start? How has it progressed (rapid versus insidious)?
- **Intensity:** How much hair is present, and how severe is it? How is it affecting your life?
- **Duration:** How long has this been going on?
- **Events associated:**
  - Virilization (PCOS, androgen-secreting tumor, CAH): Acne, oligo/amenorrhea, deepened voice, breast atrophy, male muscle pattern, temporal balding, and clitoral enlargement
  - Pituitary adenoma: Headaches, galactorrhea, bitemporal hemianopsia

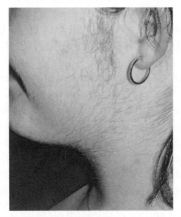

Figure 9-5 Facial hirsutism. (From Seidel HM, Dains JE, Ball JW, Benedict GW: *Mosby's guide to physical examination,* ed 5, St. Louis, 2003, Mosby, p 212, Figure 7-59.)

- Cushing's syndrome: Truncal obesity, menstrual irregularity, moon facies, striae
- Acromegaly: Thick, coarse, oily skin; acne; prognathism; increased space between teeth; increased shoe, hat, glove, and ring sizes
- Constitutional symptoms: Fever, chills, night sweats, weight loss, anorexia, and asthenia
- **Frequency:** Has this ever happened to you before? When?
- **PMH/PSH:** PCOS, pituitary tumor, adrenal tumor, ovarian cancer, or porphyria cutanea tarda
- **MEDS:** Steroids, antihypertensives, oral contraceptive pill (OCP), androgens, or cyclosporine
- **FH:** Hirsutism, ovarian cancer, adrenal/pituitary tumors, or CAH

INSTRUCTIONS TO CANDIDATE: A 53-year-old female is referred with central obesity and "stretch marks" on her abdomen and torso. Perform a focused history and physical examination.

Definition

- **Cushing's syndrome** is caused by long-term exposure to excess cortisol or exogenous cortiosteroids. Cushing's syndrome is classified as adrenocorticotropic hormone (ACTH) dependent and ACTH independent (e.g., cortisol-secreting tumor). Cushing's disease refers specifically to ACTH excess produced by the pituitary gland. In patients with excess ACTH, hyperpigmentation should be present. Cushing's syndrome is classically characterized by moon facies, central obesity, and violaceous striae.

DD$_X$ VITAMINS C

- **Metabolic:** Cushing's disease (overproduction of ACTH by the pituitary), ectopic ACTH production, and exogenous corticosteroid therapy
- **Neoplastic:** Cortisol-secreting tumor or nodule

History

- **Character:** What do these stretch marks look like? What color are they?
- **Location:** Do you feel that you carry your weight on your midriff? What about your arms and legs? Where do you notice the stretch marks? Abdomen? Axilla?
- **Onset:** When did you first notice a change in your weight or its distribution? When did you first notice the stretch marks? Under what circumstances did this come about?
- **Intensity:** How much weight have you gained? How large are the stretch marks? Length? Width? Is it getting better, worse, or staying the same? Does it limit your activities?
- **Duration:** How long has this been going on (acute versus chronic)?
- **Events associated:**
  - Muscle weakness (e.g., difficulty standing from a sitting position)?
  - Any skin changes? Acne? Easy bruising? Any change in wound healing?
  - Any change in your menstrual periods (e.g., decreased duration, frequency)? LMP?
  - Are you more emotional than usual? Increased anxiety?
  - Any difficulty sleeping? Difficulty with memory or concentration?
  - Symptoms of hyperglycemia: Polyuria, polydipsia, fatigue, polyphagia, blurred vision
  - Headache? Visual disturbance (bitemporal hemianopsia)?

- **Palliative factors:** Is there anything that makes it better? If so, what? Lifestyle modification?
- **Provocative factors:** Is there anything that makes it worse? If so, what?
- **PMH/PSH:** Pituitary adenoma, hypertension (HTN), renal colic, osteoporosis, DM, adrenal nodules, or steroid-dependent disease
- **MEDS:** Corticosteroids
- **SH:** Smoking, EtOH, street drugs, and diet
- **FH:** Endocrinopathy

Physical Examination
- **Vitals:** HR and rhythm, RR, BP, and temperature
  - HTN may be present.
- **General:** Body habitus (truncal obesity, supraclavicular fat pads, "buffalo hump," wasting of arms and legs)
- **Skin:** Hypertrichosis, violaceous striae (abdomen, axilla), skin atrophy, acne, ecchymosis, poor wound healing
- **HEENT:** Inspect the hair. Note any temporal balding. Inspect the face (plethoric "moon" facies).
- **Resp:** Chest expansion (symmetry), auscultation (breath sounds, adventitious sounds)
- **CVS:** Palpate peripheral pulses. Note pulse volume, contour, and rhythm. Auscultate the heart, looking for extra heart sounds or murmurs.
- **Abdomen:** Inspect the abdomen (note striae). Auscultate for bowel sounds. Percuss lightly in all four quadrants. Perform light and deep palpation, and identify any masses or areas of tenderness. Check for rebound tenderness. Examine the liver and spleen. Perform a DRE.
- **Neuro:** Examine the reflexes. Inspect for muscle wasting in the thighs and arms. Test muscle strength, especially proximal muscles (e.g., ask the patient to stand from a seated position). Perform a cranial nerve examination. A macroadenoma of the pituitary may cause bitemporal hemianopsia as a result of compression of the optic chiasm. Perform a funduscopic examination, and note any papilledema.

INSTRUCTIONS TO CANDIDATE: A 38-year-old male with type 1 diabetes mellitus presents to his family doctor for routine evaluation. Perform a focused history and funduscopy on this patient. Describe your findings.

Definitions
- **Diabetes mellitus (DM)** is a syndrome caused by impaired insulin secretion or effectiveness. It is characterized by hyperglycemia. Long-term sequelae include retinopathy, nephropathy, vascular disease, and neuropathies.
- Type 1 DM is primarily the result of pancreatic β-cell destruction, and patients are prone to ketoacidosis.
- Type 2 DM may include a combination of relative insulin deficiency and insulin resistance.
- Gestational DM refers to disease onset during pregnancy.

History
- **Character:** What type of diabetes do you have (type 1 or "juvenile diabetes")? Have you ever been admitted to the hospital for diabetes? Why? What happened?
- **Onset:** How old were you when you were diagnosed with DM? How were you diagnosed (how did you find out)?

- **Intensity:** How often do you monitor your "blood sugars"? What are the levels? How does diabetes affect your life?
- **Duration:** How long have you had diabetes?
- **Events associated:**
  - Do you have episodes of hypoglycemia? How often?
  - Symptoms of hypoglycemia: Pallor, sweating, anxiety, tachycardia, palpitations, tremor, headache, hunger/abdominal pain, decreased level of consciousness (LOC), syncope
  - Symptoms of hyperglycemia: Polyuria, polydipsia, fatigue, polyphagia, blurred vision
  - Foot care: Properly fitting shoes, self-inspection for wounds or ulcerations
  - Have you ever had an episode of diabetic ketoacidosis or "diabetic coma"?
  - When did you last have a HbA_{1C}? Lipid profile? Urine screen for microalbuminuria?
  - When were you last assessed by an ophthalmologist, nephrologist, or endocrinologist?
  - Education with diabetes educator and nutritionist? Support groups?
  - Use the mnemonic **BEANN** to remember the complications of DM:
    - **Bugs:** Infections
    - **Eyes:** Retinopathy, cataracts, and glaucoma
    - **Arteries:** HTN, ischemic heart disease (IHD), peripheral vascular disease (PVD), and stroke/transient ischemic attack (TIA)
    - **Nephropathy**
    - **Nerves:** Altered proprioception, mononeuropathies (CNs III, IV, and VI), peripheral neuropathy, and autonomic neuropathy (postural hypotension, gastroparesis, impotence, urinary retention)
- **PMH/PSH:** HTN, nephropathy, increased cholesterol, or retinopathy
- **MEDS:** Insulin (dosage and frequency), angiotensin-converting enzyme (ACE) inhibitors, lipid-lowering agents, or glucocorticoids
- **SH:** Smoking, EtOH, street drugs, diet, exercise, and family/peer support
- **FH:** DM, vascular disease, or endocrinopathies

Funduscopic Examination

- Darken the room. The examination may be aided by dilating the pupil. Use your left eye to examine the patient's left eye. Approach the patient from the temporal side on a 15-degree angle, eliciting the red reflex. Absence of the red reflex suggests corneal opacity (e.g., cataracts). Inspect the cornea, lens, and vitreous for opacities.
- Inspect the optic disc. Compare the discs for symmetry, and note the following:
  - Clarity of the disc outline
  - Color: Normal is yellowish orange to creamy pink.
  - Cup to disc ratio: Normal cup is <0.4.
- Inspect the retina. Follow the vessels to each of four quadrants.
  - Arteries: Light red, bright light reflex, and smaller than veins
  - Veins: Dark red, absent light reflex
  - Note exudates, hemorrhages, or other lesions.
- Inspect the macula and fovea.

Findings in Diabetic Retinopathy

- **Background retinopathy** (Figure 9-6): Microaneurysms, dot and flame hemorrhages, hard and cotton-wool exudates
- **Proliferative retinopathy:** Neovascularization on retina and vitreous and scarring (leads to vitreous hemorrhage and retinal detachment)

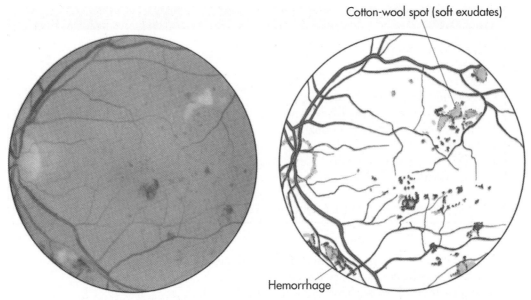

Cotton-wool spot (soft exudates)

Hemorrhage

Figure 9-6   Background retinopathy. (From Seidel HM, Dains JE, Ball JW, Benedict GW: *Mosby's guide to physical examination,* ed 5, St. Louis, 2003, Mosby, p 307, Figure 10-42.)

INSTRUCTIONS TO CANDIDATE: A 62-year-old male presents for surgical consultation. He has a "lump" in his neck anteriorly. Take a detailed history, focusing on risk factors for malignancy.

DD$_X$ VITAMINS C
- **V**ascular: Carotid aneurysm
- **N**eoplastic: Thyroid nodule
- **C**ongenital/genetic: Thyroglossal cyst
- Enlarged lymph node
- Enlarged salivary gland

History
- **Ch**aracter: What does the nodule feel like?
- **L**ocation: Where is the nodule (point to it with one finger)?
- **O**nset: When did you first notice it? How did you first come to notice it?
- **R**adiation: Any previous radiation to the neck?
- **I**ntensity: How large is the nodule? Is the size changing (getting larger or smaller or staying the same)?
- **D**uration: How long has it been there?
- **E**vents associated (Box 9-1):
  - Any pain?
  - Recent infections?
  - Dysphagia? Hoarseness?
  - Hyperthyroidism: Weight loss despite increased appetite, heat intolerance, diarrhea, and exophthalmos
  - Hypothyroidism: Weight gain despite decreased appetite, cold intolerance, and constipation
  - Constitutional symptoms: Fever, chills, night sweats, weight loss, anorexia, and asthenia
- **F**requency: Have you ever had a nodule before? How many?
- **P**alliative factors: Is there anything that makes it better? If so, what?

Box 9-1   Features of a Thyroid Nodule Suspicious for Malignancy

- Age <20 or >60 years
- Male sex
- Rapid growth
- Associated hoarseness or dysphagia
- History of radiation to the head or neck
- Firm and fixed, nontender nodule
- Nodule >2 cm
- Associated lymphadenopathy
- "Cold" nodule on thyroid scan
- Complex cystic nodule
- Family history of medullary cancer of thyroid, MEN II

- **Provocative factors:** Is there anything that makes it worse? If so, what?
  - Eating (obstructed salivary duct)?
- **Previous investigations:** Thyroid scan, biopsy
- **PMH/PSH:** Radiation to neck, thyroid disease, lymphoma, leukemia, other malignancy, or MEN
- **SH:** Smoking, EtOH
- **FH:** Thyroid disease, medullary thyroid cancer, MEN II (pheochromocytoma, hyperparathyroid hormone, thyroid cancer)

SAMPLE CHECKLISTS

> INSTRUCTIONS TO CANDIDATE: Perform a physical examination of the thyroid gland.

Key Points	Satisfactorily Carried out
Introduces self to the patient	❏
Determines how the patient wishes to be addressed	❏
Explains nature of the examination to the patient	❏
Examines the patient in a logical fashion	❏
Inspection	
• Static	❏
• On swallowing	❏
Palpation	
• Outlines isthmus	❏
• Outlines lobe margins	❏
• Movement on swallowing	❏
• Relaxation of sternocleidomastoid muscle	❏
• Size and symmetry	❏
• Consistency	❏
• Presence of nodules	❏
• Tenderness	❏
Technique	
• Examines using bimanual technique	❏
• Anterior and posterior approaches	❏
Bonus point	
• Auscultation of the gland	❏
Drapes the patient appropriately	❏
Makes appropriate closing remarks	❏

INSTRUCTIONS TO CANDIDATE: A 28-year-old female is referred for assessment of Addison's disease. Perform a focused physical examination and describe your findings.

Key Points	Satisfactorily Carried out
Introduces self to the patient	❏
Determines how the patient wishes to be addressed	❏
Explains nature of the examination to the patient	❏
Examines the patient in a logical fashion	❏
Increased pigmentation	
• Sun-exposed areas	❏
• Pressure areas	❏
• Palmar creases	❏
• Nipples	❏
• Scars	❏
• Mucous membranes	❏
Vitiligo	❏
Loss of axillary and pubic hair in females	❏
Postural hypotension	❏
Mental status examination	❏
Drapes the patient appropriately	❏
Makes appropriate closing remarks	❏

INSTRUCTIONS TO CANDIDATE: A 32-year-old male with acromegaly presents to his endocrinologist for follow-up evaluation. Examine the head, neck, and skin for clinical signs associated with this condition. Describe your findings.

Key Points	Satisfactorily Carried out
Introduces self to the patient	❏
Determines how the patient wishes to be addressed	❏
Explains nature of the examination to the patient	❏
Examines the patient in a logical fashion	❏
Skin	
• Thick and coarse	❏
• Increased body hair	❏
• Oily skin	❏
• Acanthosis nigricans	❏
• Acne	❏
Head and neck	
• Prognathism	❏
• Increased space between the teeth	❏
• Large nose	❏
• Prominent supraorbital ridge	❏
• Large tongue	❏
• Visual fields	❏
Drapes the patient appropriately	❏
Makes appropriate closing remarks	❏

CHAPTER 10

Obstetrics and Gynecology

OBJECTIVES

ANATOMY

ESSENTIAL CLINICAL COMPETENCIES
   APPROACH TO THE OBSTETRIC/GYNECOLOGIC HISTORY
   PERFORM A FOCUSED PHYSICAL EXAMINATION OF THE BREAST

SAMPLE OSCE SCENARIOS
* A 61-year-old female presents to her family doctor after finding a lump in her right breast. Take a detailed history, focusing on risk factors for malignancy.
* An 18-year-old female, G_1P_0, presents to the labor and delivery unit with "contractions." She concealed her pregnancy until recently. Take a detailed history. Determine the gestational age and presenting part using the Leopold maneuvers.
* A 32-year-old female, G_2P_1, presents to the labor and delivery unit with painless bleeding. She is 37 weeks gestation by dates. Perform a focused history and physical examination.
* A 25-year-old female, G_1P_0, presents to the labor and delivery unit with intermittent abdominal and back pain. She is 27 weeks gestation by ultrasound. Perform a focused history and physical examination.
* A 32-year-old female presents with fever and lower abdominal pain for 12 hours. She also has noted some foul smelling vaginal discharge. Perform a focused history and physical examination.
* A 21-year-old female presents to her family doctor with a history of several "missed" periods. Until last year she had regular menses. Take a detailed history, exploring possible etiologies.
* A 29-year-old female, with a 1-week-old infant, presents to her family doctor with difficulty breast-feeding. She is concerned that the baby is not getting enough milk. Take an appropriate history.

SAMPLE CHECKLISTS
- ❏ A 48-year-old female presents to your office after finding a lump during routine breast self-examination. Take a detailed history, focusing on risk factors for malignancy.
- ❏ A 32-year-old female presents to the emergency department with a fractured wrist and some facial contusions. Perform a "screen" for intimate partner violence and counsel.

OBJECTIVES

*The successful student should be able to take a **focused** obstetric and gynecologic **history**, including:*
* Menarche
* Menstrual cycle
* Premenstrual syndrome (PMS), dysmenorrhea
* Menopause, postmenopausal bleeding
* Sexual history, including sexual practices, sexual dysfunction, and number of partners
* Contraception
* Sexually transmitted infections (STIs): Vaginal discharge, labial sores/lesions
* Pelvic pain

- Breast lumps, nipple discharge
- Past Pap smears and mammography
- Pregnancy (past and current)
- Labor, contractions, and rupture of membranes
- Preterm labor
- *Per vaginam* (PV) bleeding during pregnancy: First trimester, third trimester

*The obstetric and gynecologic **examination** will include:*

Inspection
- Vulva: Labia, clitoris, and vaginal introitus
- Vaginal discharge
- Urethral meatus
- Speculum examination: cervix, vaginal walls
- Gravid abdomen
- Breast: Discharge, dimpling, skin retraction, peau d'orange, eczema/rash, and local swelling or discoloration

Auscultation
- Fetal heart tones
- Uterine soufflé

Palpation
- Vulva: Labia, Bartholin's glands
- Cervix: Open os versus closed os, cervical motion tenderness
- Bimanual examination: Adnexa, uterus
- Rectovaginal examination
- Breast: Note size, shape, symmetry, consistency, contour, warmth, and tenderness of any lesions
- Leopold maneuvers

ANATOMY

Vulva
- The external female genitalia, known as the **vulva,** consists of the mons veneris, labia majora, labia minora, clitoris, urethral meatus, vaginal introitus, Bartholin's gland, and posterior fourchette (Figure 10-1).
- The **labia majora** are wide skin folds that form the lateral margins of the vulva. It is the developmental equivalent to the male scrotum. The **labia majora** meet posteriorly to form the **posterior fourchette.**
- The **labia minora** are narrow skin folds that lie medial to the labia majora. They vary in size and may be barely noticeable in some. Contrary to the labia majora, which are covered in hair and have sebaceous glands, the labia minora have neither.
- The labia minora meet anteriorly to form the **prepuce** of the clitoris. The **clitoris** is the female equivalent to the male penis. Like the penis the clitoris is composed of erectile tissue. However, only the glans of the clitoris is visible externally.
- The female urethra is four to five times shorter than the male urethra. The **urethral meatus** is found directly inferior to the clitoris and is the opening through which urine passes externally.
- The **vaginal introitus** is the opening to the vagina and marks the division between external and internal genitalia. Inferolateral to the introitus and medial to the labia minora are **Bartholin's glands.** Secretions from these glands add lubrication during intercourse. These glands may become obstructed, infected, and painful.

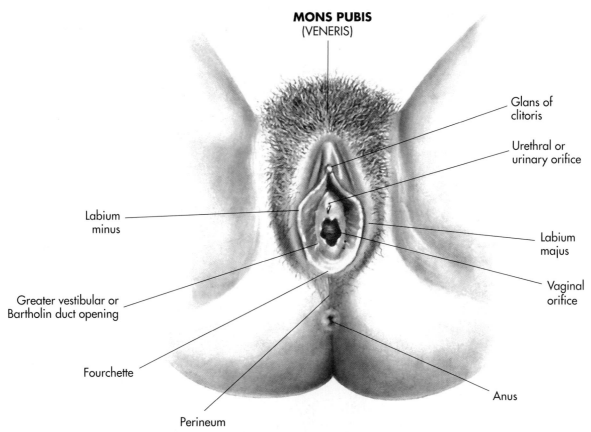

Figure 10-1 External female genitalia. (Adapted from Seidel HM, Dains JE, Ball JW, Benedict GW: *Mosby's guide to physical examination,* ed 5, St. Louis, 2003, Mosby, p 585, Figure 17-1.)

Internal Genitalia

- The internal female genitalia consist of the vagina, cervix, uterus, fallopian tubes, and ovaries (Figure 10-2).
- The **vagina** is a muscular tube that begins at the vaginal introitus and terminates at the cervix. It functions to accommodate sexual intercourse, impregnation, and childbirth.
- The **cervix** is the most inferior portion of the uterus. The cervical os is the opening to the interior of the uterus. Clinically the cervix is assessed by palpation and can be inspected with the aid of a speculum. During labor the cervix dilates to allow delivery.
- The **uterus** is a pear-shaped, hollow muscular organ. The inferior aspect is the cervix, and the superior aspect is the fundus. The innermost lining of the uterus is shed monthly in menstruating women. The uterus can be palpated in bimanual pelvic examination and its position described (Figure 10-3).
- The **fallopian tubes** emerge from the horns of the uterus and open into the peritoneal cavity. This provides a communication from the external environment through the vagina and cervix into the peritoneum.
- The fimbriae of the fallopian tube terminate at the **ovary.** The ovary is the counterpart of the testicle. It produces sex hormones and eggs that can be fertilized by sperm.

Breasts

- The **breasts,** or mammary glands, are part of the female reproductive system. They function to provide nourishment to the infant through **lactation.**

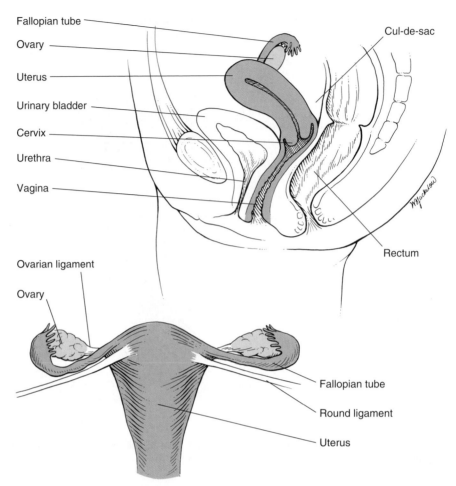

Figure 10-2 Internal female genitalia. (From Swartz M: *Textbook of physical diagnosis: history and examination,* ed 4, Philadelphia, 2002, WB Saunders, Figure 18-2.)

- Accessory breast tissue may be present along the embryonic milk lines (Figure 10-4).
- Each breast has lobules of glandular tissue that produce breast milk. These lobules are drained by **lactiferous ducts,** which drain into **lactiferous sinuses** behind the areola (Figure 10-5). The ducts open onto the **nipple,** the prominence at the center of the pigmented **areola.**
- The bulk of the breast tissue is lobular fat.
- The breast is separated from the pectoral muscle by deep fascia. **Suspensory ligaments** run from this fascia to the skin and are otherwise known as Cooper's ligaments.

ESSENTIAL CLINICAL COMPETENCIES

APPROACH TO THE OBSTETRIC/GYNECOLOGIC HISTORY

- **ID:** Age, occupation, relationship with partner, gravida, and parity
- Use **ChLORIDE FPP** to structure your approach to the presenting complaint.

Menstrual History
- Age at menarche
- Duration of menstrual cycle
- Duration and character of menses: Amount of flow (number of pads/tampons), presence of clots, and dysmenorrhea

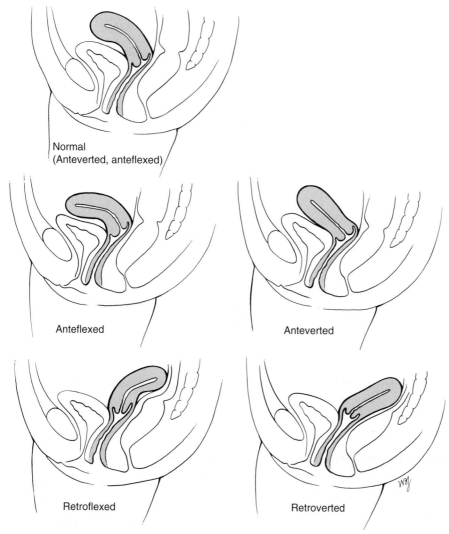

Figure 10-3 Describing uterine position. (From Swartz M: *Textbook of physical diagnosis: history and examination,* ed 4, Philadelphia, 2002, WB Saunders, Figure 18-35.)

- PMS: Bloating, breast tenderness, mood changes, decreased concentration and motivation, food cravings
- Age of menopause and associated symptoms: Fatigue, hot flashes, nervousness/irritability, headache, insomnia, depression, aches/pains, vaginal itch/dryness
- Postmenopausal bleeding
- Hormone replacement therapy (HRT)

Sexual History
- Age of first sexual intercourse
- Number of sexual partners
- Previous STIs
- Use of precautions, such as condoms (STI prevention), and use of contraceptive devices

Obstetric History
- Blood type: Rh positive versus Rh negative
- Date of last menstrual period (LMP)
- Infertility: A couple who has not conceived after attempting to conceive for 1 year

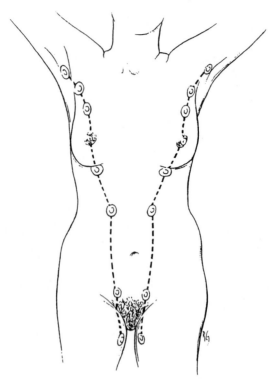

Figure 10-4 Embryonic milk line. (From Powell DE, Stelling CB: *The diagnosis and detection of breast tissue*, St. Louis, 1994, Mosby, Figure 1-1A.)

- **Nägele's rule** for estimated date of confinement (EDC)
  - EDC = date of LMP − 3 months + 7 days + 1 year
- Contraceptive use (e.g., oral contraceptive pill [OCP] may change the reliability of the LMP).
- Pregnancy history: Bleeding, discharge, premature rupture of membranes (PROM), nausea/vomiting (N/V), STIs, other infections, gestational diabetes mellitus (DM), anemia, gastroesophageal reflux (GER)
- $G_?$ $P_?$ $A_?$ (term/preterm/stillbirths/abortions): Gravida, parity, and abortions
- Date and gestation at delivery
- Onset of labor: Spontaneous versus induced
- Duration of labor: Use of augmentation
- Type of anesthetic: Oral/intravenous pain medications, NO_2, epidural
- Type of delivery: Normal spontaneous vaginal delivery (NSVD), lower segment cesarean section (LSCS), use of forceps or vacuum
- Episiotomy: Midline versus mediolateral
- Maternal complications: Tears (first degree to fourth degree), postpartum hemorrhage (PPH), infection
- Newborn: Sex, weight, breast-fed versus bottle-fed, complications, and general health

Pap History
- Date of last Pap smear
- History of abnormal Pap smears and type of follow-up evaluation and investigations
- History of human papillomavirus (HPV)
- **Past medical history (PMH):** Bleeding diathesis, DM, hypertension (HTN), cardiovascular disease, thyroid problems, renal problems, anemia, epilepsy, asthma, STIs, psychiatric problems, anesthetic problems, or malignancy

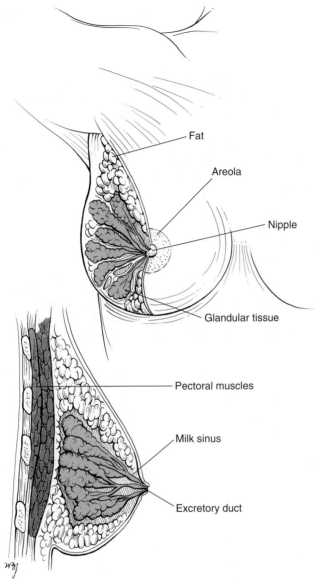

Figure 10-5   Breast anatomy. (From Swartz M: *Textbook of physical diagnosis: history and examination*, ed 4, Philadelphia, 2002, WB Saunders, p 408, Figure 15-1.)

- **Past surgical history (PSH):** Previous surgery (including cryotherapy and loop electrocautery excision procedure [LEEP]), complications, or trauma
- **Medications (MEDS):** It is important to document all medications (prescription and over the counter [OTC]) and consider all effects on pregnancy.
- **Allergies**
- **Social history (SH):** Nutrition, folic acid, smoking history, present smoking status, exposure to second-hand smoke, EtOH intake, street drugs, family support, and occupational/financial situation
- **Immunizations:** Routine immunizations and immune status/exposure to infectious diseases such as rubella, HIV, hepatitis B virus (HBV), and syphilis
- **Family history (FH):** Malformations, developmental delay, known hereditary disorders, or DM

PERFORM A FOCUSED PHYSICAL EXAMINATION OF THE BREAST

Inspection

- Inspect both breasts. Ask the patient to sit with arms at her side, arms overhead, and with hands resting on the knees (Figure 10-6). Finally ask the patient to lie supine, and inspect the breast with the ipsilateral arm resting under the head (Figure 10-7). Using these different positions helps to accentuate dimpling, skin retraction, or asymmetry between the breasts.
- Comment on breast symmetry, and note the direction to which each nipple points (it should be similar). Note dimpling, skin retraction, peau d'orange, eczema/rash, local swelling, or discoloration. Assess the color, quantity, consistency, and odor of any breast/nipple discharge.

Palpation

- With the patient supine ask her to place her ipsilateral hand behind her head (see Figure 10-7).
- Wear gloves if open lesions are present or discharge is observed.
- Begin by palpating at the junction of the clavicle and sternum. Follow a grid pattern, palpating each quadrant, medially to laterally and back (Figure 10-8). Do not neglect breast tissue in the axillary area and below the breast. Use the pads of your second, third, and fourth fingers in a rotatory motion, applying light, moderate, and deeper pressure.
- Palpate around the areola, noting the presence of discharge.
- Palpate supraclavicular, infraclavicular, and axillary lymph nodes. In large-breasted women it may be easier to examine axillary nodes in a sitting position.
- Describe the size, shape, location (Figure 10-9), consistency, and contour of any lesions (Box 10-1). Note tenderness, pulsatility, warmth, and color.
- You may be asked to simulate a breast examination using a **breast model** (synthetic). Consider the things that cannot be adequately assessed using a breast model:
  - Assessment of skin changes: Color, dimpling, skin retraction, eczema/rash, and peau d'orange
  - Assessment of nipple discharge
  - Assessment of warmth and tenderness
  - Palpation of breast tissue in axillae and axillary lymph nodes
  - Needle aspiration/core biopsy

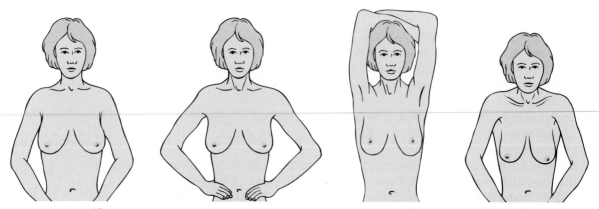

Figure 10-6 Positions for breast inspection. (From Munro JF, Campbell IW, editors: *Macleod's clinical examination,* ed 10, Edinburgh, 2000, Churchill Livingstone, p 66, Figure 2.53.)

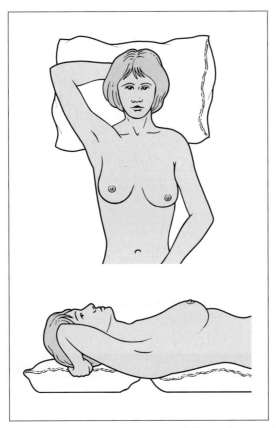

Figure 10-7   Position for breast palpation. (From Munro JF, Campbell IW, editors: *Macleod's clinical examination*, ed 10, Edinburgh, 2000, Churchill Livingstone, p 66, Figure 2.54.)

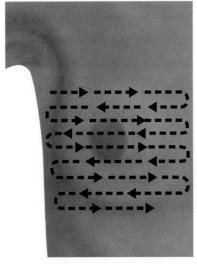

Figure 10-8   Method of breast palpation. (Based on Seidel HM, Ball JW, Dains JE, Benedict GB: *Mosby's guide to physical examination*, ed 5, St. Louis, 2003, Mosby, p 510, Figure 15-13.)

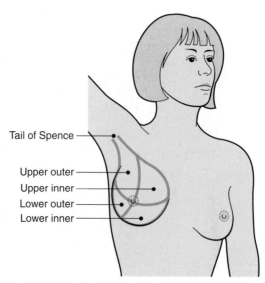

Tail of Spence

Upper outer
Upper inner
Lower outer
Lower inner

Figure 10-9 Terms to describe location of a breast lesion. (From Munro JF, Campbell IW, editors: *Macleod's clinical examination,* ed 10, Edinburgh, 2000, Churchill Livingstone, p 65, Figure 2.52.)

Box 10-1   Findings Associated with Breast Malignancy

- Hard, fixed lump with irregular borders
- Asymmetry, fixation of lesion to chest wall
- Skin changes: Retraction, dimpling, peau d'orange, and ulceration
- Nipple retraction or inversion and bloody discharge
- Lymphadenopathy: Axillary, infraclavicular, and supraclavicular
- Edema of ipsilateral arm (lymphedema or venous obstruction)
- Metastasis: Hepatomegaly, lung nodules, pleural effusion, bone pain, and seizure (central nervous system metastases)

SAMPLE OSCE SCENARIOS

> INSTRUCTIONS TO CANDIDATE: A 61-year-old female presents to her family doctor after finding a lump in her right breast. Take a detailed history, focusing on risk factors for malignancy.

DD$_X$ VITAMINS C
- **Traumatic:** Fat necrosis
- **Idiopathic/Iatrogenic:** Fibrocystic changes, cystic lesion (e.g., galactocele, abscess)
- **Neoplastic:** Breast malignancy (Box 10-2), mammary duct ectasia, intraductal papilloma, and fibroadenoma

History
- **Character:** What does the lump feel like?
  - Shape
  - Consistency: Hard versus soft, nodular versus uniform, and mobile versus fixed
  - Contour: Well-defined regular margins versus ill-defined irregular margins
  - Tenderness? Redness? Warmth?
- **Location:** Medial, lateral, superior, inferior, and central. In which breast did you find the lump (e.g., right breast)?
- **Onset:** When/how did you first notice the lump? Do you perform monthly self-examinations?
  - What was the lump like when you first noticed it?
  - Has there been any change in the size or consistency of the lump or in any other feature?
  - Does the lump change with relation to your menstrual cycle?
- **Radiation:** Have you ever had radiation therapy or been exposed to radiation?
- **Intensity:** How large is the lump? Is it a single lump or multiple lumps?
- **Duration:** How long have you had this lump in your breast?
- **Events associated:**
  - Any retraction of skin or nipple or dimpling?
  - Skin changes: Eczema/rash on the breast, ulceration, peau d'orange (like the skin of an orange)
  - Nipple discharge: Bloody, milky, serous, or purulent (green or straw-colored fluid is less worrisome)
  - Trauma (Fat necrosis)

Box 10-2   Historical Risk Factors for Breast Malignancy

- Age: >40 years, female sex
- Age of menarche: <13 years
- Age of menopause: >50 years
- Parity: Nulliparity, late first pregnancy (>30 years)
- History of breast malignancy/dysplasia/atypia
- Paget's disease of the breast
- Lynch II syndrome: Endometrial, ovarian, and colon
- Radiation therapy/exposure
- Obesity, diet high in fats, and excessive EtOH consumption
- Family history: Breast cancer in first-degree relatives, Lynch II syndrome

- Constitutional symptoms: Fever, chills, night sweats, weight loss, anorexia, and asthenia
- Frequency: Have you had any breast lumps before this one? If so, when? How frequently do you notice lumps?
- Palliative factors: Is there anything that makes the lump better? If so, what?
- Provocative factors: Is there anything that makes the lump worse? If so, what?
  - Menses?
- **Previous investigations:** Breast biopsy, mammogram, and cytology (cyst aspiration, nipple discharge)
  - What were the results?
- **PMH/PSH:** Previous breast malignancy/dysplasia, breast lumps, fibrocystic changes, other medical problems, previous surgery, or trauma
- **MEDS:** Immunosuppressive medications increase the risk of malignancy
- **SH:** Nutrition, smoking history, EtOH intake, street drugs, and family support
- **FH:** Breast cancer in first-degree relatives, Lynch II syndrome (breast, endometrial, ovarian, colon)

INSTRUCTIONS TO CANDIDATE: An 18-year-old female, G_1P_0, presents to the labor and delivery unit with "contractions." She concealed her pregnancy until recently. Take a detailed history. Determine the gestational age and presenting part using the Leopold maneuvers.

History
- **Character:** Tell me about the contractions. What are they like? Sharp? Crampy? Dull?
- **Location:** Where does the pain originate?
- **Onset:** When did it start? How did it come on (sudden versus gradual)?
- **Radiation:** Does the pain move anywhere?
- Intensity: How severe is the pain on a scale of 1 to 10, with 1 being mild pain and 10 being the worst? Is it getting better, worse, or staying the same?
- **Duration:** How long does each contraction last (quantify in seconds or minutes)?
- Events associated:
  - PV bleeding?
  - Leakage of fluid (rupture of membranes [ROM])?
  - Fetal movements?
- Frequency: Have you ever had this before? How often does the pain come (quantify in minutes)? Does it come regularly?
- **Palliative factors:** Is there anything that makes it better? If so, what?
- **Provocative factors:** Is there anything that makes it worse? If so, what?

Pregnancy History
- This aspect of the history is pivotal, especially determination of the gestational age. Because of the concealment of the pregnancy, she likely has not received prenatal care.
- **Nägele's rule:** EDC = date of LMP – 3 months + 7 days + 1 year
  - Nägele's rule depends on menstrual cycles that span 28 to 30 days and are regular.
  - Duration of menstrual cycle? Are your cycles regular? LMP?
  - Contraceptive use (e.g., OCP may change the reliability of the LMP)?
- When did you first get a positive pregnancy test?
- When did you first note fetal movement? Date of quickening is usually 18 to 20 weeks in a primigravida patient.
- Blood type: Rh positive versus Rh negative
- Pregnancy history: Bleeding, discharge, N/V, gestational DM, anemia, or GER

- STIs: Previous and current infections, especially gonococcus and herpes (may preclude vaginal delivery)
- Type of anesthetic desired for labor and delivery: Oral/IV pain medications, NO_2, epidural, or no medications at all
- **PMH:** Bleeding diathesis, DM, HTN, cardiovascular disease, thyroid problems, renal problems, anemia, epilepsy, asthma, STIs, psychiatric problems, or anesthetic problems
- **PSH:** Previous surgery (including cryotherapy and LEEP), complications, or trauma
- **MEDS:** It is important to document all medications (prescription and OTC) taken during pregnancy
- **Allergies**
- **SH:** Nutrition, folic acid, smoking history, EtOH intake and street drugs during pregnancy, family support, occupational/financial situation, and relationship with the infant's father
- **Immunizations:** Routine immunizations and immune status/exposure to infectious diseases such as rubella, HIV, HBV, and syphilis
- **FH:** Malformations, developmental delay, or known hereditary disorders

Leopold Maneuvers

- The **Leopold maneuvers** are used to determine fetal lie, presentation, and position. These maneuvers are not useful before 28 weeks gestation.
- The fetal **lie** refers to the relationship of the fetal long axis to the maternal long axis.
  - Oblique
  - Transverse
  - Longitudinal
- The fetal **presentation** refers to the part of the fetus that first passes through the birthing canal.
  - Cephalic
  - Breech
- The **position** of the fetus refers to the relationship of the fetus to the maternal pelvis. In cephalic presentations the position is defined in relation to the occiput, whereas breech presentations are defined with respect to the fetal sacrum.
- **First maneuver** (Figure 10-10, A): Facing the patient's head, palpate the fundus of the uterus to determine which part of the fetus occupies the fundus (head versus bottom). The head feels firm, round, and smooth.
- **Second maneuver** (Figure 10-10, B): Place your hands on either side of the abdomen to determine on which side the fetal back lies. The back is linear and firm, whereas the extremities are lumpy. Use one hand to steady the uterus and the other to palpate the fetus.
- **Third maneuver** (Figure 10-10, C): Place one hand just above the symphysis pubis to determine the presenting part. Grasp the presenting part between the thumb and forefinger. The vertex will feel round, firm, and ballottable, whereas the breech is irregular.
- **Fourth maneuver** (Figure 10-10, D): This maneuver is done facing the patient's feet. Place your hands on the lower abdomen just above the pelvic inlet to determine the side of cephalic prominence. Exert pressure toward the inlet. One hand usually descends further than the other, which is stopped by the cephalic prominence. If the cephalic prominence is on the same side as the fetal parts, the head is flexed. Alternatively if the prominence is on the same side as the fetal back, the head is extended.

Fundal Height

- Estimate **gestational age** by measuring **fundal height** from the pubis symphysis to the superior border of the fundus (Figure 10-11). In the third trimester this measurement in centimeters is equivalent to the gestational age in weeks.

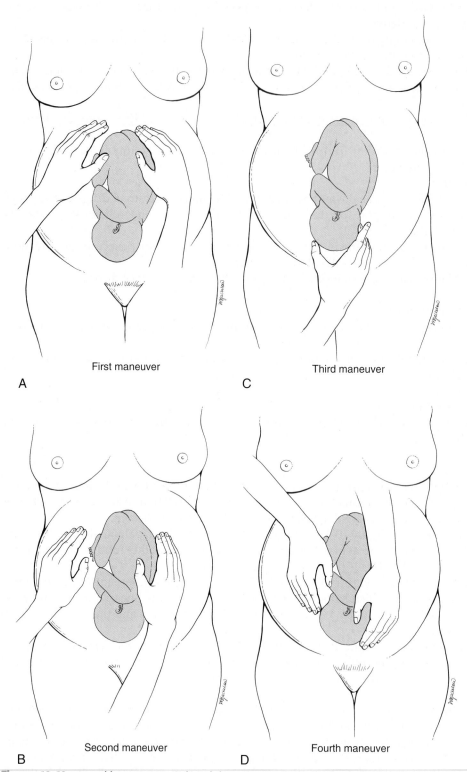

First maneuver

A

Third maneuver

C

Second maneuver

B

Fourth maneuver

D

Figure 10-10 Leopold maneuvers. (Adapted from Swartz M: *Textbook of physical diagnosis: history and examination,* ed 4, Philadelphia, 2002, WB Saunders, Figures 22-14, -15, -16, -17, *B*.)

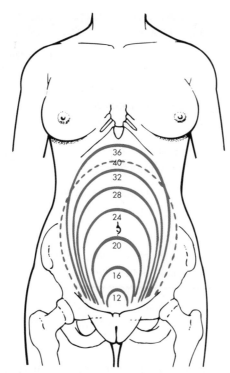

Figure 10-11   Measuring fundal height. (From Seidel HM, Ball JW, Dains JE, Benedict GB: *Mosby's guide to physical examination,* ed 5, St. Louis, 2003, Mosby, p 623, Figure 17-32.)

INSTRUCTIONS TO CANDIDATE: A 32-year-old female, G_2P_1, presents to the labor and delivery unit with painless bleeding. She is 37 weeks gestation by dates. Perform a focused history and physical examination.

DD_x VITAMINS C
- **V**ascular: Placenta previa, vasa previa
- **T**raumatic: Trauma or lesion on the external genitalia
- **I**diopathic/**I**atrogenic: Cervicitis
- **N**eoplastic: Cervical polyp, cervical malignancy
- Although her bleeding is painless, still include placental abruption in the differential diagnosis.

History
- **Ch**aracter: What color is the blood (bright red versus dark red versus brown)? Any clots? Are you still bleeding?
- **L**ocation: Where is the blood coming from (vaginal, vulvar, bowel, bladder)?
- **O**nset: How did this start (sudden versus gradual)?
- **I**ntensity: How much blood have you passed (quantify using number of pads/tampons)?
- **D**uration: How long have you been bleeding?
- **E**vents associated:
  - Fetal movements?
  - Blood type: Rh positive versus Rh negative
  - Have you had an ultrasound during this pregnancy? When?

Table 10-1   Risk Factors for Placenta Previa and Placental Abruption

	Risk Factors
Placenta previa	Previous placenta previa Grand multiparity Multiple gestation Increased maternal age Uterine scar (previous LSCS, therapeutic abortion [TA], or myomectomy)
Placental abruption	Previous placental abruption Hypertension, preeclampsia Trauma PROM Cigarette smoking, cocaine use Folate deficiency

- Placenta previa (Table 10-1): Previous bleeding with spontaneous resolution, no abdominal pain or tenderness
- Vasa previa: Painless bleeding (because it is fetal blood, even a small amount can be catastrophic)
- Pregnancy history: Bleeding, discharge, PROM, N/V, infections/STIs, gestational DM, anemia, or GER
- Placental abruption (see Table 10-1): Abdominal pain and tenderness, dark blood
- Labor: Uterine contractions
- Trauma? Recent sexual intercourse?
- **Frequency:** Has this ever happened to you before? If so, when? How often do you bleed?
- **Palliative factors:** Is there anything that seems to slow the bleeding? If so, what?
- **Provocative factors:** Is there anything that seems to make it worse? If so, what?
- **Past obstetric history:** Previous placenta previa, previous placental abruptions, preterm cesarean section, gestation at delivery, type of delivery, maternal complications (tears, PPH, infection), or complications and general health of the newborn
- **PMH/PSH:** Bleeding diathesis, liver disease, urogenital malignancy, abnormal Pap smears, or urogenital surgery
- **MEDS and Allergies**
- **SH:** Smoking, EtOH, street drugs (e.g., cocaine), and physical abuse

Physical Examination
- **Vitals:** Heart rate (HR), blood pressure (BP), respiratory rate (RR), and temperature
  - Obstetric vitals also include the fetal HR and its trends (beat-to-beat variability, accelerations).
- **General:** Apprehension, apparent distress. Check capillary refill.
- **Respiratory (Resp):** Chest expansion (symmetry), auscultation (breath sounds, adventitious sounds)
- **Cardiovascular system (CVS):** Measure the jugular venous pressure (JVP). Palpate peripheral pulses. Note pulse volume, contour, and rhythm. Auscultate the heart, looking for extra heart sounds or flow murmurs associated with hyperdynamic circulation.

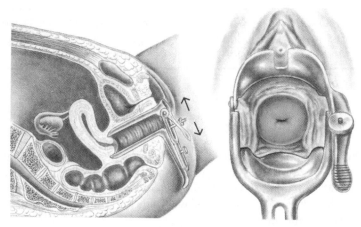

Figure 10-12   Speculum examination. (From Seidel HM, Ball JW, Dains JE, Benedict GB: *Mosby's guide to physical examination*, ed 5, St Louis, 2003, Mosby, p 605, Figure 17-16, *D*.)

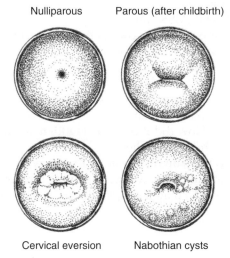

Nulliparous   Parous (after childbirth)

Cervical eversion   Nabothian cysts

Figure 10-13   Cervical descriptors. (From Wilson SF, Giddens JF: *Health assessment for nursing practice*, ed 2, St. Louis, 2001, Mosby, p 540, Figure 21-16.)

- **Abdomen:** Inspect the abdomen. Auscultate for bowel sounds. Percuss lightly. Perform light and deep palpation, and identify any masses or areas of tenderness. At 37 weeks, the uterus occupies nearly all of the palpable abdomen. In placental abruption the uterus is exquisitely tender.
- **Obstetric/Gynecologic (Obs/Gyne):** Measure the fundal height from the pubis symphysis (height in centimeters correlates with gestational age in weeks in the third trimester). Use the Leopold maneuvers to determine the position, presentation, and lie of the infant (see Figure 10-10). In placenta previa the presenting part is high riding and not engaged in the pelvis. It is important to perform a speculum examination of the cervix (Figure 10-12). Inspect the cervical os, and note any discharge, inflammation, or lesions (Figure 10-13). If the speculum examination is unremarkable, proceed with a manual PV examination. Do not perform a blind PV examination because this may incite catastrophic bleeding in placenta previa or vasa previa. Note whether the os is open or closed.

> INSTRUCTIONS TO CANDIDATE: A 25-year-old female, G_1P_0, presents to the labor and delivery unit with intermittent abdominal and back pain. She is 27 weeks gestation by ultrasound. Perform a focused history and physical examination.

Definition
- **Preterm labor** is the onset of labor before 37 weeks gestation. It is diagnosed based on documented, regular uterine contractions (four per 20 minutes) and cervical effacement of 80% or dilation of >2 cm. The onset of spontaneous preterm labor is usually idiopathic. Prematurity (20 to 37 weeks gestation) is the leading cause of perinatal morbidity and mortality.
- **Maternal risk factors:** Previous preterm delivery, uterine abnormalities, incompetent cervix, PV bleeding, bacterial vaginosis, smoking, maternal age <18 or >40 years, low socioeconomic status (SES), drug addiction, and poor nutrition

DD$_X$ VITAMINS C
- **I**nfectious: Pyelonephritis
- **T**raumatic: Musculoskeletal (MSK) injury
- **I**diopathic/**I**atrogenic: Braxton-Hicks contractions, preterm labor, and renal colic
- **S**ubstance abuse and **P**sychiatric: Cocaine use

History
- **Ch**aracter: Tell me about the pain. What is it like? Sharp? Crampy? Dull?
- **L**ocation: Where does the pain originate?
- **O**nset: When did it start? How did it come on (sudden versus gradual)?
- **R**adiation: Does the pain move anywhere?
- **I**ntensity: How severe is the pain on a scale of 1 to 10, with 1 being mild pain and 10 being the worst? Is it getting better, worse, or staying the same?
- **D**uration: How long does the pain last (quantify in seconds or minutes)?
- **E**vents associated:
  - PV bleeding?
  - Leakage of fluid (ROM)?
  - Fetal movements?
- **F**requency: Have you ever had this before? How often does the pain come (quantify in minutes)? Does it come regularly?
- **P**alliative factors: Is there anything that makes it better? If so, what?
- **P**rovocative factors: Is there anything that makes it worse? If so, what?

Pregnancy History
- This aspect of the history is pivotal, especially confirmation of the gestational age.
- **Nägele's rule:** EDC = date of LMP − 3 months + 7 days + 1 year
  - Nägele's rule depends on menstrual cycles that span 28 to 30 days and are regular.
  - Duration of menstrual cycle? Are your cycles regular? LMP?
  - Contraceptive use (e.g., OCP may change the reliability of the LMP)?
- When did you first get a positive pregnancy test?
- When did you first note fetal movement? Date of quickening is usually 18 to 20 weeks in a primigravida patient.
- Have you had an ultrasound?
- Blood type: Rh positive versus Rh negative
- Pregnancy history: Bleeding, discharge, N/V, gestational DM, anemia, or GER
- STIs: Previous and current infections, especially gonococcus and herpes (may preclude vaginal delivery)

- **PMH:** Bleeding diathesis, DM, HTN, cardiovascular disease, thyroid problems, renal problems, anemia, epilepsy, asthma, STIs, psychiatric problems, or anesthetic problems
- **PSH:** Previous surgery (including cryotherapy and LEEP), complications, or trauma
- **MEDS and Allergies**
- **SH:** Nutrition, folic acid, smoking history, EtOH intake and street drugs during pregnancy, family support, occupational/financial situation, and relationship with the infant's father
- **Immunizations:** Routine immunizations and immune status/exposure to infectious diseases such as rubella, HIV, hepatitis B virus (HBV), and syphilis
- **FH:** Malformations, developmental delay, or known hereditary disorders

Physical Examination

- **Vitals:** HR, BP, RR, and temperature
  - Obstetric vitals also include the fetal HR and its trends (beat-to-beat variability, accelerations).
- **General:** Apprehension, apparent distress. Check capillary refill.
- **Resp:** Chest expansion (symmetry), auscultation (breath sounds, adventitious sounds)
- **CVS:** Measure the JVP. Palpate peripheral pulses. Note pulse volume, contour, and rhythm. Auscultate the heart, looking for extra heart sounds or flow murmurs associated with hyperdynamic circulation.
- **Abdomen:** Inspect the abdomen. Auscultate for bowel sounds. Percuss lightly. Perform light and deep palpation, and identify any masses or areas of tenderness.
- **Obs/Gyne:** Measure the fundal height from the pubis symphysis (height in centimeters correlates with gestational age in weeks in the third trimester). Use the Leopold maneuvers to determine the position, presentation, and lie of the infant (see Figure 10-10). If there is any bleeding perform a speculum examination of the cervix (see Figure 10-12). Inspect the cervical os, and note any discharge, inflammation, or lesions. If the speculum examination is unremarkable proceed with a manual PV examination. Note whether the os is open or closed. Document effacement and dilation of the cervix.

INSTRUCTIONS TO CANDIDATE: A 32-year-old female presents with fever and lower abdominal pain for 12 hours. She also has noted some foul smelling vaginal discharge. Perform a focused history and physical examination.

DD$_X$ VITAMINS C

- **Infectious:** Pelvic inflammatory disease (PID)/tuboovarian abscess, cystitis, pyelonephritis, and psoas abscess
- **Traumatic:** MSK injury
- **Idiopathic/Iatrogenic:** Ruptured ectopic pregnancy, ovarian torsion, renal colic, appendicitis, mesenteric adenitis, diverticulitis, incarcerated hernia, and inflammatory bowel disease (IBD)

History

- **Character:** What is the pain like? Sharp? Crampy? Dull? What is the vaginal discharge like (color, consistency, odor)?
- **Location:** Where does the pain originate?
- **Onset:** When did the pain start? How did it come on (sudden versus gradual)? When did the vaginal discharge start? What is the temporal relationship to your menstrual cycle?
- **Radiation:** Does the pain move anywhere?

- **Intensity:** How severe is the pain on a scale of 1 to 10, with 1 being mild pain and 10 being the worst? How much discharge are you having (quantify using number of pads/tampons)? Are the symptoms getting better, worse, or staying the same?
- **Duration:** How long has the pain been there (12 hours)? How long have you had the discharge (acute versus chronic)?
- **Events associated:**
  - PID: Intermenstrual bleeding, vaginal discharge, fever, pain
  - Pregnancy: LMP, PV bleeding
  - Appendicitis: Fever, N/V, anorexia, initial dull central abdominal pain that later localizes to the right lower quadrant (RLQ)
  - Cystitis: Urinary frequency, dysuria, hematuria, urinary retention, urgency, strangury, incontinence
  - Intestinal obstruction/incarcerated hernia: Obstipation, feculent vomitus, pain
  - IBD: Chronic diarrhea, weight loss, extraintestinal manifestations (e.g., uveitis, erythema nodosum, peripheral arthritis)
- **Frequency:** Have you ever had this pain before? How often does the pain come (intermittent versus constant)? Have you ever had this discharge before? If so, when? How often do you notice it?
- **Palliative factors:** Is there anything that makes the pain better? If so, what?
  - Lying in one position?
- **Provocative factors:** Is there anything that makes the pain worse? If so, what?
  - Movement?
- **PMH/PSH:** STIs, PID, ectopic pregnancy, diverticular disease, previous surgeries, malignancy, IBD, or renal colic
- **MEDS:** Analgesics, antibiotics
- **SH:** Smoking, EtOH, street drugs, and sexual history

Physical Examination

- **Vitals:** HR, BP, RR, and temperature
  - Note fever and any tachycardia or hypotension.
- **General:** Check capillary refill. Note patient position on the stretcher and whether she is moving.
- **Resp:** Chest expansion (symmetry), auscultation (breath sounds, adventitious sounds)
- **CVS:** Measure the JVP. Palpate peripheral pulses. Note pulse volume, contour, and rhythm. Auscultate the heart, looking for extra heart sounds or flow murmurs associated with hyperdynamic circulation.
- **Abdomen:** Inspect the abdomen. Auscultate for bowel sounds (may be decreased in peritonitis). Percuss lightly in all four quadrants. Percussion will produce pain in a patient with peritonitis. Before palpation ask the patient to cough and point to the most tender area with one finger. Palpate the most tender area last. Perform light and deep palpation, and identify any masses or areas of tenderness. Check for rebound tenderness. Examine the liver and spleen. Perform a digital rectal examination (DRE). A retrocecal appendix may produce tenderness on palpation of the rectal walls.
- **Genitourinary (GU):** It is important to perform a pelvic examination. Inspect the cervical os, and note any discharge, inflammation, or lesions. The cervix may appear inflamed and friable in PID. If the speculum examination is unremarkable proceed with a bimanual pelvic examination. Note any discharge, cervical motion tenderness, adnexal tenderness, or pelvic masses.

INSTRUCTIONS TO CANDIDATE: A 21-year-old female presents to her family doctor with a history of several "missed" periods. Until last year she had regular menses. Take a detailed history, exploring possible etiologies.

Definition

- **Amenorrhea** is the absence of menses and may be the result of a defect at any level of the reproductive/endocrine tract. Primary amenorrhea is defined as the absence of menarche by age 16 years. Secondary amenorrhea is the absence of menses for 6 months in a woman who previously menstruated regularly or absence of menses for 1 year if she had oligomenorrhea.

DD$_X$ Secondary Amenorrhea (VITAMINS C)

- **T**raumatic: Asherman's syndrome
- **M**etabolic: Lactation, premature ovarian failure (POF), polycystic ovarian syndrome (PCOS), Cushing's syndrome, hyperthyroidism, acromegaly, Sheehan's syndrome, and malnutrition
- **I**diopathic/**I**atrogenic: Intense athletic training, systemic disease
- **N**eoplastic: Prolactinoma
- **P**regnancy, pseudocyesis

History

- **Ch**aracter: Describe your usual menstrual cycle. Amount of flow (number of pads/tampons) and presence of clots. What was your last period like? Was it normal for you?
- **O**nset: When did you start menstruating (menarche)?
- **I**ntensity: How many periods have you missed? Date of LMP? Any bleeding or spotting since then?
- **D**uration: How long does your menses usually last?
- **E**vents associated:
  - Dysmenorrhea?
  - Pregnancy? Postpartum? Breast-feeding?
  - Recent trauma, illness, or surgery (especially pelvic)?
  - Symptoms of PMS: Bloating, breast tenderness, mood changes, decreased concentration and motivation, food cravings
  - Symptoms of estrogen deficiency: Hot flashes, nervousness/irritability, insomnia, vaginal itch/dryness
  - Symptoms of virilization: Acne, hirsutism, temporal balding, deepening voice, decreased breast size
  - Lifestyle: Obesity, malnutrition (anorexia, bulimia), intense exercise, and stress
  - Hyperthyroidism: Heat intolerance, weight loss despite increased appetite, palpitations
  - Prolactinoma: Galactorrhea, bitemporal hemianopsia
  - Cushing's syndrome: Truncal obesity, moon facies, striae, and hypertrichosis
  - Acromegaly: Acne, prognathism, increased space between the teeth; increased shoe, hat, glove, and ring sizes
- **F**requency: How frequently do you usually menstruate? Have you ever missed periods before? How often?
- **P**alliative factors: Is there anything that makes things better? If so, what?
- **P**rovocative factors: Is there anything that makes things worse? If so, what?

Sexual History

- Recent sexual activity
- Current or past STIs
- Dyspareunia

- Signs of pregnancy
- Use of hormonal contraception, other contraception

Obstetric/Gynecologic History
- Previous pregnancies or abortions
- Uterine instrumentation
- Last Pap smear

- **PMH/PSH:** Oophorectomy/hysterectomy/pelvic surgery, radiation or chemotherapy, endocrinopathy, PCOS, or hepatic/renal disease
- **MEDS:** Hormonal contraception, steroids
- **SH:** Smoking, EtOH, and street drugs
- **FH:** Amenorrhea, age of onset of menopause in mother and sisters (POF), or endocrinopathies

---

INSTRUCTIONS TO CANDIDATE: A 29-year-old female, with a 1-week-old infant, presents to her family doctor with difficulty breast-feeding. She is concerned that the baby is not getting enough milk. Take an appropriate history.

DD$_X$
- Improper latch
- Perceived lack of milk
- Baby-related problem (e.g., neurologic disorder, heart failure)
- Mastitis

History
- **Character:** What kind of difficulty are you having with the breast-feeding?
  - Does the baby latch well? The baby should latch onto nearly the whole areola rather than the nipple only.
  - Is breast-feeding painful for you? Are your nipples sore (with proper latch, it should not be painful)?
- **Location:** Where do you breast-feed? At home? Public places? Is your breast-feeding position comfortable for you?
- **Onset:** When did you start to have difficulty? From the start?
- **Intensity:** What was the baby's birth weight? What is his or her weight now? It is normal to lose 10% of birth weight in the first week.
- **Events associated:**
  - Is this your first child? Have you ever breast-fed before?
  - How do you know whether the baby is getting milk? Does he or she swallow? When you watch the baby's mouth, he or she should open, pause, and close. The baby swallows during the pause.
  - Is your milk in? Do you feel your breasts filling up? Do they feel softer after each feed?
  - Do your breasts leak milk? Do you feel contractions in your uterus?
  - How many bowel movements (BMs) is the baby having each day? What color are they? The baby should have at least one BM per day, usually a loose consistency (seedy), mustard yellow stool (after meconium). The stool may appear green if the milk is not yet in.
  - How many wet diapers does the baby have each day? He or she should have at least five to six wet diapers per day.
  - Does your baby wake for feedings? Is the baby easily roused from sleep?
  - Are you sleeping when you can and eating a healthy diet? Are you drinking enough?

- Frequency: How often do you breast-feed? It is normal to breast-feed 8 to 12 times per 24 hours.
- **P**alliative factors: Is there anything that makes it better? If so, what?
- **P**rovocative factors: Is there anything that makes it worse? If so, what?

Pregnancy History
- Date and gestation at delivery
- Onset of labor: Spontaneous versus induced
- Duration of labor: Use of augmentation
- Type of delivery: NSVD, LSCS, forceps, vacuum
- Maternal complications: Tears (first to fourth degree), PPH, infection, and so on

- **PMH/PSH:** Endocrinopathies, psychiatric problems
- **MEDS:** Document all medications (prescription and OTC) and their effects on lactation
- **SH:** Nutrition, smoking history, EtOH, street drugs, family support, and occupational/financial situation
- **FH:** Malformations, developmental delay, or known hereditary disorders
- Return for reassessment if:
  - Baby sleeping for long periods or is difficult to arouse
  - Baby has <5 to 6 wet diapers per day
  - Fever/chills and a red, painful area in breast
  - Sore nipples with no improvement
- See Dr. Jack Newman's web site for excellent resource information for breast-feeding moms (it provides printable handouts for patients). http://www.breastfeedingonline.com/newman.shtml

SAMPLE CHECKLISTS

> INSTRUCTIONS TO CANDIDATE: A 48-year-old female presents to your office after finding a lump during routine breast self-examination. Take a detailed history, focusing on risk factors for malignancy.

Key Points	Satisfactorily Completed
Introduces self to the patient	❏
Determines how the patient wishes to be addressed	❏
Explains purpose of the encounter	❏
Asks about the qualities of the lump	
• Location	❏
• Size and shape	❏
• Consistency	❏
Asks about associated breast pain	❏
Asks about performance of monthly examinations	❏
Asks when this lump was first noted and whether it has changed	❏
Asks about changes in the lump throughout the menstrual cycle	❏
History of trauma to the area (fat necrosis)	❏
Skin changes	
• Skin retraction or dimpling	❏
• Eczema or rash on the breast	❏
• Ulceration	❏
• Peau d'orange	❏
• Redness	❏
Nipple discharge	❏
Constitutional symptoms	
• Fever, chills, night sweats, weight loss, anorexia, and asthenia	❏
Age of menarche (increased risk if <13 years)	❏
Age of menopause	❏
Parity: Nulliparity, late first pregnancy (>30 years)	❏
Past exposure to radiation	❏
Previous mammography	❏
Previous breast lumps	
• Malignancy	❏
• Dysplasia	❏
Paget's disease of the breast	❏
Family history	
• Breast cancer in first-degree relatives	❏
• Lynch II syndrome: Cancers in breast, endometrium, ovary, and colon	❏
Lifestyle: Smoking, EtOH use, obesity, and high-fat diet	❏
Makes appropriate closing remarks	❏

INSTRUCTIONS TO CANDIDATE: A 32-year-old female presents to the emergency department with a fractured wrist and some facial contusions. Perform a "screen" for intimate partner violence and counsel.

Key Points	Satisfactorily Completed
Introduces self to the patient	❏
Determines how the patient wishes to be addressed	❏
Explains purpose of the encounter	❏
Asks persons other than the patient to leave the room to ensure privacy	❏
Assures the patient that this encounter is confidential, although information will be recorded on her medical record	❏
Asks about her relationship with her partner	❏
Prefaces screening questions with a framing statement such as, "Domestic violence is a very common problem." OR "I have met a lot of patients who have experienced domestic violence."	❏
Asks whether her partner (or someone else close to her) has ever hit, pushed, shoved, punched, or kicked her	❏
Asks whether she is ever threatened	❏
Asks whether she feels safe at home, and clarifies any areas of concern identified by the patient	❏
Asks whether she has been involved in any abusive relationships in the past	❏
Asks about the presence of weapons in the home and specifically asks about guns	❏
Asks about hospitalizations or previous visits to the emergency department for abuse-related problems	❏
Asks whether she has ever tried to leave the relationship, and acknowledges the difficulty of leaving	❏
States that domestic assault is illegal	❏
Expresses concern for her safety (violence tends to escalate)	❏
Asks whether she has any children	❏
Informs her that you are obligated to report any suspicion of child abuse to the authorities (e.g., Child Protection Services)	❏
Asks whether the children have been abused or have witnessed any abuse	❏
Asks about support systems such as family and friends (abusers often isolate their partners)	❏

Key Points	Satisfactorily Completed
Provides contacts for community resources such as legal aid, safe houses, and counseling services	❏
Sets up a follow-up encounter	❏
Asks the patient what avenues she would like to pursue and provides support (the patient must be empowered to make these decisions herself and should also be supported even if she chooses to stay in the abusive relationship)	❏
Encourages the patient to develop and follow a safety plan	
• Have an escape plan from the home	❏
• If possible tell a neighbor to call the police in the event of a disturbance	❏
• Hide money, identification, credit cards, important documents, and important sentimental objects to take with you in the event of a quick departure	❏
• Have emergency telephone numbers nearby	❏
• Choose a safe place to go in the event of an emergency such as a women's shelter or with family or friends	❏

CHAPTER 11

Psychiatry

OBJECTIVES

CARDINAL SIGNS AND SYMPTOMS

ESSENTIAL CLINICAL COMPETENCIES
APPROACH TO THE PSYCHIATRIC HISTORY
APPROACH TO THE MENTAL STATUS EXAMINATION

SAMPLE OSCE SCENARIOS
- A 19-year-old female is brought to the emergency department by the police. Her father called the police when he found that she had written a suicide note. Take a detailed history.
- A 39-year-old male, known to have bipolar disorder, is brought to the emergency department by his sister because he has stopped taking his medications. He has missed work for the past 3 days because he has been working fervently on projects at home. Take a detailed history.
- A 52-year-old female presents to her family doctor with "anxiety." She says she just "worries about everything." She is requesting a tranquilizer to help her sleep. Take a detailed history.
- A 49-year-old male is brought into the emergency department by a friend because he has "nowhere else to go." He has recently quit his job, sold all of his things, and given up his apartment. He was going to travel to another city to stay with family but could not get on the bus because it was "infested with bugs." He wanted to leave town to get away from the infestation. Take a detailed history.

SAMPLE CHECKLIST
- ❏ A 33-year-old male presents for evaluation of depression. Take a detailed history.

OBJECTIVES

*The successful student should be able to take a **focused** psychiatric **history**, including:*
- Mood: Depressed, expansive/elevated
- Suicidal ideation, homicidal ideation
- Delusions
- Hallucinations
- Anxiety
- Obsessions and compulsions
- Panic attacks
- Eating disorders: Binge-purge behaviors, body image disturbance
- Addictions: Alcohol, other substances, gambling, sex, and theft
- Sleep disturbance: Insomnia, hypersomnia
- Feelings of worthlessness
- Somatization

The student should be familiar with:
- Major depression
- Bipolar disorder
- Generalized anxiety disorder

- Panic disorder
- Phobias (including agoraphobia)
- Obsessive-compulsive disorder
- Posttraumatic stress disorder
- Schizophrenia, schizoaffective disorder, and schizophreniform disorder
- Substance abuse/dependence
- Anorexia nervosa, bulimia
- Somatization, somatoform disorder
- Factitious syndrome (Munchausen's syndrome)
- Personality disorders

CARDINAL SIGNS AND SYMPTOMS

Perception
- A **hallucination** is a subjective sensory perception in the absence of an external stimulus. These can be visual, auditory, gustatory (taste), or olfactory in nature. **Hypnagogic** and **hypnopompic** hallucinations occur on falling asleep and waking, respectively, and are not considered pathologic.
- **Formication** is a tactile hallucination of insects crawling on or under the skin.
- An **illusion** is the misperception of an actual external stimulus (e.g., mistaking a billowing curtain for a person).
- **Depersonalization** is a state in which a person loses the sense of his or her own identity in relation to others and their environment.
- **Derealization** is a state in which a person perceives his or her environment and ordinarily familiar things as strange or unreal.

Thought Content
- A **delusion** is a fixed, false belief not shared by other individuals of the same religious/cultural background. Some common delusions are **delusions of reference** (delusional belief that insignificant comments, objects, or events have special meaning or reference to the patient), **delusions of grandeur** (delusional belief of a special talent, power, or identity), and **delusions of persecution** (delusional belief that one is being followed, monitored, or conspired against in some way by others).
- **Thought broadcasting** is the delusional belief that one's thoughts are being broadcast and can be heard by others.
- **Thought insertion** is the delusional belief that one's thoughts are not one's own, having been placed or inserted into one's mind by an external person or force.

Thought Process
- **Circumstantiality** is a disturbance in thought process evident when speech takes a circuitous route, providing excessive detail (circumstances) before finally getting to the point.
- **Tangentiality** is a disturbance in thought process evident when speech takes a tangential route, providing detail about associated thoughts as they arise without ever reaching the point.

Affect
- **Affect** is the observed or perceived emotional state of an individual, whereas **mood** is the emotional state as experienced and reported by an individual.
- **Anhedonia** is lack of pleasure in performing activities that are normally enjoyable.

Negative Symptoms
- **Avolition** is the inability to perform goal-directed activities.
- **Alogia** is poverty of speech.

- **Flat affect** is the complete lack of emotional expression, as if one is conversing with an inanimate object.

Miscellaneous
- **La belle indifference** is typically noted in conversion disorder. It is an inappropriate lack of emotion or concern about one's own disability or affliction.
- An **obsession** is a recurrent, intrusive thought, idea, or impulse that cannot be voluntarily suppressed.
- A **compulsion** is an uncontrollable impulse to perform an act, often repetitively, as a means of neutralizing anxiety caused by obsessive thoughts.

ESSENTIAL CLINICAL COMPETENCIES

APPROACH TO THE PSYCHIATRIC HISTORY

Starting the Interview
- Start the interview by introducing yourself to the patient and stating your role in this patient's evaluation and subsequent care.
- It may be helpful to tell the patient how long you expect the interview to last.
- Confirm the identity of the patient, and determine how the patient would like to be addressed.
- Start the interview in an open-ended fashion (e.g., "So tell me, what brings you in here today?"), and allow the patient to speak uninterrupted or with minimal prompting for the first 5 to 10 minutes (for a 45- to 60-minute interview).
- Be sure that there is a clear path between you and the door (means of escape as necessary) and the patient and the door (do not be caught between the bolting patient and his or her means of escape).
- In the interest of safety do not wear things around your neck like a stethoscope or identification badge.

History
- **ID:** Age, sex, source, and reliability of the historian
- **Chief complaint (CC):** Document the patient's chief complaint in his or her own words.
- **History of presenting illness (HPI):** Review the current complaint and associated symptoms in detail. You may need to seek supplemental information from family members, friends, or police.

Psychiatric Symptom Screen
- When screening for symptoms that may carry a stigma such as delusions and hallucinations, it may be helpful to put the symptom in context and normalize it before asking the question. For example, "Some people tell me that when they watch television, they get special messages from God. Have you ever experienced something like that?"
- Depression: Depressed mood + **SIGE CAPS**
  - **S**leeplessness
  - Loss of **I**nterest
  - **G**uilt
  - Decreased **E**nergy
  - Inability to **C**oncentrate
  - Loss of **A**ppetite
  - **P**sychomotor retardation: Do you feel as if you are slowed down?
  - **S**uicidal ideation
- Mania: **ImPAIRED**
  - **Im**pulsivity

- Pressured speech
- Increased **A**ctivity: Have you taken on any new projects or tasks recently? Do you find it hard to sit still?
- **I**nsomnia: Do you need less sleep than usual?
- **R**acing thoughts: Do you feel like your thoughts are racing?
- **E**steem inflation: Do you feel more self-confident than usual? Do you have any special talents or abilities?
- **D**istractible
- Psychosis:
  - Hallucinations: Do you ever see things or hear things that other people do not see or hear? Do you ever feel like there is something crawling or creeping on your skin?
  - Delusions: Do you ever get special messages while watching TV or reading the newspaper that are intended especially for you? Do you feel like anyone or anything is out to get you? Do you ever get the sense that other people can read your thoughts? Or that thoughts are being inserted into your mind against your will?
  - Negative symptoms: Flat affect, alogia, and avolition
  - Disorganized speech
- Anxiety:
  - Panic attacks
  - Recent traumatic event
  - Obsessions and compulsions: Are you ever bothered by persistent thoughts that you cannot get out of your mind? What do you do about it? Do you ever feel the need to repeat certain activities over and over again even though you do not want to?
- Suicidal thoughts
- Homicidal thoughts
- Substance abuse/dependence: Establish amount and frequency of alcohol consumption and other recreational drugs. Administer the CAGE questionnaire as a screen for alcohol abuse. Some research supports using a cutoff of two affirmative answers as a positive screening test.
  - **C**ut down: Have you ever tried to cut down on your drinking?
  - **A**nnoyed by criticism: Are you annoyed by criticism about your drinking?
  - **G**uilty about drinking: Do you ever feel guilty about drinking?
  - **E**ye-opener: Do you ever need to drink first thing in the morning (eye-opener)?
- **Past psychiatric history:** Past psychiatric diagnoses and treatments, past psychiatric admissions, and past suicide attempts
- **Past medical history (PMH)/past surgical history (PSH):** Previous surgeries, current and past medical problems
- **Medications (MEDS):** Include all current medications (over the counter [OTC], herbal/natural remedies, and prescriptions)
- **Allergies**
- **Social history (SH):** Smoking, EtOH, street drugs, and sexual history
- **Family history (FH):** Psychiatric illnesses, medical illnesses (It is useful to draw a small pedigree, including grandparents, parents, siblings, and children.)
- **Review of systems (ROS):** Ask about common symptoms in each major body system.

Psychosocial History

- Where were you born and raised?
- Were there any problems, that you known of, with your mother's pregnancy with you or with your delivery?
- Did you reach developmental milestones (such as walking and talking) on time?
- Who did you feel close to while you were growing up?
- What was your family like?
- Was there any violence in your home?

- When did you start school? Did you like school? Did you have any troubles in school (e.g., needing to repeat a grade)?
- What were you like as a child? As a teenager?
- Do you have any children of your own? What is your relationship like with your children?
- Tell me about your relationship with your family (siblings, parents, and grand-parents) now.
- Do you have any close relationships right now? Tell me about that.
- Are you or have you been married? Describe what your marriage is like.
- Where do you live now? What is it like?
- Are you working right now? Tell me about your job or your trade.
- What kinds of jobs have you had in the past?
- What kinds of things do you do for fun?
- How satisfied are you with your life right now?

APPROACH TO THE MENTAL STATUS EXAMINATION

- The mental status examination begins as soon as you enter the room to begin the patient encounter. The majority of the data can be gleaned during the interview from observation only rather than direct questioning (Box 11-1).
- Observe the patient's **appearance**, noting hygiene, makeup, jewelry, clothing, body habitus, and any distinctive physical features.
- Characterize the patient's **behavior**, noting body language (e.g., elaborate hand gestures), mannerisms (e.g., lip smacking), attentiveness, and psychomotor retardation or agitation. Note whether the patient appears to be responding to cues in the room (e.g., visual or auditory hallucinations).
- Observe the rate and volume of **speech**. The way the patient talks to you and responds to your questions may be equally as important as the content of his or her speech.
- Note the range and stability of the patient's **affect**. Describe the affect (an observed phenomenon) and its intensity (e.g., flat versus inflated). Elicit the patient's description of his or her **mood**, and note whether it is congruent with your observations.
- The **thought content** of the patient is inferred from the content of his or her speech. Note any delusions, obsessions, phobias, and thoughts of suicide or homicide.
- Similarly ideas about **thought process** also are inferred from the patient's speech. Note whether the patient's speech appears to be coherent and follows a logical progression. Characterize the speech for tangentiality, circumstantiality, loose associations, and perseveration.
- Note any **hallucinations** reported by the patient or any apparent hallucinations experienced by the patient during your encounter.

Box 11-1   Outline for the Mental Status Examination

- General appearance
- Behavior
- Speech
- Affect and mood
- Thought content
- Thought process
- Perceptual disturbances
- Judgment
- Insight
- Orientation

- Assess **judgment** by asking the patient to respond to some questions. For example, ask the patient what he or she would do if he or she woke up in his or her home and found it to be on fire. Other such scenarios could be used instead if preferred.
- Document whether the patient appears to have any **insight** into his or her illness or current problem.
- Finally determine whether the patient is **oriented** to person, place, and time. This may be done in the context of a Folstein Mini-Mental State Examination (see pp 346-347).

SAMPLE OSCE SCENARIOS

INSTRUCTIONS TO CANDIDATE: A 19-year-old female is brought to the emergency department by the police. Her father called the police when he found that she had written a suicide note. Take a detailed history.

Collateral History
- Ask the police about their interaction with the patient. Is she known to them? Did they find any pill bottles or weapons in the home? Did they bring the suicide note?
- Ask the father about the suicide note and its content. Was there any stated plan? Where did he find it? Was there an argument or some type of confrontation? Has this ever happened before? Describe stressors in the home. Is there anything new of which you are aware?
- Are there any guns in the home?

History
- Tell me what happened. Why are you here?
- Did you take any pills, or do something else to harm yourself today?
- What were you planning to do? Were you planning to kill yourself?
- How long have you been thinking about suicide (acute versus chronic)?
- How did things come about today (planned in advance or impulsive)?
- Ask the patient why she wanted to kill herself.
- Are you still thinking about killing yourself? By what means? It is important to be direct in your questioning on this manner and determine whether she has a suicide plan.
- How are things at home? How are things at school? At work? With your relationships?
- Assessment of suicidal risk using **SAD PERSONS** mnemonic (risk factors):
  - **Sex:** Male
  - **Age:** <19 or >45 years
  - **Depression**
  - **Previous attempts**
  - **EtOH**
  - **Rational thinking loss**
  - **Separated, divorced, or widowed**
  - **Organized plan**
  - **No social support**
  - **Stated future intent**
- Perform a psychiatric symptom screen as outlined in the **approach to the psychiatric history** (see pp 287-289).
- **Past psychiatric history:** Past psychiatric diagnoses and treatments, past psychiatric admissions, and past suicide attempts
- **PMH/PSH:** Any illnesses requiring hospital admission or surgery, endocrine disease
- **MEDS:** Antidepressants, steroids, anxiolytics, antipsychotics, or other medications
- **Allergies**
- **SH:** Smoking, EtOH, street drugs, and sexual history
- **FH:** Psychiatric illnesses, suicide, or medical illnesses
- **ROS:** Ask about common symptoms in each major body system.

Involuntary Commitment
- Suicidal patients who refuse treatment or hospitalization may need to be held in the hospital involuntarily for their own safety. Although this is considered an acceptable

intervention in the acutely suicidal patient, involuntary hospitalization has not been proven to prevent future suicide.

- Laws surrounding involuntary commitment vary from province to province and state to state; therefore, be aware of the laws in your region and the policies at your institution.
- Generally patients must have a mental illness and be deemed a danger to themselves or to others (some jurisdictions also include risk of harm to property).
- Patients who are certified but retain decision-making capacity (see p 363) cannot be treated against their wishes.

PEARLS

- Most completed suicides are committed with guns. The presence of a gun in the household is an independent risk factor for suicide, especially in adolescents.
- Most suicide attempts are executed with ingested toxins.
- Women attempt suicide more often than men, but men are more likely to complete suicide.

INSTRUCTIONS TO CANDIDATE: A 39-year-old male, known to have bipolar disorder, is brought to the emergency department by his sister because he has stopped taking his medications. He has missed work for the past 3 days because he has been working fervently on projects at home. Take a detailed history.

DD$_x$

- Bipolar disorder
- Acute psychosis
- Cyclothymia
- Substance ingestion or withdrawal
- Schizoaffective disorder

Collateral History

- What about your brother's behavior worries you? What type of projects is he working on? Does he sleep?
- How would you describe his mood?
- How long has he been off his medications?
- Any changes in his speech?

History

- Tell me what brings you here today.
- Are you here voluntarily?
- How are things going at home? At work?
- Have you missed work recently? Why? What have you been doing instead? Are you worried that you might lose your job?
- Tell me your plans for these home projects you are working on.
- Have you been doing anything outside of the home?
- Your sister is concerned that you have stopped taking your pills. Is this true? How long have you been off your medication? What do you normally take (include dosing schedule)?
- How would you describe your mood now?
- Have you been sleeping? How much?
- Do you find yourself irritable or distractible lately?
- Have you made any investments recently?
- Mania: **ImPAIRED**
  - **Im**pulsivity
  - **P**ressured speech

- Increased **A**ctivity: Have you taken on any new projects or tasks recently? Do you find it hard to sit still?
  - Insomnia: Do you need less sleep than usual?
  - **R**acing thoughts: Do you feel like your thoughts are racing?
  - **E**steem inflation: Do you feel more self-confident than usual? Do you have any special talents or abilities?
  - **D**istractible
- Perform a psychiatric symptom screen as outlined in the **approach to the psychiatric history** (see pp 287-289), including assessment of suicide risk (see p 291).
- **Past psychiatric history:** Past psychiatric diagnoses and treatments (bipolar disorder), past psychiatric admissions, and past suicide attempts
- **PMH/PSH:** Any illnesses requiring hospital admission or surgery, endocrine disease
- **MEDS:** Antidepressants, mood stabilizers, steroids, anxiolytics, antipsychotics, or other medications
- **Allergies**
- **SH:** Smoking, EtOH, street drugs, and sexual history
- **FH:** Bipolar disorder, other psychiatric disease, suicide, or medical illnesses
- **ROS:** Ask about common symptoms in each major body system.

PEARLS
- Bipolar disorder is a life-long illness punctuated by episodic deteriorations.
- Judgment is often impaired in acute manic episodes.

INSTRUCTIONS TO CANDIDATE: A 52-year-old female presents to her family doctor with "anxiety." She says she just "worries about everything." She is requesting a tranquilizer to help her sleep. Take a detailed history.

DD$_x$
- Generalized anxiety disorder
- Panic disorder
- Agoraphobia
- Obsessive-compulsive disorder (OCD)
- Post-traumatic stress disorder (PTSD)
- Adjustment disorder
- Anxiety secondary to a general medical condition
- Anxiety secondary to substance use
- Drug seeking

History
- Tell me what brings you here today.
- What are your major worries? What kinds of things do you worry about?
- When did this trouble with anxiety start up?
- Is it getting better, worse, or staying the same?
- What is making you seek medical attention right now?
- Have you ever had this trouble before? When?
- How are things going at home? At work?
- Have you missed work recently? Are you functioning well in your current job?
- Tell me about a typical day for you.
- Do you go out to grocery shop? Do you go out to socialize?
- How are your relationships? Do you get along well with people?
- Any stressful events recently?
- Do you avoid certain types of situations to get around your anxiety?
- Have you ever had panic attacks?

Box 11-2   Predictors of Anxiety with Organic Etiology

- Onset of anxiety after age 35 years
- Lack of a personal history or family history of anxiety disorder
- Lack of a childhood history of significant anxiety, phobia, or separation anxiety
- Absence of significant life events generating or exacerbating anxiety symptoms
- Lack of avoidance behaviors
- Poor response to anxiolytics

Adapted from Marx JA, Hockberger RS, Walls RM, editors: *Rosen's emergency medicine: concepts and clinical practice,* ed 5, St. Louis, 2002, Mosby, p 1558, Box 106-2.

Box 11-3   Some Organic Etiologies of "Anxiety"

- Myocardial infarction
- Tachyarrhythmia
- Hyperthyroidism
- Pheochromocytoma
- Pulmonary emboli
- Seizure disorders (e.g., temporal lobe epilepsy)
- Alcohol withdrawal, benzodiazepine withdrawal
- Drug intoxication

- How would you describe your mood?
- Perform a psychiatric symptom screen as outlined in the **approach to the psychiatric history** (see pp 287-289), including assessment of suicide risk (see p 291).
- **Past psychiatric history:** Past psychiatric diagnoses and treatments (panic disorder, anxiety disorder), past psychiatric admissions, and past suicide attempts
- **PMH/PSH:** Any illnesses requiring hospital admission or surgery, endocrine disease
- **MEDS:** Antidepressants, mood stabilizers, steroids, anxiolytics, antipsychotics, or other medications
- **Allergies**
- **SH:** Smoking, EtOH, street drugs, and sexual history
- **FH:** Anxiety disorder, other psychiatric disease, or suicide
- **ROS:** Ask about common symptoms in each major body system.

PEARL
- Anxiety disorders may present with symptoms of physical disease, and organic disease may present with symptoms of anxiety. See Box 11-2 for predictors of anxiety of organic origin and Box 11-3 for some items to consider in the differential diagnosis of organic anxiety.

INSTRUCTIONS TO CANDIDATE: A 49-year-old male is brought into the emergency department by a friend because he has "nowhere else to go." He has recently quit his job, sold all of his things, and given up his apartment. He was going to travel to another city to stay with family but could not get on the bus because it was "infested with bugs." He wanted to leave town to get away from the infestation. Take a detailed history.

DD$_X$
- Brief psychotic disorder
- Schizophrenia

- Bipolar disorder
- Psychosis secondary to a medical condition
- Substance ingestion or withdrawal
- Schizoaffective disorder
- Organic brain syndrome

Collateral History

- Tell me what has been going on with your friend. How long have you known him?
- When did you first notice this change in his behavior? How long has he been concerned about bugs? Has he had any other strange concerns?
- Has this ever happened before?
- Does he have any psychiatric or medical problems of which you are aware?
- Does he drink EtOH or use recreational drugs?

History

- Tell me what brings you here today.
- Are you here voluntarily?
- How are things going at home? At work?
- Did you quit your job? Why? Were there any bugs in your workplace?
- What happened with your apartment? Why were you leaving town?
- Were there bugs in your apartment? What did you do to get rid of them?
- How long has this been going on? Has this ever happened before? When?
- Have you been sleeping? How much?
- How would you describe your mood?
- Check orientation to person, place, and time.
- Do you ever see or hear things that other people do not see or hear?
- Do you ever feel like there is something crawling or creeping on your skin?
- Do you ever get special messages while watching TV or reading the newspaper that are intended especially for you?
- Do you feel like anyone or anything is out to get you?
- Do you ever get the sense that other people can read your thoughts? Or that thoughts are being inserted into your mind against your will?
- Perform a psychiatric symptom screen as outlined in the **approach to the psychiatric history** (see pp 287-289), including assessment of suicide risk (see p 291).
- **Past psychiatric history:** Past psychiatric diagnoses and treatments (schizophrenia, bipolar disorder), past psychiatric admissions, and past suicide attempts
- **PMH/PSH:** Any illnesses requiring hospital admission or surgery, endocrine disease
- **MEDS:** Antidepressants, mood stabilizers, steroids, anxiolytics, antipsychotics, or other medications
- **Allergies**
- **SH:** Smoking, EtOH, street drugs, and sexual history
- **FH:** Schizophrenia, bipolar disorder, other psychiatric disease, or suicide
- **ROS:** Ask about common symptoms in each major body system.

PEARL

- Psychosis can be caused by organic brain syndrome (Table 11-1). There is a wide range of organic etiologies for psychosis, including (but not limited to) central nervous system (CNS) tumor or infection, electrolyte disturbances, toxic ingestion, and drug withdrawal.

Table 11-1   Differentiating Organic from Functional Psychosis (MAD FOCS)

	Organic	Functional
Memory deficits	Recent impairment	Remote impairment
Activity	Psychomotor retardation	Repetitive activity
	Tremor	Posturing
	Ataxia	Rocking
Distortions	Visual hallucinations	Auditory hallucinations
Feelings	Emotional lability	Flat affect
Orientation	Disoriented	Oriented
Cognition	Islands of lucidity	Continuous scattered thoughts
	Attends occasionally	Unable to attend (focus)
		Unfiltered perceptions
Some other findings	Age >40 years	Age <40 years
	Sudden onset	Gradual onset
	Abnormal physical examination	Normal physical examination
	Abnormal vital signs	Normal vital signs
	Social immodesty	Social modesty
	Aphasia	Intelligible speech
	Impaired consciousness	Awake and alert

Adapted from Marx JA, Hockberger RS, Walls RM, editors: *Rosen's emergency medicine: concepts and clinical practice*, ed 5, St. Louis, 2002, Mosby, p 1544, Box 104-1.

SAMPLE CHECKLIST

INSTRUCTIONS TO CANDIDATE: A 33-year-old male presents for evaluation of depression. Take a detailed history.

Key Points	Satisfactorily Carried out
Introduces self to the patient	❏
Determines how the patient wishes to be addressed	❏
Explains the purpose of the encounter	❏
Develops good patient rapport	❏
Asks about depressed mood	❏
Inquires about sleep patterns (**S**leeplessness)	❏
Asks about normal daily activities (loss of **I**nterest)	❏
Asks about feelings of **G**uilt	❏
Inquires about level of energy (decreased **E**nergy)	❏
Asks about inability to **C**oncentrate	❏
Asks about loss of **A**ppetite	❏
Observes for **P**sychomotor retardation	❏
Suicidal ideation • Do you feel like life is not worth living? • Have you thought about killing yourself? • Do you have any suicidal plan?	❏ ❏ ❏
Social supports	❏
How are things at home?	❏
How are things at work? Have you been able to function properly?	❏
Past psychiatric problems	❏
History of medical or surgical problems	❏
Prescription medications	❏
Use of alcohol and recreational drugs	❏
Makes appropriate closing remarks	❏

CHAPTER 12

Pediatrics

OBJECTIVES

ANATOMY

ESSENTIAL CLINICAL COMPETENCIES

APPROACH TO THE PEDIATRIC PATIENT

PERFORM A FOCUSED PHYSICAL EXAMINATION OF A CHILD'S EARS AND THROAT

PERFORM A FOCUSED PHYSICAL EXAMINATION OF A CHILD'S EYES

PERFORM A FOCUSED PHYSICAL EXAMINATION FOR DEVELOPMENTAL DYSPLASIA OF THE HIP IN A NEWBORN

PERFORM A DENVER DEVELOPMENTAL SCREENING TEST

SAMPLE OSCE SCENARIOS

- A 15-year-old female presents with malaise and "swollen glands." Perform a focused physical examination.
- A 14-month-old girl is brought to the emergency department by her parents because of diarrhea. Perform a focused history and physical examination.
- A 10-year-old girl with a history of asthma is brought to the emergency department from gym class. At the triage desk she is tachypneic and has an audible wheeze. Perform a focused history and physical examination.
- A 7-year-old boy is brought to his family doctor by his father. He is complaining of a sore throat and fever for 2 days. Perform a focused history and physical examination.
- A 2-year-old boy is brought to the emergency department by his parents because of cough, fever, and rapid breathing. Perform a focused history and physical examination.
- A 31-month-old boy is brought to the emergency department via ambulance because of a seizure. His parents say that he was "shaking all over" and his eyes rolled back in his head. The paramedic tells you that he has a temperature of 39.3° C. Perform a focused history and physical examination.
- A 13-year-old male presents to the emergency department with a headache and fever. He recently returned from army cadet camp. Perform a focused history and physical examination.
- A 1-month-old boy is brought to the emergency department because of a 5-day history of vomiting. His mother is concerned that he is becoming dehydrated because he "can't keep anything down." Take a detailed history, exploring possible etiologies.
- A 5-year-old girl is brought to her family doctor by her mother because of ongoing bedwetting. Take a detailed history, exploring possible etiologies.
- A 30-month-old boy is brought to his pediatrician by his mother who is concerned about his small vocabulary. Take a detailed history, exploring possible etiologies.
- A 3-year-old male is brought in by his parents because of a very swollen right eye, which he can no longer open voluntarily. Perform a focused history and physical examination.
- A 28-month-old female is brought to her family physician by her mother for the first time. They have recently immigrated to this country. Take an immunization history.
- You are a senior medical student on your neonatology rotation. The nurse in charge asks you to measure the height, weight, and head circumference of a newborn baby boy and plot them on the growth charts provided. Perform a routine newborn examination.

Continued

- The next day the nurse in charge asks you to reassess the boy because he appears jaundiced. Take a detailed history from his mother, exploring possible etiologies. What is the differential diagnosis?
- A 2-year-old female is brought in by her parents because she is having episodes of screaming, complaining that she has a "sore belly." Between episodes she is playing with her toys. The triage nurse asks you to come and assess this patient as she is having another episode of screaming.
- A 4-year-old male is brought in by his mother because she has noticed him limping for the past 2 days. Perform a focused history, exploring possible etiologies.

SAMPLE CHECKLISTS

❑ A 4-year-old female is under observation in the emergency department after experiencing an anaphylactic reaction to peanut butter. Counsel the girl's mother about peanut allergy.

❑ An 8-month-old female is brought to the emergency department by her grandmother because she is not as active as usual. She cries whenever her grandmother tries to change her diaper and seems to be in pain. Interpret the x-ray. What are your responsibilities in this case?

OBJECTIVES

*The successful student should be able to take a **focused** pediatric **history**, including:*
- Abdominal pain
- Nausea, vomiting (N/V)
- Diarrhea, constipation
- Diet
- Cough
- Wheeze, shortness of breath (SOB)
- Sore throat, runny nose
- Lymphadenopathy
- Ear pain
- Headache, stiff neck
- Fever
- Seizures: Epilepsy, febrile seizure
- Allergic reactions
- Exanthem
- Ataxia
- Limp
- Arthritis
- Strabismus, amblyopia
- Developmental delay: Verbal, social, and motor (gross and fine)
- Failure to thrive
- Perinatal history
- Jaundice
- Nocturnal enuresis, encopresis
- Trauma, injury, and burns

*The pediatric **examination** will include:*
- Vitals (account for age-appropriate differences)

Inspection
- Level of interaction with parent/caregiver
- Level of activity, gait, and coordination
- Cry: Stridor, consolability
- Respiratory distress: Tachypnea, pursed lips, nasal flare, tripod positioning, tracheal tug, accessory muscle use, intercostal/subcostal retractions, and thoracoabdominal dissociation
- Cyanosis, pallor, jaundice, and mottling

- Abdomen: Distension, asymmetry, and peristalsis
- Eyes, ears, nose, and pharynx (including funduscopy and otoscopy)
- Gait, joints

Percussion
- Abdomen
- Chest
- Costovertebral angle

Palpation
- Fontanelles
- Tracheal position, thoracic deformities
- Abdomen: Tenderness, liver, spleen, and hernias
- Joints
- Testicles (identify cryptorchism)

Auscultation
- Chest:
  - Heart sounds, murmurs
  - Breath sounds, adventitious sounds
- Abdomen: Bowel sounds
- Bruits

ANATOMY

- Children are not merely "small adults"; there are many anatomic differences between them, and just a few key differences are outlined below.

General
- Children have a large head-to-body ratio compared with adults, which raises their center of gravity and makes them more prone to head trauma in falls and motor vehicle collisions.
- The larger body surface area-to-mass ratio predisposes children to hypothermia. It is important to bear this in mind when children are disrobed for examination in a chilly emergency department, especially in trauma or resuscitation situations.
- Heart rate (HR), blood pressure (BP), and respiratory rates (RR) vary with age (Table 12-1).

Airway
- Children have a relatively larger tongue in relation to the size of the oral cavity (common cause of upper airway obstruction).
- The epiglottis is larger and floppier, and the larynx is more anterior and cephalad than that of an adult.
- The cricoid ring is the narrowest part of the pediatric airway, which allows for the use of an uncuffed endotracheal tube in children aged <8 years (in adults the larynx is the narrowest part of the airway).

Breathing
- The chest wall of a child is very compliant. As such chest wall injury is uncommon, but the underlying lung parenchyma, heart, kidneys, spleen, and liver are susceptible to injury nonetheless.

Circulation
- Pediatric blood volume is approximately 8% of total body weight versus 6% of body weight in adults.

Table 12-1   Normal Ranges for Vital Signs by Age

Age	Heart Rate (beats/min)	Systolic Blood Pressure (mm Hg)	Respiratory Rate (breaths/min)
Infant	120-160	>60	30-50
6 months to 1 year	120-140	70-80	30-40
2-4 years	100-110	80-95	20-30
5-8 years	90-100	90-100	14-20
8-12 years	80-100	100-110	12-20
>12 years	60-90	100-120	12-16

Adapted from Marx JA, Hockberger RS, Walls RM, editors: *Rosen's emergency medicine: concepts and clinical practice,* ed 5, St. Louis, 2002, Mosby, p 2221, Table 160-3.

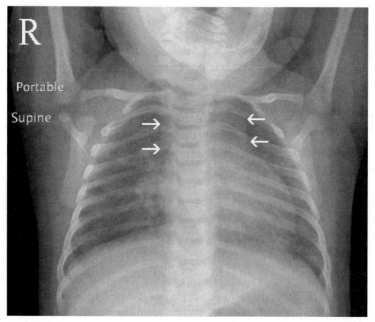

Figure 12-1   Portable anteroposterior chest-x-ray in a neonate. Arrows point out left and right margins of the thymus.

- Because the absolute blood volume in a child is less than that of an adult, the hemodynamic consequences of a given volume of blood loss are greater in a child.

Musculoskeletal (MSK)

- The presence of growth plates in children sometimes makes the interpretation of radiographs challenging. It may be helpful to take a comparative radiograph of the contralateral joint to identify the normal anatomy.
- The growth plate is the weakest part of the bone. Children are more likely to sustain a growth plate injury than a sprain (relatively speaking the ligamentous connective tissue is stronger than the cartilaginous growth plate).

Thymus

- Relative to the body the thymus is largest at birth. This is evident on the infant chest x-ray as a "mediastinal mass" (Figure 12-1).
- It reaches its largest absolute mass during puberty and begins to involute thereafter.

ESSENTIAL CLINICAL COMPETENCIES

APPROACH TO THE PEDIATRIC PATIENT

Communication

- Children are often accompanied by one or both parents or another family member. Although it is important to get information from the caregiver about the reasons for the visit, do not ignore the importance of communicating directly with the child because he or she is a valuable source of clinical data.
- Address the caregivers' concerns. It may be helpful to ask a question such as, "What is your biggest worry or concern today?" This will help to identify expectations for the visit and perceptions about the child's complaint or illness.
- Avoid using technical jargon. Establishing a good rapport with the caregiver will be important to your encounter with the child, who is likely to pick up on the discomfort of his or her caregiver.
- Follow the lead of the caregiver to ensure that you communicate with the child at an appropriate level. When addressing a child ensure that your eyes are on the same horizontal plane by sitting, kneeling, or crouching as necessary. Engage the child by talking about things he or she likes such as a favorite toy or activity, friends, or school.
- An older child or adolescent should be addressed primarily in the interview, garnering supplemental information from the caregiver afterward.
- In children the prenatal, natal, and neonatal history may be relevant to differentiate their current presentation. This type of history should definitely be sought in children aged <2 years.

Physical Examination

- A great deal can be learned by simply observing the pediatric patient. Watching the parent-child interaction and watching the child play, socialize, and interact with his or her environment provide valuable data about development. Furthermore, observation can identify respiratory distress, cry, or physical limitations such as a limp or handedness. Overall a great deal of the neuromuscular examination and developmental assessment can be documented without laying hands on the child.
- The remainder of the physical examination is largely opportunistic in nature. The order of the examination is not important, and you should routinely leave the most invasive or uncomfortable parts for last. For example, if the child is quiet take the opportunity to auscultate the chest.
- To improve the comfort level of the child and increase cooperation, it is helpful to examine the child on his or her parent's lap or with the parent nearby.

PEARL

- Always consider abuse. The majority of children are well cared for, but if you fail to keep this possibility in the back of your mind, you are likely to overlook it.

PERFORM A FOCUSED PHYSICAL EXAMINATION OF A CHILD'S EARS AND THROAT

Inspection

- Are both ears present and normally formed and are they normally positioned (Figure 12-2)?
  - Small, malformed, and low-set ears may be associated with genetic syndromes.
- Inspect the pinnae and tragi (Figure 12-3). Note signs of trauma, eczema, redness, swelling, or tenderness.

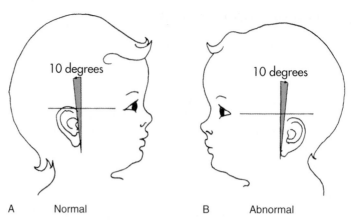

A   Normal   B   Abnormal

Figure 12-2   Ear alignment. (From Barkauskas VH, Baumann LC, Darling-Fisher CS: *Health and physical assessment*, ed 3, St Louis, 2002, Mosby, p 656, Figure 26-41.)

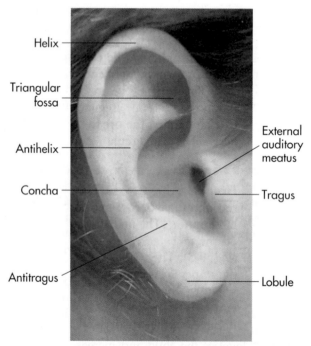

Figure 12-3   External ear. (From Seidel HM, Ball JW, Dains JE, Benedict GB: *Mosby's guide to physical examination*, ed 5, St. Louis, 2003, Mosby, p 315, Figure 11-3.)

- Inspect the palate and pharynx (Figure 12-4). Look at the size of the tonsils. "Kissing" tonsils may be large enough to cause airway obstruction. Note any petechiae, erythema, exudate, or vesicles.
  - Petechiae and exudate may be present in streptococcal pharyngitis.
  - Vesicles may suggest herpangina, a painful condition, usually caused by Coxsackie virus.
  - "Cobble stoning" of the posterior pharynx may be seen in postnasal drip.

Palpation
- Palpate the external ear. Movement of the pinna and tragus is painful in acute otitis externa.
- Palpate the mastoid. Tenderness may suggest mastoiditis.
- Examine the lymph nodes of the head and neck (see pp 228-229).

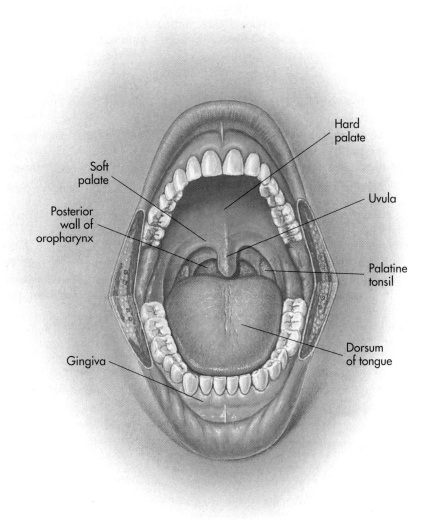

Figure 12-4   Oropharynx. (From Seidel HM, Ball JW, Dains JE, Benedict GB: *Mosby's guide to physical examination*, ed 5, St. Louis, 2003, Mosby, p 320, Figure 11-10.)

Otoscopic Examination

- Explain the examination to the parent and child. You may allay anxiety in the child by seating him or her on the parent or caregiver's lap. If the child needs to be restrained, ask the parent or caregiver to turn the child's head to one side, holding the head against the parent's body. Protect the ear by bracing your hand between the child's head and the otoscope.
- Grasp the auricle, and pull it upward, backward, and slightly away from the head to straighten the external auditory canal. Hold the otoscope between your thumb and fingers. Gently insert the speculum of the otoscope into the ear canal. Describe any abnormalities such as discharge, erythema, or swelling. Inspect for foreign bodies and cerumen.
- Examine the tympanic membrane, and identify landmarks (see Figure 5-6). The normal tympanic membrane has a lucent appearance. Opacification is usually caused by thickening or effusion. Note its color, contour, and any bulging or retraction. Note any perforation, scars, or the presence of "tubes."
- Acute otitis media usually presents with a hyperemic, opaque, bulging tympanic membrane with loss of normal landmarks. A middle ear effusion may give a bluish (serous) or yellow (pus) appearance to the tympanic membrane.

- **Pneumootoscopy:** Using a bulb attached to the otoscope, apply positive and negative pressure in the ear canal. Decreased compliance with positive pressure suggests a bulging tympanic membrane, whereas decreased compliance with negative pressure suggests a retracted tympanic membrane.

Auditory Acuity

- If a parent believes his or her child cannot hear, it should be assumed correct until proven otherwise.
- Occlude one ear with a finger and whisper softly into the other ear using words or numbers of equally accented syllables.
- **Acoustic blink test:** To test an infant's hearing observe blinking in response to a sudden sharp sound produced approximately 12 inches from the ear (e.g., snapping fingers, clapping).
- If acuity is decreased use Weber's and Rinne's tests to distinguish sensorineural from conductive hearing loss. These tests are not useful in young children.
- **Weber's test:** Place a vibrating tuning fork (512 Hz or 1024 Hz) firmly on top of the patient's head. Ask the patient whether he or she hears it in one or both ears. Normally the sound is heard midline. In conductive hearing loss sound will be lateralized to the impaired ear. In sensorineural hearing loss the sound lateralizes to the good ear.
- **Rinne's test:** Place a vibrating tuning fork (512 Hz or 1024 Hz) on the mastoid bone, behind the ear, level with the external auditory canal. When the patient can no longer hear the sound place the tuning fork close to the ear canal ("U" facing forward), and ask whether the sound is now audible. In conductive hearing loss sound is best transmitted by bone conduction. In sensorineural hearing loss sound is best transmitted through air.

PERFORM A FOCUSED PHYSICAL EXAMINATION OF A CHILD'S EYES

Inspection

- **Alignment:** Check the eyes for position and alignment with each other, noting any deviation or protrusion.
- **Lids:** Inspect the lids, noting their position in relation to the eye itself. Document any swelling or redness in the area of the lacrimal glands.
  - **Ptosis** is drooping of the upper lid and may be related to myasthenia gravis, Horner's syndrome, or cranial nerve (CN) III palsy (congenital and acquired).
  - **Retracted lid** is noted with the visualization of a rim of sclera between the upper lid and the iris. When the lids are retracted, also look for **lid lag**. Ask the child to follow an object from midline up to down. Normally the lid overlaps the iris slightly throughout this movement. In lid lag a rim of sclera is seen between the upper lid and iris when the patient gazes downward. The presence of retracted lids and lid lag may suggest hyperthyroidism.
- **Eyes:** Note any excessive tearing or dryness. Inspect the sclerae, noting any icterus or redness. Injection of the conjunctiva should be qualified by noting the pattern (e.g., peripheral versus ciliary). Look at the iris; its margins should be clearly defined.
- **Pupils:** Inspect size, shape, and symmetry of the pupils. If the pupils are large (>5 mm), small (<3 mm), or unequal, measure them. Use the swinging flashlight test to assess the direct and consensual response to light. Pupillary constriction can also be observed during accommodation; ask the child to look at your finger or an object, and bring it progressively closer until the eyes cross.
  - **Miosis** refers to constriction of the pupil.
  - **Mydriasis** refers to dilation of the pupil.
  - **Anisocoria** refers to pupillary inequality (up to 1 mm of asymmetry is considered within normal limits).

Visual Acuity

- Test visual acuity using the Snellen eye chart. In young children use a Snellen E chart, and ask them to identify which way the letter is facing. It is difficult to quantify visual acuity in children aged <3 years. Patients who have prescription glasses should wear them. Position the child 20 feet from the chart. Cover one eye using a "pirate's patch," and ask them to read the smallest print possible. Visual acuity is expressed as two numbers (e.g., 20/20), in which the first number indicates the distance of the patient from the chart, and the second, the distance at which the average person can read the line of letters. Normal visual acuity at age 3 is 20/40 and usually reaches 20/20 by age 6. A discrepancy in visual acuity between the eyes is abnormal and may lead to amblyopia. Refractive errors improve when looking through a pinhole.
  - **Myopia** refers to impaired far vision (i.e., near sighted).
  - **Hyperopia** refers to impaired near vision (i.e., far sighted).
  - **Amblyopia** refers to unilateral decreased visual acuity without any detectable cause. It most commonly relates to suppression of vision in patients with strabismus.

Visual Fields

- Seat the child on the parent's lap. Hold the child's head in midline position, and bring a brightly colored object into the child's field of vision from behind (upper and lower temporal fields). Eye deviation toward the object indicates that the child has seen it. The blind spot is 15 degrees temporal.

Extraocular Movements

- Using a light or an object assess the extraocular eye movements (Figure 12-5). Note any dysconjugate movement or nystagmus at the extremes of gaze. Dysconjugate movements may be caused by a CN palsy (CNs III, IV, and VI) or muscular problem (strabismus). Brief nystagmus (<3 beats) on extreme lateral gaze is normal.

Strabismus Screening

- Shine a light on the patient's eyes, and ask the patient to look at it. Observe the reflection of the light on the corneas. Normally the reflection is visible slightly nasally with respect to the center of the pupil and is symmetrical (Figure 12-6).

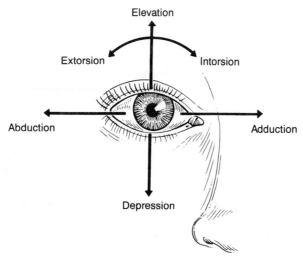

Figure 12-5 Extraocular movements. (From Swartz M: *Textbook of physical diagnosis: history and examination,* ed 4, Philadelphia, 2002, WB Saunders, Figure 9-4.)

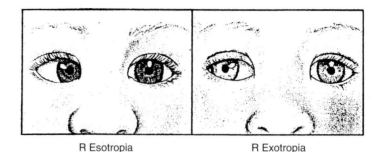

R Esotropia   R Exotropia

Figure 12-6   Asymmetric corneal light reflex. (Adapted from Jarvis CJ: *Physical examination and health assessment,* ed 2, Philadelphia, 1996, WB Saunders, p 340, Table 12-2.)

Funduscopic Examination

- Darken the room. Tell the child you are going to shine a light in his or her eyes. Have the child pick which eye he or she would like you to look in first. Use your left eye to examine the patient's left eye. Approach the patient from the temporal side on a 15-degree angle, eliciting the red reflex. Absence of the red reflex suggests corneal opacity (e.g., cataracts) or retinoblastoma. Inspect the cornea, lens, and vitreous for opacities.
- Inspect the optic disc. Compare the discs for symmetry, and note the following:
  - Clarity of the disc outline and color. Papilledema is rarely seen in children aged <3 years because the sutures can open to accommodate increased intracranial pressure (ICP).
  - Inspect the retina. Follow the vessels to each of four quadrants. Note exudates, hemorrhages, or other lesions. Inspect the macula and fovea.

PERFORM A FOCUSED PHYSICAL EXAMINATION FOR DEVELOPMENTAL DYSPLASIA OF THE HIP IN A NEWBORN

Anatomy

- The hip is a ball (femoral head) and socket (acetabulum) joint. The components of the joint are interdependent for normal growth and development. The etiology of developmental dysplasia of the hip (DDH) is multifactorial.

Definition

- **Developmental dysplasia of the hip** refers to congenitally dislocated hips. The etiology is multifactorial and is progressive unless corrected; thus every newborn should be examined for DDH. Beyond 2 months of age DDH becomes more difficult to detect clinically because of increased muscle strength and increased soft tissue.

Inspection

- Inspect the contour of the legs while the infant is lying supine. **Count the skin folds** on the medial aspect of the thigh (Figure 12-7). Asymmetry suggests femoral head dislocation (increased skin folds ipsilaterally).
- **Visualization of the perineum** in this position suggests bilateral hip dislocations. The normal position of the thighs should cover most of the perineum.
- Flex the infant's knees and hips. Place the infant's feet side by side with the plantar aspects of the feet against the examination table. Observe the relative heights of the knees. If the knees are symmetrical either both hips are normal or both are dislocated. If the knee height is asymmetric, suspect either femoral head dislocation on the side of the shorter knee **(Galeazzi sign)** or a congenitally short femur.

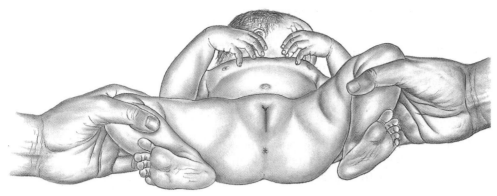

Figure 12-7 Asymmetric gluteal folds. (From Seidel HM, Ball JW, Dains JE, Benedict GB: *Mosby's guide to physical examination,* ed 5, St. Louis, 2003, Mosby, p 743, Figure 20-58.)

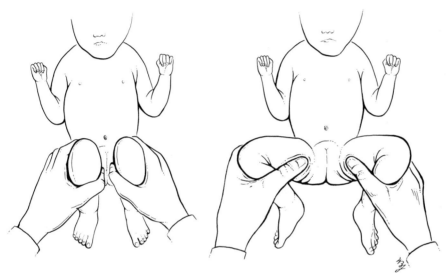

Figure 12-8 Ortolani test. (From Swartz M: *Textbook of physical diagnosis: history and examination,* ed 4, Philadelphia, 2002, WB Saunders, Figure 23-14.)

Range of Motion (ROM)
- Test the passive ROM of the hip: flexion, extension, abduction, adduction, and internal and external rotation. Limitation of abduction is abnormal and may indicate DDH. The neonatal joints are agile; normal infants should readily abduct to nearly 90 degrees.

Special Tests
- Perform these tests with the infant supine, legs pointing toward you.
- **Ortolani test** (Figure 12-8): Flex the knees and hips to 90 degrees. Place your index finger over the greater trochanter and your thumb over the lesser trochanter. Simultaneously abduct both hips until the lateral aspect of each knee touches the examination table. When DDH is present you will feel and sometimes hear a "clunk" as the dislocated femoral head reenters the acetabulum.
- **Barlow test:** Place your index finger over the greater trochanter and your thumb over the lesser trochanter. Using the opposite hand to stabilize the pelvis, push your thumb posterolaterally and feel for movement of the femoral head as it slips out onto the posterior lip of the acetabulum. Then with your index finger press the greater trochanter anteromedially. Feel for movement of the femoral head as it reenters the acetabulum. Normally no movement is felt. Movement in both directions constitutes a positive Barlow test (hip instability).

PERFORM A DENVER DEVELOPMENTAL SCREENING TEST

- The **Denver Development Screening Test (DDST)** assesses development of children from birth to 6 years of age using four categories:
  - Personal-social
  - Fine motor-adaptive
  - Language
  - Gross motor
- The DDST is not a test of intelligence. The criteria for passing the DDST are set low to minimize labeling normal children as abnormal, making it more specific than sensitive. Children with "borderline" or "questionable" scores should be followed closely.
- **To use the DDST** (Figure 12-9): Draw a line from top to bottom according to the age of the child. Test each of the milestones crossed by this line. Failure to perform an item passed by 90% of children is significant. Two failures in any of the four categories are indicative of a developmental delay in that domain.

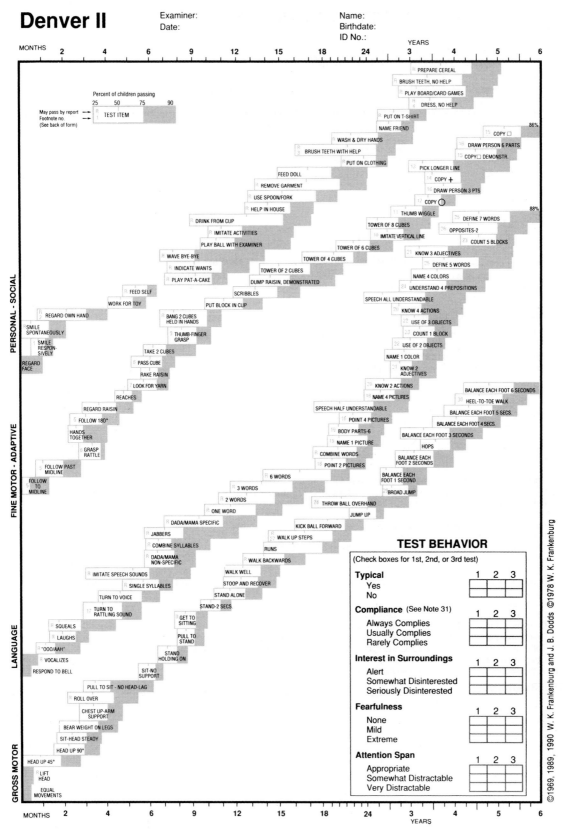

Figure 12-9 Denver Developmental Screening Test. (From Swartz M: *Textbook of physical diagnosis: history and examination,* ed 4, Philadelphia, 2002, WB Saunders, Figure 23-1.)

DIRECTIONS FOR ADMINISTRATION

1. Try to get child to smile by smiling, talking, or waving. Do not touch him/her.
2. Child must stare at hand several seconds.
3. Parent may help guide toothbrush and put toothpaste on brush.
4. Child does not have to be able to tie shoes or button/zip in the back.
5. Move yarn slowly in an arc from one side to the other, about 8" above child's face.
6. Pass if child grasps rattle when it is touched to the backs or tips of fingers.
7. Pass if child tries to see where yarn went. Yarn should be dropped quickly from sight from tester's hand without arm movement.
8. Child must transfer cube from hand to hand without help of body, mouth, or table.
9. Pass if child picks up raisin with any part of thumb and finger.
10. Line can vary only 30 degrees or less from tester's line.
11. Make a fist with thumb pointing upward and wiggle only the thumb. Pass if child imitates and does not move any fingers other than the thumb.

12. Pass any enclosed form. Fail continuous round motions.
13. Which line is longer? (Not bigger.) Turn paper upside down and repeat. (pass 3 of 3 or 5 of 6)
14. Pass any lines crossing near midpoint.
15. Have child copy first. If failed, demonstrate.

When giving items 12, 14, and 15, do not name the forms. Do not demonstrate 12 and 14.

16. When scoring, each pair (2 arms, 2 legs, etc.) counts as one part.
17. Place one cube in cup and shake gently near child's ear, but out of sight. Repeat for other ear.
18. Point to picture and have child name it. (No credit is given for sounds only.)
    If less than 4 pictures are named correctly, have child point to picture as each is named by tester.

 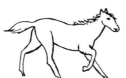   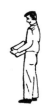

19. Using doll, tell child: Show me the nose, eyes, ears, mouth, hands, feet, tummy, hair. Pass 6 of 8.
20. Using pictures, ask child: Which one flies?... says meow?... talks?... barks?... gallops? Pass 2 of 5, 4 of 5.
21. Ask child: What do you do when you are cold?... tired?... hungry? Pass 2 of 3, 3 of 3.
22. Ask child: What do you do with a cup? What is a chair used for? What is a pencil used for?
    Action words must be included in answers.
23. Pass if child correctly places <u>and</u> says how many blocks are on paper. (1, 5).
24. Tell child: Put block **on** table; **under** table; **in front of** me, **behind** me. Pass 4 of 4.
    (Do not help child by pointing, moving head or eyes.)
25. Ask child: What is a ball?... lake?... desk?... house?... banana?... curtain?... fence?... ceiling? Pass if defined in terms of use, shape, what it is made of, or general category (such as banana is fruit, not just yellow). Pass 5 of 8, 7 of 8.
26. Ask child: If a horse is big, a mouse is __? If fire is hot, ice is __? If the sun shines during the day, the moon shines during the __? Pass 2 of 3.
27. Child may use wall or rail only, not person. May not crawl.
28. Child must throw ball overhand 3 feet to within arm's reach of tester.
29. Child must perform standing broad jump over width of test sheet (8 1/2 inches).
30. Tell child to walk forward, ∞∞ ∞∞→ heel within 1 inch of toe. Tester may demonstrate.
    Child must walk 4 consecutive steps.
31. In the second year, half of normal children are non-compliant.

OBSERVATIONS:

Figure 12-9 *Continued*

SAMPLE OSCE SCENARIOS

> INSTRUCTIONS TO CANDIDATE: A 15-year-old female presents with malaise and "swollen glands." Perform a focused physical examination.

DD$_X$ VITAMINS C
- **Infectious:** Mononucleosis, other viral illness, tuberculosis (TB), and HIV
- **Neoplastic:** Lymphoma (Hodgkin's and non-Hodgkin's types), leukemia, and other malignancies

Physical Examination
- **Vitals:** HR, RR, BP, and temperature (may find low-grade fever)
- **General:** Cachexia, diaphoresis
- **Skin:** Jaundice, pallor (lips, buccal mucosa, conjunctiva, palmar creases), petechiae, or ecchymosis
- **Lymphatic system:** Note size, shape, mobility, consistency, tenderness, warmth, and number of enlarged nodes. Seat the patient in a chair, and stand behind him or her. Flex the neck slightly. Palpate using the pads of the fingers in a rotatory motion (moving the skin over the underlying tissues).
  - Occipital: Base of skull posteriorly
  - Postauricular: Superficial to mastoid process
  - Preauricular: Anterior to ear
  - Tonsillar: Angle of mandible
  - Submandibular: Midway between the angle and the tip of the mandible
  - Submental: Midline behind the tip of the mandible (helpful to palpate with one hand while bracing the top of the head with the other hand)
  - Anterior cervical: Along the anterior border of the sternocleidomastoid (SCM) muscle
  - Superficial cervical: Superficial to the SCM muscle
  - Posterior cervical: Along the anterior edge of the trapezius muscle
  - Deep cervical: Deep to the SCM muscle and often inaccessible (hook your thumb and fingers around the SCM muscle, and roll the muscle between your fingers)
  - Supraclavicular: Deep in the angle between the clavicle and SCM muscle
  - Infraclavicular: Inferior to the clavicle
  - Axillary
  - Epitrochlear
  - Inguinal
- **Respiratory (Resp):** Inspect for thoracic deformity and chest expansion (symmetry). Auscultate for breath sounds and adventitious sounds. Note any signs of infection, pleural effusion, or tracheobronchial compression.
- **Cardiovascular system (CVS):** Check capillary refill. Palpate the peripheral pulses. Note pulse volume, contour, and rhythm. Auscultate the heart, looking for extra heart sounds or murmurs. Look for signs of anemia such as hyperdynamic precordium and aortic flow murmur.
- **Abdomen:** Inspect the abdomen. Auscultate for bowel sounds, noting borborygmus. Percuss lightly in all four quadrants. Perform light and deep palpation, and identify any masses or areas of tenderness. Check for rebound tenderness. Examine the liver and spleen (looking for organomegaly).
- Note any signs or sources of infection.

> INSTRUCTIONS TO CANDIDATE: A 14-month-old girl is brought to the emergency department by her parents because of diarrhea. Perform a focused history and physical examination.

Definition

- **Diarrhea** is abnormally frequent passage of poorly formed or watery stool. Quantified it is the passage of >300 ml of liquid feces in a 24-hour period.

DD$_X$ Diarrhea (VITAMINS C)

- Infectious: Bacterial/parasitic/viral infection, pseudomembranous colitis
- **A**utoimmune/**A**llergic: Celiac disease
- **M**etabolic: Drugs (e.g., laxative abuse)
- **I**diopathic/**I**atrogenic: Inflammatory bowel disease (IBD), irritable bowel syndrome (IBS)
- **C**ongenital/genetic: Cystic fibrosis (CF), lactose intolerance

History

- **Character:** Describe your bowel movements (BMs).
  - Are the stools frequent, voluminous, and poorly formed (diarrhea)? Are there any food particles?
  - Are the stools large, oily, malodorous, but somewhat formed (steatorrhea)?
  - Are the stools frequent and formed but small?
  - Any blood, pus, or mucus in the stool? Describe the color of the stool.
  - Does diarrhea persist despite fasting?
  - Does she experience nocturnal diarrhea?
  - Describe her usual BMs.
- **Location:** Where was she when this started? Any recent travel?
- **Onset:** When did the diarrhea start (sudden versus insidious)?
- **Intensity:** How severe is it (number of stools per day and approximate volume of stool)? Has it gotten worse?
- **Duration:** How long has the diarrhea been going on (acute versus chronic)?
- **Events associated:**
  - N/V? Fever/chills? Abdominal pain? Appetite?
  - Consumption of dairy or meat products in the 72 hours preceding onset of diarrhea (undercooked hamburger or chicken, shellfish, lactose intolerance)? Excessive cereal/prunes/roughage? Artificial sweeteners?
  - Periods of constipation (IBS)?
  - Travel to tropical/subtropical regions? Infectious contacts? Contaminated water ingestion?
  - IBD: Chronic diarrhea, abdominal pain, weight loss, perianal disease, and extraintestinal manifestations
  - Constitutional symptoms: Fever, chills, night sweats, weight loss, anorexia, and asthenia
- **Frequency:** Has this ever happened before? Is every BM like diarrhea (intermittent versus constant)?
- **Palliative factors:** Is there anything that makes it better? If so, what?
  - Fasting?
- **Provocative factors:** Is there anything that makes it worse? If so, what?
  - Dairy products?
  - Solid foods?
- **Previous investigations:** Stool analysis
- **Past medical history (PMH)/past surgical history (PSH):** IBD, celiac disease, hyperthyroidism, previous gastrointestinal (GI) surgery, CF, HIV/AIDS, or malignancy

- **Medications (MEDS):** Laxatives, antidiarrheal agents, recent antibiotics, or corticosteroids
- **Allergies:** Medications, food allergies or intolerances
- **Social history (SH):** Diet
- **Family history (FH):** IBD, CF, GI malignancy, celiac disease, or HIV/AIDS

Prenatal, Natal, and Neonatal History
- Did you have prenatal care? Any difficulties during the pregnancy?
- Use of alcohol or recreational drugs during the pregnancy? Smoking?
- Singleton versus multiple gestation
- Date and gestation at delivery
- Onset of labor, duration of labor, and type of delivery (normal spontaneous vaginal delivery [NSVD], lower segment cesarean section [LSCS], forceps, or vacuum)
- Birth weight? Breast-fed versus bottle-fed?
- Apgar scores at 1 and 5 minutes?
- Any health problems as a baby? Any hospital admissions?
- Any delay in speech, language, or motor development?

Examination
- **Vitals:** HR, RR, BP (lying and standing), and temperature
- **General:** Inspect for signs of dehydration (sunken eyes, dry buccal mucosa, loss of skin turgor, delayed capillary refill, lethargy). Note distress, diaphoresis, or pallor.
- **Head, eyes, ears, nose, and throat (HEENT):** Inspect the sclerae. Note any aphthous oral ulcers (IBD), glossitis, or cheilosis (anemia).
- **Resp:** Inspect for thoracic deformity and chest expansion (symmetry). Auscultate for breath sounds and adventitious sounds.
- **CVS:** Check capillary refill. Palpate the peripheral pulses. Note pulse volume, contour, and rhythm. Auscultate the heart, looking for extra heart sounds or murmurs.
- **Abdomen:** Inspect the abdomen. Hyperperistalsis may be evident in a thin person. Auscultate for bowel sounds, noting borborygmus. Percuss lightly in all four quadrants. Perform light and deep palpation, and identify any masses or areas of tenderness. Check for rebound tenderness. Examine the liver and spleen. Inspect the perianal area for fissures, fistulas, skin tags, or other lesions. Perform a digital rectal examination (DRE).
- **Examine the stool:** Note the proportion of water to solids and the presence of pus, mucus, fat globules, and food particles. Note any fresh blood, and test for the presence of occult blood.
- **Neurologic (Neuro):** Mental status (interaction with parent/caregiver, level of activity, consolability)

INSTRUCTIONS TO CANDIDATE: A 10-year-old girl with a history of asthma is brought to the emergency department from gym class. At the triage desk she is tachypneic and has an audible wheeze. Perform a focused history and physical examination.

Definition
- **Wheeze** is produced by partial obstruction of the lower airway and is heard on expiration. High-pitched, musical wheezes come from small, peripheral airways.

DD$_x$ VITAMINS C
- "All that wheezes is not asthma," although it is the most common cause of wheeze in children.
- **V**ascular: Cardiac wheeze

- Infectious: Bronchiolitis
- Traumatic: Foreign body (FB) aspiration
- Autoimmune/Allergic: Angioedema
- Idiopathic/Iatrogenic: Asthma, gastroesophageal reflux (GER)
- Congenital/genetic: CF

- **First evaluate A**irway, **B**reathing, and **C**irculation. It may be necessary to perform an immediate intervention, such as supplemental O_2, IV access, or intubation.
  - Is the patient able to talk? Swallow? Cough?
  - Signs of respiratory distress: Tachypnea, pursed lips, nasal flare, tripod positioning, tracheal tug, accessory muscle use, intercostal/subcostal retractions, and thoracoabdominal dissociation
  - Are both lungs ventilated? Is the patient oxygenating (mentation, pulse oximetry)?
  - Abnormal vitals? Peripheral circulation (pulses, capillary refill)?
  - If no immediate interventions are required, proceed to perform an appropriate history and physical examination.

History
- **Character:** Describe the "wheeze." What time of day is the wheeze at its worst?
  - High-pitched versus low-pitched, inspiratory versus expiratory
  - Do you feel SOB? Describe the nature of your breathing difficulty.
- **Location:** Where were you when this started? What were you doing?
- **Onset:** How did the wheeze begin (sudden versus insidious onset)? How did the SOB start?
- **Intensity:** How severe is the wheeze right now on a scale of 1 to 10, with 10 being the most severe? How severe has the wheeze been in the past? How is it affecting your daily activities? How severe is the SOB?
- **Duration:** How long have you had this wheeze (acute versus chronic)? How long have you been SOB?
- **Events associated:**
  - Asthma: Nocturnal cough, decreased exercise tolerance, atopy, acetylsalicylic acid (ASA)/nonsteroidal antiinflammatory drug (NSAID) sensitivity, and nasal polyps
  - FB aspiration: Choking spell, cyanosis, cough, and wheeze localized to one area of the chest
  - GER: Heartburn, nonspecific chest pain, dysphagia, pharyngitis/laryngitis, and symptoms aggravated by lying or bending and specific foods (e.g., peppermint, fatty foods)
  - Anaphylaxis: Exposure to allergen, anxiety and apprehension, urticaria and edema, choking sensation/cough/bronchospasm or laryngeal edema, abdominal pain, N/V, and hypotension
- **Frequency:** Have you had this wheeze before? Have you been SOB before? If so, when? How frequently does it occur (continuous versus intermittent)?
- **Palliative factors:** Is there anything that makes the wheeze/SOB better? If so, what?
  - Inhalers?
  - Steroids?
- **Provocative factors:** Is there anything that makes the wheeze/SOB worse? If so, what?
  - Exposure to known allergens: Animal dander, dust mites, pollen, and feathers
  - Pets or stuffed animals? Carpets? Pillow?
  - Environment: Exposure to cold air, type of heating system in the home, industrialized area, air pollution/smog, and scented products
  - Do you smoke? Any smokers in your home?
  - Infections: Upper respiratory tract infection (URTI), pneumonia, and influenza
  - Exercise: Change in exercise habits, exposure to cold air
  - Emotional stress: Crying, screaming, or hard laughing

- **PMH/PSH:** Asthma, atopy, GER, or congenital anomalies
- **MEDS:** NSAIDs, ASA, or sulfa drugs
  - Any increase/decrease in medication dosage? More frequent use of inhalers?
  - Noncompliance?
  - Have you been prescribed any new medications?
- **FH:** Asthma, allergic rhinitis, atopy, or eczema

Physical Examination

- **Vitals:** HR and rhythm, RR (depth, effort, and pattern), BP, pulsus paradoxus, and temperature
- **General:** Respiratory distress (e.g., inability to speak), diaphoresis, or anxiety
  - Respiratory distress: Tachypnea, pursed lips, nasal flare, tripod positioning, tracheal tug, accessory muscle use, intercostal/subcostal retractions, and thoracoabdominal dissociation
- **Skin:** Peripheral edema, cyanosis, clubbing, or eczema
- **HEENT:** Central cyanosis, tracheal position (tug may be noted), lymphadenopathy, nasal polyps, or rhinitis
- **Resp (Table 12-2):** Inspect for thoracic deformity and chest expansion (symmetry). Perform tactile fremitus and chest percussion. Auscultate for breath sounds and adventitious sounds.
- **CVS:** Jugular venous pressure (JVP) and hepatojugular reflux (signs of venous congestion may herald a pneumothorax), peripheral pulses; palpate the apical impulse, and auscultate, looking for a loud P_2, an S_3, or any murmurs.
- **Neuro:** Mental status (adequate brain oxygenation)

PEARLS

- **Asthma** is a pulmonary disease characterized by reversible airway obstruction, airway inflammation, and increased airway responsiveness to a variety of stimuli. Airway obstruction in asthma is caused by spasm of airway smooth muscle, edema of airway mucosa, increased mucus secretion, cellular infiltration of airway walls, and injury and desquamation of the airway epithelium.
- **Asthma triad:** Atopy, ASA sensitivity, and nasal polyps
- A quiet-sounding chest in a patient having an asthma attack may be a *warning* of patient fatigue or obstruction of small airways. It can quickly become *life threatening*.
- The most reliable signs of a severe attack are dyspnea at rest, inability to speak, accessory muscle use, cyanosis, and pulsus paradoxus. An asthma attack may begin with cough and wheezing, rapidly progressing to dyspnea. Confusion and lethargy may indicate respiratory failure and CO_2 narcosis. A normal or increased $PaCO_2$ may indicate respiratory failure (hyperventilation should result in a decreased $PaCO_2$).

Table 12-2 Expected Findings in an Acute Exacerbation of Asthma

Examination	Expected Findings
Thoracic deformity	Barrel chest: hyperinflation
Chest movement	May be asymmetric in case of associated pneumothorax
Trachea	Midline, may note tracheal tug
Tactile fremitus	Decreased
Percussion	Hyperresonant, flattened diaphragms
Breath sounds	Prolonged expiratory phase; localized disappearance of breath sounds can occur temporarily from bronchial plugging
Adventitious sounds	High-pitched wheezes

INSTRUCTIONS TO CANDIDATE: A 7-year-old boy is brought to his family doctor by his father. He is complaining of a sore throat and fever for 2 days. Perform a focused history and physical examination.

Definitions
- **Pharyngitis** refers to inflammation of the pharynx.

DD$_X$ Pharyngitis (VITAMINS C)
- Infectious: Viral infection (e.g., adenovirus, herpangina), bacterial infection (e.g., strep throat), pharyngeal abscess, and epiglottitis
- Traumatic: Ingestion of a caustic substance

History
- **Character:** What is your sore throat like? Does it hurt when you swallow? Does your neck hurt?
- **Location:** Point to where it hurts.
- **Onset:** How did it come on (sudden versus insidious)?
- **Intensity:** Use a pain scale to rate the discomfort (Figure 12-10). Are the symptoms preventing you from sleeping? From attending school? From playing?
- **Duration:** When did this begin (2 days ago)? How long has this been going on (acute versus chronic)?
- **Events associated:**
  - Strep throat: Fever >38.3° C, macular exanthem, adenopathy, and infectious contacts
  - URTI: Clear rhinorrhea, cough, myalgia, headache, ± fever, decreased appetite, and infectious contacts
  - Adenovirus: Rhinorrhea, conjunctivitis, and GI symptoms (e.g., diarrhea)
- **Frequency:** Has your child ever had this before? If so, when? How frequently does it occur?
- **Palliative factors:** Is there anything that makes it better? If so, what?
- **Provocative factors:** Is there anything that makes it worse? If so, what?
- **PMH/PSH:** URTIs, atopy, and tonsillectomy
- **MEDS:** Antibiotics, decongestants
- **SH:** Smokers in the home, pets, carpets, wood stove, teddy bears, and so on.
- **FH:** Infectious contacts

Physical Examination
- **Vitals:** HR and rhythm, RR (depth, effort, and pattern), BP, and temperature
- **General:** Diaphoresis, flushed appearance, anxiety, drooling, or respiratory distress
- **Skin:** Inspect for macular exanthem, other lesions.
- **HEENT:** Determine tracheal position, and ensure the neck is supple. Inspect the conjunctiva, noting any injected appearance. Inspect the nasal mucosa for inflammation or polyps. Note any discharge (e.g., clear versus purulent). Inspect the mouth. Note any erythema, petechiae, or vesicles on the palate. Note the size of the tonsils and the presence of any exudate (Figure 12-11). Examine for cervical lymphadenopathy.

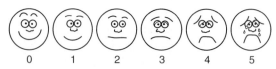

Figure 12-10 Adapted version of Wong-Baker FACES Pain Rating Scale. (From Magaret ND, Clark TA, Warden CR, Magnusson AR, Hedges JR: Patient satisfaction in the emergency department: a survey of pediatric patients and their parents. *Acad Emerg Med* 9:1388, 2002, Appendix A.)

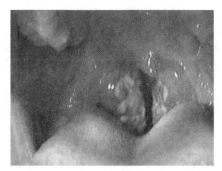

Figure 12-11   Enlarged tonsils with exudate. (Used with permission of Dr. Brett Taylor, Dalhousie University.)

- **Resp:** Inspect for thoracic deformity and chest expansion (symmetry). Percuss the chest wall. Auscultate for breath sounds and adventitious sounds.
- **CVS:** Check capillary refill. Palpate the peripheral pulses. Note pulse volume, contour, and rhythm. Auscultate the heart, looking for extra heart sounds or murmurs.
- **Abdomen:** Inspect the abdomen. Auscultate for bowel sounds. Percuss lightly in all four quadrants. Identify any masses or areas of tenderness. Examine the liver and spleen.
- **Neuro:** Mental status (orientation, level of interaction with father, level of activity)

PEARL
- Modified Centor criteria for streptococcus pharyngitis: Fever >38.3° C, absence of cough, presence of pharyngeal exudate and cervical lymphadenopathy

> INSTRUCTIONS TO CANDIDATE: A 2-year-old boy is brought to the emergency department by his parents because of cough, fever, and rapid breathing. Perform a focused history and physical examination.

Definition
- **Cough** is a sudden, noisy expulsion of air from the lungs. It is a nonspecific reaction to irritation anywhere from the pharynx to the lungs. Cough may be voluntary or stimulated by inhaled agents (e.g., dust), internal agents, or external pressure on air passages. Stimulation in the external auditory meatus may also precipitate cough.

DD$_X$ Acute Cough (VITAMINS C)
- **Vascular:** Congestive heart failure (CHF; pulmonary edema)
- **Infectious:** Pneumonia, bronchiolitis, croup, bronchitis, tracheitis, pertussis, and sinusitis
- **Traumatic:** FB aspiration, thermal or chemical inhalation
- **Idiopathic and Iatrogenic:** Asthma, GER
- **Neoplastic:** Tracheobronchial tree neoplasm or neoplasm compressing the tracheobronchial tree (e.g., lymphoma, thymoma)
- **First evaluate Airway, Breathing, and Circulation.** It may be necessary to perform an immediate intervention, such as supplemental O$_2$, IV access, or intubation.

History
- **Character:** What is the cough like?
  - Clearing of the throat: GER and postnasal drip
  - Barking cough (like a seal): Croup
  - Hacking cough: Pharyngitis, tracheobronchitis, and early pneumonia
  - Whooping cough: Pertussis
  - Any sputum production? If so, what color and how much (mucus, blood, pus)?

- **Onset:** How did it start (sudden versus gradual)?
- **Intensity:** How severe is the cough? At what time of day (if any) is the cough most severe? Is the child too weak to eat or play? Any difficulty breathing? Have you taken the child's temperature? By what means? How high has the temperature been?
- **Duration:** How long has it been going on (acute versus chronic versus paroxysmal versus seasonal versus perennial)? If the cough is chronic, how has it changed recently? Is it getting better, worse, or staying the same?
- **Events associated:**
  - Exposure to irritants? Sudden paroxysmal onset of cough (FB aspiration)?
  - Any difficulty breathing? Any noisy breathing?
  - Infectious contacts: Day care, recent parties, school, and baby-sitter
  - URTI: Malaise, sore throat, rhinorrhea, myalgias, headache, ear pain
  - Pneumonia: Fever, chills, rigors, increased sputum production
  - Tracheitis: Retrosternal pain
  - Asthma: SOB on exertion (SOBOE), exercise/cold-induced cough, wheeze, and nocturnal cough
  - CHF: Exertional dyspnea, orthopnea, cyanosis
- **Frequency:** Has your child ever had this cough before? When? How often?
- **Palliative factors:** Is there anything that makes the cough and fever better? If so, what?
  - Inhalers?
  - Cough suppressants?
  - Acetaminophen? Ibuprofen?
- **Provocative factors:** What brings on the cough? What makes the cough worse?
  - Exercise?
  - Cigarette smoke?
  - Exposure to known allergens?
- **PMH/PSH:** Asthma, allergies or eczema, whooping cough, CF, congenital heart disease, bronchopulmonary dysplasia, tracheomalacia, or HIV/AIDS
- **MEDS:** Antibiotics, other medications (e.g., angiotensin-converting enzyme [ACE] inhibitors are known to have cough as a side effect)
- **Allergies:** Medications, foods, and environmental
- **SH:** Smokers in the home, pets, carpets, wood stove, teddy bears, and so on.
- **Immunizations:** Especially pertussis and *Haemophilus influenzae* type b (Hib) vaccine
- **FH:** Asthma, allergies/eczema/rhinitis, CF, or α_1-antitrypsin deficiency

Prenatal, Natal, and Neonatal History

- Did you have prenatal care? Any difficulties during the pregnancy?
- Use of alcohol or recreational drugs during the pregnancy? Smoking?
- Singleton versus multiple gestation
- Date and gestation at delivery
- Onset of labor, duration of labor, and type of delivery (NSVD, LSCS, forceps, vacuum)
- Birth weight? Breast-fed versus bottle-fed?
- Apgar scores at 1 and 5 minutes?
- Any health problems as a baby? Any hospital admissions?
- Any delay in speech, language, or motor development?

Physical Examination

- **Vitals:** HR and rhythm, RR (depth, effort, and pattern), BP, pulsus paradoxus, and temperature
- **General:** Respiratory distress, stridor. Observe for coughing during the history and examination.
- **HEENT:** Central cyanosis, tracheal position, lymphadenopathy, conjunctiva, tympanic membranes, pharynx, and tonsils

Box 12-1   Rochester Criteria

Infant appears well (no signs of toxicity)
No skin, soft tissue, bone, joint, or ear infection
Previously healthy infant
- Term birth
- No perinatal antibiotic therapy
- No history of unexplained hyperbilirubinemia
- No previous or current antibiotic therapy
- Not previously hospitalized except for birth (not hospitalized for longer than the mother
- No chronic or underlying illness
Laboratory values
- Peripheral WBC count of 5,000–15,000/mm^3
- Total band count of <1,500/mm^3
- ≤10 WBCs per high-power field (×40) on microscopic examination of spun urine sediment
- ≤5 WBCs per high-power field (×40) on microscopic examination of a stool smear (in infants with diarrhea)

Adapted from Lopez JA, McMillin KJ, Tobias-Merrill EA, Chop WM: Managing fever in infants and toddlers. *Postgrad Med* 101:242, 1997 (Table 1).

- **Resp:** Inspect for thoracic deformity and chest expansion (symmetry). Auscultate for breath sounds and adventitious sounds.
- **CVS:** Check capillary refill. Palpate the peripheral pulses. Note pulse volume, contour, and rhythm. Auscultate the heart, looking for extra heart sounds or murmurs.
- **Abdomen:** Inspect the abdomen. Auscultate for bowel sounds. Percuss lightly in all four quadrants. Identify any masses or areas of tenderness. Examine the liver and spleen.

PEARLS

- **Croup** is the most common cause of infectious upper airway obstruction affecting children aged 6 months to 3 years. Obstruction is caused by inflammation and swelling in the subglottic space. Most causative agents are viral.
- The **Rochester criteria** can be used to help identify febrile infants at low risk for serious bacterial infections (Box 12-1). To be considered at low risk all criteria must be met.

INSTRUCTIONS TO CANDIDATE: A 31-month-old boy is brought to the emergency department via ambulance because of a seizure. His parents say that he was "shaking all over" and his eyes rolled back in his head. The paramedic tells you that he has a temperature of 39.3° C. Perform a focused history and physical examination.

Definition

- A **seizure** is a spontaneous, transient brain disturbance, manifesting as motor, somatosensory, autonomic, or psychic impairment (or a combination thereof). It is often accompanied by alternation or loss of consciousness.
- Criteria for **febrile seizures**:
  - Age: 3 months to 5 years
  - Temperature >38.8° C
  - Non–central nervous system (CNS) source of infection

DD$_X$ of Seizure (VITAMINS C)

- **V**ascular: Intracranial hemorrhage (e.g., arteriovenous malformation [AVM])
- **I**nfectious: CNS infection (meningitis, encephalitis, abscess)
- **T**raumatic: Toxic ingestion, head injury
- **M**etabolic: Disturbance in sodium, calcium, magnesium, glucose, or renal function
- **I**diopathic/**I**atrogenic: Febrile seizure, epilepsy
- **N**eoplastic: Intracranial malignancy
- **S**ubstance abuse and **P**sychiatric: Pseudoseizure
- **C**ongenital/genetic: Congenital structural defects

History

- **Character:** What happened? What did you see? Did he fall? Was there any trauma? Was he well before this episode? What was happening at the time of this episode? Were there any movements (e.g., automatisms, tonic-clonic activity)? Was he able to talk to you? What was he like afterward? How long did it take to get back to normal (post-ictal period)?
- **Location:** Where did this happen?
- **Onset:** Was there any warning? An aura (lights, sounds, smells)? Has this ever happened before? If so, what was the age of onset? How did it start?
- **Duration:** How long did this episode last? How long did it take to get back to normal?
- **Events associated:**
  - Fever: URTI, headache, urinary tract infection (UTI)
  - Salivation, cyanosis, tongue biting, or incontinence
  - Post-ictal symptoms: Muscle aches, tongue soreness, headache, drowsiness, and confusion
- **Frequency:** Has this ever happened before? When? How often?
- **Palliative factors:** Did anything seem to help? If so, what (e.g., medications)?
- **Provocative factors:** Is there anything that seemed to have brought on the "seizure"? If so, what?
  - Fever? Illness? How high was the fever? How quickly did it come on?
  - Head injury?
- **PMH/PSH:** Birth injury, head trauma, stroke, CNS infection, or previous seizures
- **MEDS:** Prescription or over-the-counter (OTC) medications (antipyretics), or anticonvulsants
- **FH:** Seizures

Prenatal, Natal, and Neonatal History

- Did you have prenatal care? Any difficulties during the pregnancy?
- Use of alcohol or recreational drugs during the pregnancy? Smoking?
- Singleton versus multiple gestation
- Date and gestation at delivery
- Onset of labor, duration of labor, and type of delivery (NSVD, LSCS, forceps, vacuum)
- Birth weight? Breast-fed versus bottle-fed?
- Apgar scores at 1 and 5 minutes?
- Any health problems as a baby? Any hospital admissions?
- Any delay in speech, language, or motor development?

Physical Examination

- **Vitals:** HR and rhythm, RR (depth, effort, and pattern), BP, and temperature
- **General:** Diaphoresis, flushed appearance
- **Skin:** Inspect for exanthem, other lesions (e.g., infectious exanthem, petechiae)
- **HEENT:** Ensure the neck is supple (Figure 12-12). Inspect the conjunctiva, noting any injected appearance. Inspect the nasal mucosa. Note any discharge. Inspect the mouth. Note any erythema, petechiae, or vesicles on the palate. Note the size of the

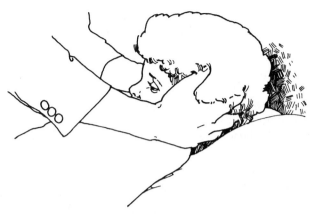

Figure 12-12   Examination for neck stiffness. (From Gill D, O'Brien N: *Paediatric clinical examination made easy,* ed 4, London, 2002, Churchill Livingstone, p 146, Figure 5.16.)

tonsils and the presence of any exudate. Examine for cervical lymphadenopathy. Perform funduscopy, looking for papilledema (increased ICP) or hemorrhage.

- **Resp:** Inspect for thoracic deformity and chest expansion (symmetry). Percuss the chest wall. Auscultate for breath sounds and adventitious sounds.
- **CVS:** Check capillary refill. Palpate the peripheral pulses. Note pulse volume, contour, and rhythm. Auscultate the heart, looking for extra heart sounds or murmurs.
- **Abdomen:** Inspect the abdomen. Auscultate for bowel sounds. Percuss lightly in all four quadrants. Identify any masses or areas of tenderness. Examine the liver and spleen.
- **Neuro:** Mental status (orientation, level of interaction with parents, level of activity). Look for focal neurologic deficits to suggest a space-occupying lesion. Most of the neurologic examination can be performed by simply observing the child play (motor function, CNs).

PEARLS
- Febrile seizures are common in children.
- Most infections arise from the middle ear, upper respiratory tract, and lymph nodes.
- Features that increase the risk of recurrent seizures include:
  - >1 seizure in 24 hours
  - Seizure duration >15 minutes
  - Focal seizure (most febrile seizures are generalized tonic-clonic type)
  - Age <1 year
  - FH of seizure disorder

> INSTRUCTIONS TO CANDIDATE: A 13-year-old male presents to the emergency department with a headache and fever. He recently returned from army cadet camp. Perform a focused history and physical examination.

Definition
- **Meningitis** is inflammation of the membranes (pia, arachnoid, and dura) in the CNS. To some degree the inflammation involves all intracranial structures. The etiology is usually infectious (bacterial, viral, fungal).

DD$_X$ Headache and Fever (VITAMINS C)
- **Vascular:** Cavernous sinus thrombosis, vasculitis
- **Infectious:** CNS infection (meningitis, encephalitis, intracranial abscess)

- Idiopathic/Iatrogenic: Collagen vascular disease
- Coincidental fever: Migraine, tension headache, intracranial hemorrhage, increased ICP, and trauma

History

- **Character:** Describe the headache. Bandlike? Pulsatile? Nonspecific? Did you take your temperature at home? By what means (e.g., axillary, oral, tympanic)?
- **Location:** Where is the headache? Bilateral? Unilateral? Occipital? Does it involve your neck?
- **Onset:** How did it start (sudden maximal intensity versus gradual buildup)?
- **Radiation:** Does the pain move anywhere (e.g., neck)?
- **Intensity:** What is the severity of the pain on a scale of 1 to 10, with 1 being mild and 10 being the worst? How high is your temperature?
- **Duration:** How long have you had the headache and fever (acute versus chronic)? Which came on first?
- **Events associated:**
  - Malaise? Lethargy? Loss of appetite?
  - N/V? Skin lesions (e.g., petechiae)?
  - Head injury? Previous neurosurgery? Shunt?
  - Facial cellulitis (venous drainage to cavernous sinus)? Sinusitis, retropharyngeal abscess (extension into CNS)?
  - Infectious contacts: Family, cadet camp
- **Frequency:** Have you ever had a headache like this before? When? How frequently (intermittent versus constant)?
- **Palliative factors:** Is there anything that makes it better? If so, what?
  - NSAIDs?
  - Acetaminophen?
- **Provocative factors:** Is there anything that makes it worse? If so, what?
  - Movement?
  - Bright light (photophobia)?
  - Loud noises (phonophobia)?
- **PMH/PSH:** Head trauma, CNS infection, HIV or other immunosuppression, asplenia, migraines, previous neurosurgery, or shunt
- **MEDS:** Antibiotics, antipyretics, or immunosuppressants
- **FH:** Seizures

Physical Examination

- **Vitals:** HR and rhythm, RR (depth, effort, and pattern), BP, and temperature
- **General:** Diaphoresis, flushed appearance
- **Skin:** Inspect for exanthem, other lesions (e.g., infectious exanthem, petechiae).
- **HEENT:** Ensure the neck is supple (see Figure 12-12). Inspect the conjunctiva, noting any injected appearance. Inspect the nasal mucosa. Note any discharge. Inspect the mouth. Note any erythema, petechiae, or vesicles on the palate. Note the size of the tonsils and the presence of any exudate. Examine for cervical lymphadenopathy. Perform funduscopy, looking for papilledema (increased ICP).
- **Resp:** Inspect for thoracic deformity and chest expansion (symmetry). Percuss the chest wall. Auscultate for breath sounds and adventitious sounds.
- **CVS:** Check capillary refill. Palpate the peripheral pulses. Note pulse volume, contour, and rhythm. Auscultate the heart, looking for extra heart sounds or murmurs.
- **Abdomen:** Inspect the abdomen. Auscultate for bowel sounds. Percuss lightly in all four quadrants. Identify any masses or areas of tenderness. Examine the liver and spleen.
- **Neuro:** Mental status (orientation, level of activity). Look for focal neurologic deficits to suggest a space-occupying lesion.

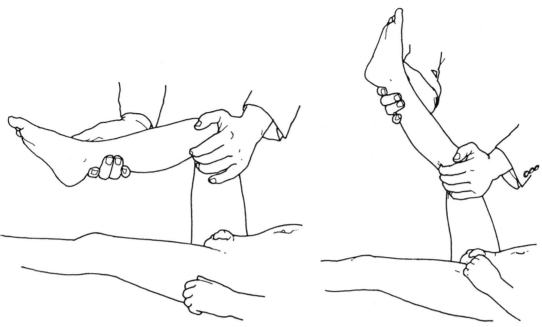

Figure 12-13   Kernig's sign. (From Gill D, O'Brien N: *Paediatric clinical examination made easy,* ed 4, London, 2002, Churchill Livingstone, p 148, Figure 5.17.)

- **Kernig's sign** (Figure 12-13): With the patient supine flex the hip and knee to 90 degrees. Attempt to extend the knee. In patients with meningeal irritation, full extension may be impossible because of resistance and pain (extension increases meningeal stretch).
- **Brudzinski's sign:** With the patient supine gently attempt to flex the neck. Brudzinski's sign is said to be present when this produces neck pain and simultaneous flexion of the knees (to decrease meningeal stretch).

PEARL
- In true meningism when testing neck suppleness, you will find it to be stiff (board-like rigidity), enabling you to lift the upper body off the bed as well.

INSTRUCTIONS TO CANDIDATE: A 1-month-old boy is brought to the emergency department because of a 5-day history of vomiting. His mother is concerned that he is becoming dehydrated because he "can't keep anything down." Take a detailed history, exploring possible etiologies.

Definition
- **Vomiting** is the forceful ejection of gastric contents. **Regurgitation** is different from vomiting and is generally nonforceful reflux.

DD$_X$ VITAMINS C
- **I**nfectious: Gastroenteritis
- **A**utoimmune/**A**llergic: Food allergy (milk protein intolerance)
- **I**diopathic/**I**atrogenic: GER, GI obstruction (e.g., malrotation and volvulus), necrotizing enterocolitis, systemic illness, and increased ICP
- **C**ongenital/genetic: Inborn errors of metabolism, pyloric stenosis
- Overfeeding

History

- **Character:** What is the vomiting like? Projectile? Spitting up? What is the temporal relationship to feeds?
  - Describe vomitus: Color (clear, bilious, bloody, feculent), quantity, and smell
  - Bilious vomiting suggests obstruction distal to the ampulla of Vater
  - Hematemesis: Bright red blood versus coffee grounds
  - Did the child retch before vomiting or retch without vomiting at all?
- **Location:** Where were you when this started? Has the family been traveling?
- **Onset:** How did the vomiting begin (sudden versus gradual)? Does it come on after a meal (postprandial)? What time of day does it occur (morning vomiting may be related to increased ICP)?
- **Intensity:** How severe is the vomiting? Number of episodes of vomiting per day? Small or large volumes?
- **Duration:** When did the vomiting begin? Is it getting better, worse, or staying the same?
- **Events associated:**
  - Fever/chills? Lethargy? Weight loss?
  - Appetite? Does he eat readily? Any change in volume of feeding?
  - Does he appear to have any pain? Jaundice?
  - Any change in BMs (diarrhea, constipation, melena, hematochezia, steatorrhea)?
  - Any noticeable change in the size of the baby's head (hydrocephalus, space occupying lesion [SOL])?
  - Diet: Formula-fed versus breast-fed? Any other foods?
  - Infectious contacts: Day care, recent parties, school, and baby-sitter
- **Frequency:** Has this ever happened to your child before? When? How frequently (intermittent versus constant)?
- **Palliative factors:** Is there anything that makes it better? If so, what?
- **Provocative factors:** Is there anything that makes it worse? If so, what?
- **PMH/PSH:** IBD, CF, or gastric obstruction
- **MEDS:** Erythromycin, antibiotics, antidepressants, chemotherapy, anticholinergics, or narcotics
- **SH:** Other children at home, stressors (e.g., financial, relationships)
- **FH:** IBD, CF, or intestinal cancers

Prenatal, Natal, and Neonatal History

- Did you have prenatal care? Any difficulties during the pregnancy?
- Use of alcohol or recreational drugs during the pregnancy? Smoking?
- Singleton versus multiple gestation
- Date and gestation at delivery
- Onset of labor, duration of labor, and type of delivery (NSVD, LSCS, forceps, vacuum)
- Birth weight? Breast-fed versus bottle-fed?
- Apgar scores at 1 and 5 minutes?
- Any health problems as a baby? Any hospital admissions?
- Any delay in speech, language, or motor development?

INSTRUCTIONS TO CANDIDATE: A 5-year-old girl is brought to her family doctor by her mother because of ongoing bedwetting. Take a detailed history, exploring possible etiologies.

Definition

- **Nocturnal enuresis** refers to nighttime urinary incontinence. It is **primary** when the child has never been continent for a prolonged period and **secondary** when incontinence recurs after a 6- to 12-month period of continence.

DD$_x$ of Primary Enuresis (VITAMINS C)

- **I**diopathic/**I**atrogenic: Idiopathic enuresis, delayed maturation of the urethral sphincter
- **C**ongenital/genetic: Congenital anomalies

DD$_x$ of Secondary Enuresis (VITAMINS C)

- **I**nfectious: UTI
- **T**raumatic: Chemical distal urethritis (bubble bath)
- **M**etabolic: DM
- **I**diopathic/**I**atrogenic: Polydipsia, fecal impaction
- **S**ubstance abuse and **P**sychiatric: Psychological stress

History

- **Ch**aracter: Tell me about the bedwetting. Is there any incontinence during the daytime?
- **L**ocation: Does this happen at home? Does it happen at sleepovers?
- **O**nset: When did the bedwetting begin? Has the child ever been continent?
- **I**ntensity: How frequently does this occur? Every night? More than once a night? Is it getting better, worse, or staying the same? Does it interfere with any of her activities?
- **D**uration: How long has this been going on?
- **E**vents associated:
  - UTI: Urinary frequency, dysuria, hematuria, urinary retention, urgency
  - Chemical urethritis: Bubble bath, perfumed soaps
  - Does she need to strain to urinate? Any dribbling or small-caliber stream?
  - Stress incontinence? Continuous dampness?
  - Polydipsia?
  - Gait disturbance? Change in behavior?
  - Any encopresis? Constipation?
  - What do you do when she wets the bed? Is she punished? Have you tried any reward systems?
- **F**requency: How often does it occur (times per night, times per week)?
- **P**alliative factors: Is there anything that makes it better? If so, what?
  - Behavior modification, such as emptying the bladder before sleep?
  - Limiting fluid intake before bed?
- **P**rovocative factors: Is there anything that makes it worse? If so, what?
  - Drinking before bed?
  - Caffeine?
  - Soft drinks?
  - Use of bubble bath or perfumed soaps?
  - Constipation?
- **PMH/PSH:** Diabetes, spina bifida, fecal impaction, or genitourinary (GU) malformations
- **MEDS:** Imipramine, desmopressin (DDAVP)
- **SH:** Psychologically stressful situations in the home
- **FH:** Bedwetting

INSTRUCTIONS TO CANDIDATE: A 30-month-old boy is brought to his pediatrician by his mother who is concerned about his small vocabulary. Take a detailed history, exploring possible etiologies.

DD$_x$ of Language Delay

- Global developmental delay
- Isolated language delay
- Hearing impairment

- Social deprivation
- Autism
- Oral-motor abnormalities

History

- **Character:** Tell me about your concern about your son's language.
  - What have you noticed? What is your biggest concern?
  - Does he understand you? Does he follow instructions?
  - Does he have trouble expressing his wants? Does he get frustrated?
- **Onset:** When did you notice his trouble with words? Has he taken any steps backward? Is he continuing to gain words? Has he stopped progressing?
- **Radiation:** Any social or motor troubles (gross and fine)?
- **Intensity:** How many words does he use? How many words does he know?
- **Duration:** How long has this been going on (acute versus chronic)?
- **Frequency:** Is his language difficulty constant, or does it fluctuate?
- **Palliative factors:** Is there anything that makes it better? If so, what?
- **Provocative factors:** Is there anything that makes it worse? If so, what?
  - Unfamiliar situations or people?
- **PMH/PSH:** Meningitis, prematurity, or birth defects
- **MEDS:** Aminoglycosides, loop diuretics
- **Immunizations**
- **SH:** Other children in the home, day care, and stress or tension in the home
- **FH:** Speech/language delay, hearing deficit, autism, or Tourette's syndrome

Prenatal and Natal History

- Did you have prenatal care? Any difficulties during the pregnancy?
- Bleeding, discharge, premature rupture of membranes (PROM), and abdominal trauma
- N/V, malnutrition, gestational DM, anemia, and GER
- Infections: STI, UTI, and **T**oxoplasmosis, **O**ther agents, **R**ubella, **C**ytomegalovirus, **H**erpes simplex (TORCH) infections
- Use of alcohol or recreational drugs during the pregnancy? Use of OTC and prescription drugs? Smoking?
- Singleton versus multiple gestation
- Date and gestation at delivery
- Onset of labor: Spontaneous versus induced
- Duration of labor: Use of augmentation
- Type of delivery: NSVD, LSCS, forceps, or vacuum
- Complications at delivery?

Neonatal History

- Birth weight? Breast-fed versus bottle-fed?
- Apgar scores at 1 and 5 minutes?
- Any health problems as a baby? Any hospital admissions?

Growth and Development

- Has the child reached normal developmental milestones?
- Use the DDST to screen for language items.

Hearing

- Do you have any concerns about your child's hearing? Has his or her hearing ever been tested?
- Risk factors for hearing loss: Congenital hearing loss in a family member, high bilirubin (neonatal), congenital rubella, congenital defects in the ears, nose, or throat (ENT), very low birth weight (<1500 g), meningitis, and ototoxic medications

Environmental Stimulation

- Does your child play with other children? Do you read or talk/interact with your child? Has your child ever been abused (physical, verbal, sexual) or witnessed/experienced a traumatic event?

INSTRUCTIONS TO CANDIDATE: A 3-year-old male is brought in by his parents because of a very swollen right eye, which he can no longer open voluntarily (Figure 12-14). Perform a focused history and physical examination.

DD$_X$ (VITAMINS C)

- Infectious: Orbital cellulitis, periorbital cellulitis
- Trauma
- Allergic reaction (likely to be bilateral)

History

- **Ch**aracter: Describe the swelling. Is it painful? Is he otherwise well?
- Location: Which eye is swollen? Any troubles with the other eye?
- **O**nset: How did it start (did it come about suddenly, or has it been worsening over several hours/days)?
- Intensity: What is the severity of the pain, if present (see Figure 12-10)? Is the pain worse with eye movement?
- **D**uration: How long has this been going on?
- Events associated:
  - Malaise? Lethargy? Loss of appetite? N/V?
  - Head/face injury? Recent infection? Sinusitis? Dental surgery?
  - Change in vision? Fever?
- **F**requency: Has this ever happened before? When?
- **P**alliative factors: Is there anything that makes it better? If so, what?
  - NSAIDs?
  - Acetaminophen?
- **P**rovocative factors: Is there anything that makes it worse? If so, what?
  - Eye movement?
  - Bright light (photophobia)?
- **PMH/PSH:** Sinusitis, recent penetrating trauma, or facial fractures
- **MEDS:** Antibiotics, antipyretics, or immunosuppressants

Physical Examination

- **Vitals:** HR and rhythm, RR (depth, effort, and pattern), BP, and temperature
- **General:** Activity level, eye contact with his parents

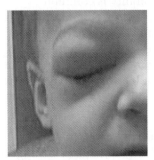

Figure 12-14   Swollen, erythematous right eye in a 3-year-old male. (Used with permission of Dr. Brett Taylor, Dalhousie University.)

- **HEENT:** Ensure the neck is supple. Inspect the eye, noting erythema and whether he is able to open it. Palpate the periorbital tissues, noting warmth and any tenderness. Gently retract the eyelid, and inspect the conjunctiva. Note any proptosis (protrusion of the eye). Using a brightly colored object observe ocular mobility (extraocular movements). Check the pupillary responses to light. Inspect the nasal mucosa for discharge, and palpate the maxillary sinuses (frontal sinuses do not form until about age 6 years). Inspect the mouth. Note the size of the tonsils and the presence of any exudate. Examine for cervical lymphadenopathy.
- **Resp:** Observe chest expansion for symmetry with breathing. Auscultate for breath sounds and adventitious sounds.
- **CVS:** Check capillary refill. Palpate the peripheral pulses. Note pulse volume, contour, and rhythm. Auscultate the heart, looking for extra heart sounds or murmurs.
- **Skin:** Inspect for exanthem, other lesions (e.g., infectious exanthem, petechiae).
- **Neuro:** Most of the neurologic examination can be performed by simply observing the child play (motor function, CNs).

PEARL

- It is vital to distinguish periorbital from orbital cellulitis. Periorbital cellulitis is associated with swelling, erythema, and warmth with normal ocular mobility and vision. Orbital cellulitis may appear similar, but there may be change in vision, proptosis, pain with eye movement, and systemic symptoms such as fever. Although these conditions may appear similar, the management varies considerably.

INSTRUCTIONS TO CANDIDATE: A 28-month-old female is brought to her family physician by her mother for the first time. They have recently immigrated to this country. Take an immunization history.

Immunization History

- From where did you immigrate? Specific immunization schedules vary from country to country.
- Has your child had any vaccinations? If so, determine the age at immunization and type of immunizations received.
- Do you have an immunization record or a copy of your daughter's health records?
- Describe any adverse reactions to past vaccinations.
    - Local reactions: Induration, tenderness, and redness at the injection site. Edema and abscess formation occasionally occur.
    - Systemic reactions: Fever, exanthem, joint or muscle pains, fainting, seizures, and other CNS symptoms. Irritability is common.
    - Allergic reactions (rare): Urticaria, rhinitis, bronchospasm, anaphylaxis
- Persons lacking written documentation of immunization should be started on an age-appropriate immunization schedule (Table 12-3).
- Minor illnesses such as the common cold are not contraindications to immunization (Table 12-4). Infections do not increase the risk of adverse effects from immunization and do not interfere with immune responses to vaccines.

Prenatal, Natal, and Neonatal History

- Did you have prenatal care? Any difficulties during the pregnancy?
- Use of alcohol or recreational drugs during the pregnancy? Smoking?

Table 12-3   Routine Immunization Schedule for Children <7 Years Not Immunized in Infancy

Age	DTaP	IPV	Hib	MMR	Hep B	Td	Comments
First visit	✓	✓	✓	✓	✓		
2 months later	✓	✓	✓	(✓)	✓		MMR optional.
2 months later	✓	(✓)					IPV is not needed but may be included for convenience.
6-12 months later	✓	✓	(✓)		✓		Hib not needed if child >5 years.
4-6 years	✓	✓					
14-16 years						✓	Td booster should be given every 10 years after this vaccination. Further polio boosters are not required.

Varicella, pneumococcal, and meningococcal vaccines also may be given at the first visit. Subsequent schedule and doses depend on the age of the child.

Adapted from National Advisory Committee on Immunization: *Canadian immunization guide,* ed 6, Ottawa, 2002, Canadian Medical Association, p 56, Table 2.

Table 12-4   Some Contraindications and Precautions

Vaccine	True Contraindications	Precautions
All vaccines	Anaphylactic reaction to previous dose of vaccine or to a constituent of the vaccine	Moderate to severe illness with or without fever
DTaP	Anaphylactic reaction to previous dose of vaccine	Hypotonic-hyporesponsive state within 48 hr after previous dose of DTaP
IPV	Anaphylactic reaction to previous dose of vaccine or to neomycin	
MMR	Anaphylactic reaction to previous dose of vaccine or to neomycin	Recent administration of immunoglobulin
	Pregnancy	
	Severe immunodeficiency	
Influenza	Anaphylactic reaction to previous dose of vaccine or egg ingestion	

Adapted from National Advisory Committee on Immunization: *Canadian immunization guide,* ed 6, Ottawa, 2002, Canadian Medical Association, pp 5-6, Table 2.

- Singleton versus multiple gestation
- Date and gestation at delivery
- Onset of labor, duration of labor, and type of delivery (NSVD, LSCS, forceps, vacuum)
- Birth weight? Breast-fed versus bottle-fed?
- Apgar scores at 1 and 5 minutes?
- Any health problems as a baby? Any hospital admissions?
- Any delay in speech, language, or motor development?

> INSTRUCTIONS TO CANDIDATE: You are a senior medical student on your neonatology rotation. The head nurse asks you to measure the height, weight, and head circumference of a newborn baby boy and plot them on the growth charts provided (Figure 12-15). Perform a routine newborn examination.

- Height, weight, and head circumference should be plotted on standardized **growth charts** at routine health encounters. Serial measurements are much more valuable than single measurements, reflecting changes in the child's growth pattern. The commonest reason for deviation from the growth curve is measuring error. Take every measurement at least twice, and do a third measurement if there is a discrepancy.

Head Circumference
- Use a measuring tape that is not stretchable to measure the head circumference. Place the tape over the occipital, parietal, and frontal prominences to get the greatest circumference of the head.

DD$_X$ Decreased Head Circumference (VITAMINS C)
- Idiopathic/Iatrogenic: Premature closure of the sutures
- Congenital/genetic: Familial microcephaly

DD$_X$ Increased Head Circumference (VITAMINS C)
- Idiopathic/Iatrogenic: Hydrocephalus (obstructive and nonobstructive)
- Neoplastic: Space occupying lesion in CNS
- Congenital/genetic: Familial megalocephaly

Height
- Use a measuring board to quantify the height. It is inaccurate to use a measuring tape. Hold the infant's head against the upper board, and adjust the lower board. Ensure that both feet are flat against the base.

Weight
- Use an infant scale to measure the weight. Remove all clothing, including the diaper, and ensure that the infant is not touching the wall.
- When caloric intake is inadequate the weight percentile decreases first, followed by height and finally head circumference. The World Health Organization (WHO) recommends that **weight for height** be used as an index of acute malnutrition and **height for age** be used as an index of chronic malnutrition.

Newborn Examination
- **Vitals:** Observe the baby undressed for 1 to 2 minutes. A normal RR is 30 to 50 breaths/min. Note any signs of respiratory distress, such as grunting, nasal flare, intercostal/subcostal retractions, tracheal tug, and thoracoabdominal dissociation. Use a well-lubricated rectal thermometer to determine temperature. Determine the HR by auscultation. The average HR is 120 to 140 beats/min (<90 beats/min is abnormal).
- **General:** The limbs should be moving in a random and asymmetric manner. Jerky or symmetric movements are abnormal.
- **Skin:** Inspect the skin, noting the color and any lesions. Note any signs of birth trauma, especially if instrumentation was used in the delivery.
  - **Acrocyanosis** refers to the presence of cyanosis in the extremities while the trunk is pink and warm.
  - **Pallor** may be associated with anemia, vasoconstriction, or edema.

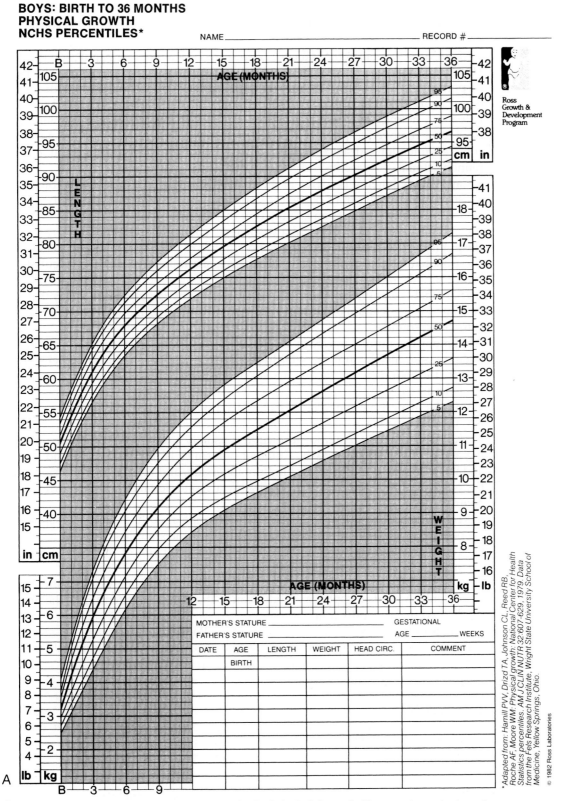

BOYS: BIRTH TO 36 MONTHS
PHYSICAL GROWTH
NCHS PERCENTILES*

NAME _____ RECORD # _____

Ross
Growth &
Development
Program

Figure 12-15   Growth chart. (From Swartz M: *Textbook of physical diagnosis: history and examination,* ed 4, Philadelphia, 2002, WB Saunders, Figure 23-16, *A.*)

- The yellow discoloration of **jaundice** is common in newborns and most noticeable on the brow and face. Jaundice occurring in the first 24 hours of life is considered abnormal.
  - **Milia** are sebaceous retention cysts, appearing as small white papules on the face.
- **HEENT:** Examine the fontanelles, and assess the shape and symmetry of the head. Inspect the face for symmetry, and note the presence of epicanthal folds or low-set ears. Ensure that the nares are patent. Inspect the palate. Use your gloved finger to palpate it, noting any clefts. Inspect the gums for neonatal teeth (these will likely need to be removed to prevent aspiration). Inspect the eyes, and perform a funduscopic examination. Absence of the red reflex may connote congenital cataracts or retinoblastoma.
  - **Caput succedaneum** is edema of the soft tissues of the vertex related to the birth.
  - **Esophageal atresia** may be detected by the presence of excessive saliva in the mouth as saliva production is limited in the neonate.
  - **Coloboma** is any defect of ocular tissue (e.g., coloboma iridis).
- **Resp:** Inspect for thoracic deformity and symmetry of chest expansion. Percuss the chest bilaterally. The chest should be hyperresonant and symmetric. Auscultate for breath sounds and adventitia.
- **CVS:** Palpate the radial and femoral pulses, noting any radial-femoral delay that may be related to coarctation of the aorta. Auscultate the heart, and note any murmurs or extra heart sounds.
- **Abdomen:** The normal newborn abdomen is protuberant. Inspect for umbilical herniation (associated with congenital hypothyroidism). Auscultate for bowel sounds. Palpate the abdomen, noting any masses or apparent tenderness. Attempt to palpate the liver and spleen.
- **Genitalia:** Inspect the genitalia for ambiguity. Look at the urethral meatus, and identify any hypospadias.
- **MSK:** Inspect the feet. Forefoot adduction is usually a result of intrauterine positioning and resolves spontaneously. Clubfoot deformity is more extensive and serious and includes forefoot adduction, hindfoot inversion, and internal tibial torsion. Note the position of the head and neck. Tilting toward one side may indicate torticollis.
- **Neuro:**
  - **Rooting reflex:** Touch the corner of the infant's mouth. A normal response is opening the mouth and turning the head toward the stimulus.
  - **Palmar grasp:** Place your finger or an object in the palm of the infant's hand. A normal response is a complete grasp.
  - **Moro's reflex (startle reflex):** Supporting the infant's head, allow the infant to drop suddenly. A normal response is abduction of the arms and extension of the fingers, followed by arm adduction.
  - Plantar reflexes are usually upgoing (positive **Babinski**).
  - **Plantar grasp:** With the infant's knee and hip flexed, press your thumb into the sole of the foot. Normally the toes flex, as if to grasp the thumb.

INSTRUCTIONS TO CANDIDATE: The next day the nurse in charge asks you to reassess the boy because he appears jaundiced. Take a detailed history from his mother, exploring possible etiologies. What is the differential diagnosis?

Definition

- **Jaundice** refers to the yellowish staining of skin and other tissues with bile pigment. The presence of jaundice correlates reliably with hyperbilirubinemia. Bilirubin is normally taken up by liver cells and excreted in the bile. Physiologic jaundice is the most common cause of neonatal jaundice occurring in normal newborns. Jaundice occurs with bilirubin concentrations of 40 to 45 µmol/L. It is best observed in natural light.

DD$_x$ Neonatal Jaundice (VITAMINS C)

- **I**nfectious: TORCH infections, sepsis
- **T**raumatic: Hematoma resorption (birth trauma)
- **A**utoimmune/**A**llergic: Blood group incompatibility
- **M**etabolic: Gilbert syndrome, Crigler-Najjar syndrome
- **I**diopathic/**I**atrogenic: Physiologic jaundice, breast milk jaundice, and meconium ileus
- **C**ongenital/genetic: Hereditary hemolytic anemia (e.g., spherocytosis), sickle cell anemia, thalassemia, biliary atresia, and Hirschsprung's disease
- There are many more diagnoses associated with neonatal jaundice!

Prenatal History

- Did you have prenatal care?
- Any difficulties during the pregnancy?
- Bleeding? PROM? Gestational DM?
- STIs? TORCH infections?
- Use of alcohol or recreational drugs during the pregnancy?
- Smoking?
- Singleton versus multiple gestation?
- Establish Rh status.

Birth History

- Date and gestation at delivery
- Onset of labor: Spontaneous versus induced
- Duration of labor: Use of augmentation
- Type of delivery: NSVD, LSCS, forceps, or vacuum
- Birth trauma (e.g., cephalohematoma)?

Newborn History

- Birth weight?
- Apgar scores at 1 and 5 minutes?
- Breast-fed versus bottle-fed?
- Describe the color of the baby now. On what part of the baby was this color change noted (e.g., trunk, face)? When was the change in color first noted?
- Has he passed any stools yet (meconium)?
- Any systemic symptoms?
  - Fever? Lethargy?
  - Vomiting?
  - Poor feeding?
- **Maternal PMH:** Hepatitis, hemolytic disorders, or metabolic disorders (e.g., Gilbert's)
- **Maternal MEDS:** Hepatotoxic drugs (ASA, anticonvulsants, antipsychotics, herbals)
- **FH:** Jaundice, metabolic disorders, or unexplained infant deaths

PEARLS

- Jaundice appearing in the first 24 hours of life is usually pathologic.
- Direct hyperbilirubinemia in a neonate is always pathologic.

INSTRUCTIONS TO CANDIDATE: A 2-year-old female is brought in by her parents because she is having episodes of screaming, complaining that she has a "sore belly." Between episodes she is playing with her toys. The triage nurse asks you to come and assess this patient as she is having another episode of screaming.

DD$_X$ Abdominal Pain (VITAMINS C)
- **V**ascular: Henoch-Schönlein purpura (HSP)
- **I**nfectious: UTI, pneumonia
- **T**raumatic: Occult trauma (abuse)
- **M**etabolic: Diabetic ketoacidosis (DKA)
- **I**diopathic/**I**atrogenic: Intussusception, incarcerated hernia, appendicitis, and pancreatitis
- **S**ubstance abuse and **P**sychiatric: Toxic ingestion
- **C**ongenital/genetic: Meckel's diverticulum, malrotation with volvulus, and sickle cell crisis

History
- **Ch**aracter: Tell me about these screaming episodes. How long do they last? How is she between episodes?
- **L**ocation: Where is the pain in her belly?
- **O**nset: When did this start? How did it come on (sudden versus gradual)?
- **R**adiation: Does it hurt anywhere else?
- **D**uration: How long has this been going on?
- Events associated:
  - Fever? Recent infection?
  - Vomiting (bilious versus nonbilious)?
  - How is her appetite? Any recent weight loss or gain?
  - Change in stools: Diarrhea, steatorrhea, constipation, melena, or hematochezia
  - Change in urine: Hematuria, dysuria
  - Possible toxic ingestion?
- **F**requency: Has this ever happened before? How many episodes has she had (how often do they occur)?
- **P**alliative factors: Is there anything that seems to make it better? If so, what?
- **P**rovocative factors: Is there anything that seems to make it worse? If so, what?
- **PMH/PSH:** Previous surgery, sickle cell anemia, and DM
- **MEDS, Allergies**
- **SH:** Living arrangements, recent changes at home
- **FH:** Sickle cell anemia, DM

Physical Examination
- **Vitals:** HR and rhythm, RR (depth, effort, and pattern), BP, and temperature
- **General:** Appearance, anxiety/crying/screaming (duration), position of comfort, and interaction with her parents; observe behavior between episodes of apparent discomfort.
- **Skin:** Inspect for exanthem, other lesions.
- **HEENT:** Ensure the neck is supple. Inspect the conjunctiva and mouth. Note any erythema, petechiae, or vesicles on the palate. Examine for cervical lymphadenopathy.
- **Resp:** Inspect for thoracic deformity and chest expansion (symmetry). Auscultate for breath sounds and adventitious sounds.
- **CVS:** Check capillary refill. Palpate the peripheral pulses. Note pulse volume, contour, and rhythm. Auscultate the heart, looking for extra heart sounds or murmurs.
- **Abdomen:** Inspect the abdomen. Auscultate for bowel sounds. Percuss lightly in all four quadrants. Perform light and deep palpation, and identify any masses or areas

of tenderness. Check for rebound tenderness. Examine the liver and spleen. Check diaper area for any blood or perianal lesions.
- **Neuro:** Mental status (orientation, level of interaction with parents, level of activity)

Instructions to Candidate: A 4-year-old male is brought in by his mother because she has noticed him limping for the past 2 days. Perform a focused history, exploring possible etiologies.

DD$_X$ Limp (VITAMINS C)
- **V**ascular: Avascular necrosis of the femoral head (Legge-Calvé-Perthes), hemarthrosis (e.g., hemophilia)
- **I**nfectious: Septic arthritis
- **T**raumatic: Injury to bone or soft tissue (known traumatic history or occult trauma, as in abuse)
- **A**utoimmune/**A**llergic: Juvenile rheumatoid arthritis
- **I**diopathic/**I**atrogenic: Toxic synovitis
- **N**eoplastic: CNS malignancy (ataxia)
- **C**ongenital/genetic: DDH, sickle cell crisis

History
- **Ch**aracter: Describe the limp. Is it painful? What is the pain like?
- **L**ocation: Where does the pain originate?
- **O**nset: When did the limp start? When did the pain start (before or after the limp)? How did it come on (sudden versus gradual)?
- **R**adiation: Does the pain move anywhere?
- **I**ntensity: What is the severity of the pain, if present (see Figure 12-10)?
  - How does it affect his activities (getting dressed, going to the bathroom, participating in sports, playing with his friends)?
  - Is it getting better, worse, or staying the same?
- **D**uration: How long has the limp or pain been there (acute versus chronic)?
- **E**vents associated:
  - Trauma? Describe the mechanism of injury.
  - Sports? New activities?
  - Fever, chills? Weight loss? Night pain?
  - Is there limitation of movement?
  - Morning stiffness? Swelling? Redness?
  - Muscle pain (thigh, calf)? Wasting? Weakness?
- **F**requency: Has this ever happened before? How often (intermittent versus constant)?
- **P**alliative factors: Is there anything that makes the pain better? If so, what?
  - Rest? What is the position of comfort?
  - Activity?
  - NSAIDs? Acetaminophen?
- **P**rovocative factors: Is there anything that makes the pain worse? If so, what?
  - Rest?
  - Activity? Particular movements?

Motor Development
- Sits unsupported at 6 months.
- Crawls and pulls to standing position at 9 months.
- Walks alone at 12 to 15 months.
- Runs at 18 months.

- **PMH/PSH:** DDH, hemophilia, sickle cell anemia, arthritis, connective tissue disease, past injuries, and previous surgeries
- **MEDS:** NSAIDs, acetaminophen, narcotics, ASA, steroids, or immunosuppressants
- **Allergies:** Cefaclor hypersensitivity is associated with serum sickness with migratory arthritis.
- **SH:** Living arrangements, family dynamics
- **FH:** Arthritis, connective tissue disease

PEARLS

- A child with a hip effusion may prefer to lie with the hip flexed, abducted, and externally rotated to minimize intraarticular pressure.
- Be sure to differentiate a painless "limp" from ataxia, which may be caused by a posterior fossa tumor.
- Beware of the painful limp that is worsening, limits activity, and is unrelieved by NSAIDS; it may herald serious pathology.

SAMPLE CHECKLISTS

> INSTRUCTIONS TO CANDIDATE: A 4-year-old female is under observation in the emergency department after experiencing an anaphylactic reaction to peanut butter. Counsel the girl's mother about peanut allergy.

Key Points	Satisfactorily Carried out
Introduces self to the parent	❏
Determines how the parent wishes to be addressed	❏
Develops a rapport with the parent	❏
States that nut allergy (peanuts, tree nuts) is relatively common (affects approximately 1.1% of Americans)	❏
Often a lifelong allergy	❏
States that peanut allergy can be life threatening	❏
States that she will be referred to an allergist for further evaluation	❏
Counsels on strategies for allergen avoidance	
• Check all food labels for the presence of peanuts in the ingredients	❏
• Avoid high-risk situations such as buffets, ice cream parlors, and unlabeled candy or desserts	❏
Counsels the parent to avoid tree nuts such as walnuts, cashews, and pistachios because cross-reactivity is common	❏
States that symptoms of allergy may develop minutes to hours after ingesting the allergen	❏
Describes early symptoms associated with food-related anaphylaxis	
• Itching and tingling in the mouth	❏
• Itching at the back of the throat	❏
• Sensation of tightening in the airways	❏
• Abdominal pain, nausea/vomiting	❏
• Flushed appearance	❏
• Hives	❏
• Swelling of the lips and tongue	❏
Advises parent to contact Food Allergy and Anaphylaxis Network for more educational materials (www.foodallergy.org)	❏
Advises the parent that in case of exposure to peanuts and early symptoms and signs of a reaction	
• Administer 1 mg/kg of liquid oral diphenhydramine	❏
• Administer injectable epinephrine (IM in thigh)	❏
• Transport to an emergency facility	❏

Key Points	Satisfactorily Carried out
Informs the parent about the importance of educating their child's school/day care personnel about avoidance of nuts and provide them with a written emergency plan	❏
Ensures that the parent understands the emergency instructions (in case of exposure)	❏
Provides an opportunity for the parent to ask questions	❏
Provides written instructions for avoiding allergen exposure and an emergency plan in case of reaction	❏
Ensures that the parent has the appropriate prescription for injectable epinephrine	❏
Makes appropriate closing remarks	❏

INSTRUCTIONS TO CANDIDATE: An 8-month-old female is brought to the emergency department by her grandmother because she is not as active as usual. She cries whenever her grandmother tries to change her diaper and seems to be in pain. Interpret the x-ray (Figure 12-16). What are your responsibilities in this case?

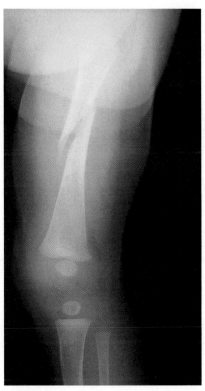

Figure 12-16   Anteroposterior x-ray of left femur. (From Hobbs CJ, Wynne JM: *Physical signs of child abuse,* ed 2, London, 2001, WB Saunders, p 107, Figure 11.29.)

Key Points	Satisfactorily Carried out
Checks the name and date on the x-ray film	❏
Comments on the type of view and adequacy of film	❏
Names spiral fracture of the femoral shaft	❏
Looks for other fractures or abnormalities	❏
Comments on need for skeletal survey to detect other acute or healing injuries	❏

Obligations
- Examine the child ❏
- Ensure adequate pain control ❏
- Treat the fracture ❏
- Take an appropriate history from the child's grandmother about potential mechanism of injury ❏
- Ascertain the social history, including information about the child's caregivers ❏ ❏
- Explain the finding on the x-ray ❏
- Explain that you will be required to report the child's injury ❏
- Contact Child Protection Services to investigate possible abuse ❏

CHAPTER 13

Geriatrics

OBJECTIVES

ESSENTIAL CLINICAL COMPETENCIES
APPROACH TO THE GERIATRIC PATIENT
PERFORM A FOLSTEIN MINI-MENTAL STATE EXAMINATION

SAMPLE OSCE SCENARIOS
- An 80-year-old male presents to your office with complaint of decreased hearing in his right ear. Perform a focused history and physical examination.
- A 72-year-old male is brought to the hospital by his wife with increasing confusion and troubles with memory. She states that he has been found wandering outside, and she is very concerned for his safety. Differentiate between delirium, dementia, and depression.
- An 88-year-old female presents via ambulance from her home with a complaint of "weakness." Take a detailed history, exploring possible etiologies.
- A 79-year-old male presents to the emergency department via ambulance after falling at home. Take a detailed history, exploring possible etiologies.
- A 75-year-old female is brought to your office by her daughter for a checkup. This patient has been dependent on her family for her care since having a stroke last year. Before you see the patient the nurse tells you that she noted several bruises and decubitus ulcers. Take a detailed history, focusing on risk factors for abuse and neglect.

SAMPLE CHECKLIST
- ❏ A 76-year-old female presents to her family doctor with a history of leaking urine. This limits her activities outside of the home. Take a detailed history, exploring possible etiologies.

OBJECTIVES

*The geriatric history includes all aspects of the systems-based histories discussed in Chapters 1 through 11. Aspects of the history that require special attention in the geriatric population are highlighted in these objectives. The successful student should be able to take a **focused** geriatric **history**, including:*

- Cognitive decline: Dementia, depression, and delirium
- Social isolation
- Immobility, instability, and falls
- Functional status: Activities of daily living (ADLs)
- Incontinence: Urinary, fecal
- Bowel dysfunction: Constipation, diarrhea
- Malnutrition
- Sensory impairment: Hearing, vision, and taste
- Immune deficiency, infection, and immunization status
- Insomnia
- Sexual dysfunction
- Polypharmacy

- Elder abuse and neglect
- Weakness
- Pain

*The geriatric examination includes all aspects of the systems-based examinations discussed in Chapters 1 through 11. Aspects of the examination that require special attention in the geriatric population are highlighted in these objectives. The geriatric **examination** will include:*
- Orthostatic vitals
- Posture
- Characterization of gait and coordination
- Visual acuity
- Hearing
- Primitive reflexes
- Proprioception, peripheral sensation
- Complete skin examination (peripheral vascular disease, decubitus ulcers/skin breakdown, bruises, malignancy, hygiene)
- Digital rectal examination (DRE; prostate enlargement, rectal masses, fecal impaction)
- Peripheral pulses
- Folstein Mini-Mental State Examination (MMSE; for cognitive impairment)
- Complete mental status examination (see pp 289-290)
- Functional status assessment

ESSENTIAL CLINICAL COMPETENCIES

APPROACH TO THE GERIATRIC PATIENT

History Taking
- Approach the history of a presenting complaint in the same way as outlined in previous chapters, using the **ChLORIDE FPP** method. However, many medical problems in elderly patients present in "atypical" fashion compared with "classic" descriptions. For example, an elderly person may have a serious systemic infection without mounting a fever.
- Your ability to take a detailed history is sometimes hindered by cognitive decline, speech difficulties, and sensory impairment such as decreased hearing. In these cases you can optimize data gathering by speaking slowly with increased volume as necessary. Ensure that there is good lighting in the room (e.g., some elderly persons adapt by lip reading). Sometimes you may have to resort to communicating through pen and paper. Allow the patient adequate time to respond to questions.

Past Medical/Surgical History
- Current medical problems for which the patient is being treated or investigated
- Past medical problems
- Previous hospitalizations
- Previous surgeries
- Consider health maintenance issues, such as mammography, Pap smears, and DRE ± hemoccult testing.

Medications
- Establish a complete list of all current medications and dosing schedule, including prescription, over-the-counter (OTC), and herbal medications.

- Ask whether there have been any recent changes to the medication schedule or whether new medications have been added.
- Ask the patient whether he or she takes the medications regularly.
- Do you have any concerns about your medications? Any side effects?
- In elderly persons medication use, particularly polypharmacy, is a significant source of iatrogenic health problems. Generally medical problems should be treated without medications when possible. Be conscientious about drug-drug interactions. Adjust renally excreted drugs according to the patient's creatinine clearance. Do not prescribe a drug to manage a side effect of another drug.
- Consult a resource such as the Beers criteria for specific recommendations on medication use in the elderly (Fick DM, Cooper JW, Wade WE, Waller JL, MacLean R, Beers MH: Updating the Beers criteria for potentially inappropriate medication use in older adults: results of a US consensus panel of experts. *Arch Intern Med* 163:2716-2724, 2003).

Social History

- Ask the patient about his or her living conditions. What type of home does the patient have (apartment versus house)? Are there stairs?
- Do you live alone? If not, with whom do you live? Are you taking care of anyone (e.g., spouse)? Is someone taking care of you (e.g., dependent or semi-dependent on a caregiver)?
- Do you have any financial concerns? Many elderly persons live on a fixed income. This may impact their ability to get to medical appointments or fill prescriptions.
- What is your primary means of transportation (e.g., driving, caregiver, public transit)?
- Do you smoke cigarettes? Drink alcohol (quantify)? Use recreational/street drugs?
- Do you currently work outside the home? What is/was your occupation? What is the highest level of education you have received?
- Do you have an advance directive? Do you have a substitute decision maker? See pp 361 and 364 for specific discussion on advance care directives. In elderly patients it is particularly important to establish their definition or perception of an acceptable quality of life.

Basic Activities of Daily Living
- Grooming, bathing
- Getting dressed
- Toileting, continence
- Feeding oneself
- Ambulating

Instrumental Activities of Daily Living
- Cooking and cleaning
- Using a telephone
- Managing medications and money
- Shopping
- Reading and writing
- Ability to travel (e.g., drive a car, use public transportation)

Immunization History
- Specifically address whether the patient has received tetanus, influenza, and pneumococcal vaccines.

Symptom Screen
- Sensory impairment: Decreased vision, decreased hearing
- Mobility: Ability to ambulate, ability to transfer from bed/chair to toilet, and ability to mobilize outside the home
- Incontinence: Urinary, fecal
- Malnutrition: Weight loss, dietary habits
- Memory disturbance: Folstein MMSE
- Depression: Mood, satisfaction with life
- Social isolation: Spending time with family or friends, activities outside the home, recreation, and hobbies

Review of Systems
- Perform a detailed review of systems as outlined in the **Introduction**.

PERFORM A FOLSTEIN MINI-MENTAL STATE EXAMINATION

- The Folstein MMSE tests orientation, registration, attention, recall, comprehension, language, and constructional ability.
- Prompted answers do not count.
- The test is scored out of 30. Mild cognitive impairment is considered to be present with a score of 20 to 25, moderate impairment with a score of 10 to 20, and severe impairment with a score of 0 to 10. These cutoff scores are not useful if the patient has less than the equivalent of a grade nine education.

Orientation
- What is the year, season, day of week, date, and month? (5 points)
- What is the country, province/state, city, hospital, and floor? (5 points)

Registration
- Name three objects (e.g., "apple, table, penny"), and ask the patient to repeat the three items. Give one point for each correct item (3 points).
- If necessary repeat the items until the patient learns them. Record the number of trials necessary to achieve this.
- Instruct the patient that you will ask about these three items again later.

Attention
- After ensuring that the patient can spell "world" forward, ask him or her to spell it backward. Give 1 point for each correct letter (5 points).
- **OR** ask the patient to count serial 7s back from 100, giving 1 point for each correct answer (5 points).

Memory
- Ask the patient to name the three items you asked him or her to remember from above (registration). Give 1 point for each item recalled correctly (3 points). You cannot test memory if the patient failed to register the items in the first place.

Language
- Show the patient two objects, and ask the patient to name them (e.g., pencil, watch). One point is given for each correctly named item (2 points).
- Ask the patient to repeat the following statement: "No ifs, ands, or buts." (1 point)
- Ask the patient to "Take this piece of paper in your right hand, fold it in half, and put it on the floor." Give 1 point for each stage of the command correctly executed (3 points).

- Ask the patient to read a written command ("Close your eyes."), and do what it says (1 point).
- Ask the patient to write a complete sentence (1 point).

Visual-Spatial Functioning

- Ask the patient to copy the design below (two overlapping pentagons). Give 1 point for a correctly completed copy; the intersection of the pentagons must form a four-sided figure (1 point).

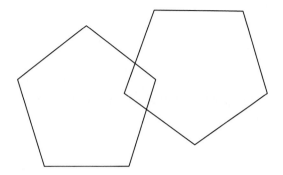

SAMPLE OSCE SCENARIOS

> INSTRUCTIONS TO CANDIDATE: An 80-year-old male presents to your office with complaint of decreased hearing in his right ear. Perform a focused history and physical examination.

DD$_X$ VITAMINS C

- **I**nfectious: Otitis media
- **T**raumatic: Foreign body obstructing external canal, ossicular disruption, and noise trauma (loss of hair cells from organ of Corti)
- **A**utoimmune/**A**llergic: Multiple sclerosis (MS)
- **I**diopathic/**I**atrogenic: Cerumen obstructing external canal, otosclerosis, ototoxic medications (e.g., aminoglycosides, furosemide, acetylsalicylic acid [ASA]), Paget's disease, and presbyacusis
- **N**eoplastic: Tumor obstructing external canal, cerebellopontine angle (CPA) tumor
- **S**ubstance abuse and **P**sychiatric: Pseudo-deafness (depression)
- **C**ongenital/genetic: Hereditary deafness (unlikely in this age group)

Definition

- **Presbyacusis** is sensorineural hearing loss associated with advanced age (decreased ability to perceive or discriminate sound). Although it affects the majority of elderly persons (aged >65 years), only a fraction of these have a functional deficit.

History

- **C**haracter: Other than decreased hearing, have you noticed anything else? Tinnitus? Hyperacusis? Do you have difficulty localizing sound in noisy environments?
- **L**ocation: Is the hearing loss in the right ear only? In what situations have you noticed the hearing loss?
- **O**nset: When and how did the loss start?
- **R**adiation: Are there any problems with hearing in the other ear?
- Intensity: How severe is the hearing loss?
- **D**uration: How long has the hearing impairment been going on?
- **E**vents associated:
  - Any pain in your ears? Headache?
  - Any discharge from your ears?
  - Any difficulties with speech?
- **F**requency: How often does your hearing pose a problem for you (constant versus intermittent)?
- **P**alliative factors: Is there anything that seems to help? If so, what (e.g., quiet surroundings, hearing aid)?
- **P**rovocative factors: Is there anything that seems to make your hearing worse? If so, what (e.g., background noise)?
- **Past medical history (PMH)/past surgical history (PSH):** Previous surgeries, malignancy, MS, or otitis media
- **Medications (MEDS):** Ototoxic medications such as aminoglycosides
- **Social history (SH):** Smoking, EtOH, recreational drugs, and occupation and recreational activities
- **Family history (FH):** Deafness, MS

Physical Examination

- **Vitals:** Heart rate (HR), respiratory rate (RR), blood pressure (BP), and temperature
  - Fever may be associated with otitis media, inner ear, or central nervous system [CNS] infection

- **General:** Cachexia (malignancy or systemic illness)
- **Skin:** Café au lait spots, neurofibromas
- **Head, eyes, ears, nose, and throat (HEENT):**
  - **Inspect** external ear (auricle, tragus) and auditory canal.
  - **Otoscopy:** Grasp auricle, and pull it upward, backward, and slightly away from the head. Gently insert the speculum of the otoscope into the ear canal (hold otoscope between thumb and fingers, and brace your hand against the patient's face). Examine the tympanic membrane, and identify landmarks (see Figure 5-6). Describe any abnormalities such as discharge, erythema, swelling, or loss of landmarks.
  - **Auditory acuity** should be assessed in a quiet room. Occlude one ear, and ask the patient to speak out loudly. Whisper softly into the other ear, using words or numbers of equally accented syllables. Use a normal voice or a shout, depending on the degree of hearing loss.
  - **Weber's test** (lateralization): Place a vibrating tuning fork (512 Hz or 1024 Hz) firmly on top of the patient's head. Ask the patient whether he hears it in one or both ears. Normally the sound is heard midline. In conductive hearing loss sound will be lateralized to the impaired ear. In sensorineural hearing loss the sound lateralizes to the good ear.
  - **Rinne's test** (compare air conduction with bone conduction): Place a vibrating tuning fork (512 Hz or 1024 Hz) on the mastoid bone, behind the ear, level with the external auditory canal. When the patient can no longer hear the sound, place the tuning fork close to the ear canal ("U" facing forward), and ask whether the sound is now audible. In conductive hearing loss sound is best transmitted by bone conduction. In sensorineural hearing loss sound is best transmitted through air.
- **Neurologic (Neuro):** Test the motor and sensory aspects of cranial nerve (CN) V, as well as the corneal reflex. Test the muscles of facial expression (CN VII). Observe balance, gait, and speech. Perform tests of coordination (rapid alternating movements, finger-nose testing) and fine motor control (pick up a dime from the table top). Inspect the extraocular movements, and characterize any nystagmus (by the direction of the fast phase).

INSTRUCTIONS TO CANDIDATE: A 72-year-old male is brought to the hospital by his wife with increasing confusion and troubles with memory. She states that he has been found wandering outside, and she is very concerned for his safety. Differentiate between delirium, dementia, and depression.

Definitions (Table 13-1)

- **Delirium** is acute cognitive dysfunction secondary to an underlying medical illness. It may otherwise be known as an organic brain syndrome. It is characterized by clouded consciousness and reduced ability to focus, maintain, or shift attention.
- **Dementia** is a progressive deterioration of cognitive function without impairment of consciousness. It affects memory, judgment, intellect, and mood.
- **Depression** in elderly persons may cause a dementia-like syndrome (pseudodementia). Major symptoms associated with depression (SIGE CAPS) are discussed on pp 287 and 297. The decreased concentration and psychomotor retardation are two of the symptoms that may cause depression to be mistaken for dementia.

History

- Interview the patient separately from his wife. Obtain collateral history from the wife afterward (to corroborate the history obtained from the patient and delineate her specific concerns that precipitated this medical visit).
- Have you noticed any memory loss? Any difficulty recalling recent events or conversations?

Table 13-1 Differentiate Between Delirium, Dementia, and Depression

	Delirium	Dementia	Depression
Onset	Hours to days (acute)	Months to years (insidious)	Weeks to months
Duration	Variable	Remainder of life	Short
Mood	Labile	Fluctuates	Consistent
Disabilities	New disabilities appear (acute)	May conceal deficits	Recognizes
Answers	May be incoherent (acute)	Offers responses that are not correct (but may be close to correct, concealing the deficit)	"Don't know."
MMSE	Acute fluctuations	Acutely stable with downward trajectory over time	Performance fluctuates
Progression	Resolves with treatment	Ongoing	Resolves with treatment

- Have you begun to have trouble remembering people's names?
- Difficulty finding the words you want to say in conversation?
- Do you ever get lost or forget where you are going?
- Are you ever confused about the date or place? This is a good time to check orientation to person, place, and time.
- When did you first notice these troubles?
- How have these symptoms changed or progressed during the past weeks and months (rapid versus gradual versus stepwise versus static)?
- Screen for difficulties performing basic and instrumental ADLs, namely, reading, writing, using the telephone, and managing money and medications.
- Associated symptoms:
  - Incontinence
  - Wandering
  - Agitation or disruptive behavior
  - Paranoia
- The Folstein MMSE is a useful screening test that looks at orientation, registration, attention, recall, comprehension, language, and constructional ability. Mild cognitive impairment is considered to be present with a score of 20 to 25, moderate impairment with a score of 10 to 20, and severe impairment with a score of 0 to 10. These cutoff scores are not useful if the patient has less than the equivalent of a grade nine education.
- Administer a brief depression-screening questionnaire such as the **Geriatric Depression Scale (very short form)**. The answer in parentheses is suggestive of depression, giving 1 point for each suggestive answer. A score > 2 is considered a positive screening test for depression.
  - Are you basically satisfied with your life? (No)
  - Do you often get bored? (Yes)
  - Do you often feel helpless? (Yes)
  - Do you prefer to stay at home rather than going out and doing new things? (Yes)
  - Do you feel pretty worthless the way you are now? (Yes)
- Perform a thorough mental status examination as outlined on pp 289-290.
- Safety concerns (as per wife): Does he ever wander or get lost? Does he go outside without appropriate clothing (e.g., going outside in winter without coat and shoes)? Has he ever left the stove on or the water running? Do you have concerns about him driving? Any other concerns?
- **Review of systems (ROS):** The ROS may help you to further delineate the contribution of organic disease to the entity of "confusion."

- **PMH/PSH:** Hypertension, stroke, transient ischemic attack (TIA), depression, malignancy, falls, head trauma, or previous surgeries
- **MEDS:** Complete list of medications (prescription, OTC, herbals) and dosing schedule, recent medication changes, or new medications
- **SH:** Smoking, EtOH, recreational drugs, educational level, and occupation and recreational activities
- **FH:** Dementia, depression, or neurovascular disease

INSTRUCTIONS TO CANDIDATE: An 88-year-old female presents via ambulance from her home with a complaint of "weakness." Take a detailed history, exploring possible etiologies.

DD$_X$ VITAMINS C
- **V**ascular: TIA, stroke, and temporal arteritis
- **I**nfectious: Pneumonia, urinary tract infection (UTI)
- **T**raumatic: Subdural hemorrhage
- **A**utoimmune/**A**llergic: Myasthenia gravis, Guillain-Barré syndrome
- **M**etabolic: Hypoxia, hyponatremia/hypernatremia, hypoglycemia, hypocalcemia/hypercalcemia, hypomagnesemia, hypokalemia/hyperkalemia, and anemia
- **I**diopathic/**I**atrogenic: Adverse medication effects, orthostatic hypotension
- **N**eoplastic: Constitutional symptoms from neoplasm such as cachexia and asthenia, paraneoplastic syndrome (e.g., Eaton-Lambert syndrome)
- **S**ubstance abuse and **P**sychiatric: Drug intoxication or withdrawal
- The differential diagnosis for such a nonspecific complaint in the geriatric age group is broad and may reflect metabolic derangement, systemic illness, infection, neurologic disease, or something else!

History
- **Ch**aracter: Describe what you mean by weakness. Muscular weakness? Fatigue? Presyncope?
- **L**ocation: Is the weakness localized? If so, where is your weakness?
- **O**nset: How did the weakness come on (sudden versus gradual)?
- **R**adiation: Is the weakness spreading (ascending versus descending)?
- **I**ntensity: How severe is the weakness? Are you able to walk? Can you accomplish ADLs (feeding yourself, cooking, toileting, dressing)?
- **D**uration: How long has this been going on?
- **E**vents associated:
  - Has the weakness caused you to fall? Elicit a history of falls, if present.
  - Any difficulty swallowing, chewing, talking, or breathing?
  - Any changes in bowel or bladder habit? Nausea/vomiting (N/V)?
  - Bleeding: Hematuria, hematochezia, melena, hematemesis, hemoptysis, or vaginal bleeding
  - Constitutional symptoms: Fever, chills, night sweats, weight loss, and anorexia
- **F**requency: Has this ever happened to you before? When? How often (constant versus intermittent)?
- **P**alliative factors: Is there anything that seems to help? If so, what?
- **P**rovocative factors: Is there anything that seems to make it worse? If so, what?
- **ROS:** The ROS may help you to further delineate the etiology of this confusing symptom by looking at the whole picture.
- **PMH/PSH:** Diabetes, malignancy, vascular disease, falls, or previous surgeries
- **MEDS:** Anticholinergic medications, diuretics, sedatives, insulin, diabetic medications (hypoglycemia), recent medication changes, or new medications
- **SH:** Smoking, EtOH, recreational drugs, and occupation and recreational activities
- **FH:** Malignancy, neurovascular disease

INSTRUCTIONS TO CANDIDATE: A 79-year-old male presents to the emergency department via ambulance after falling at home. Take a detailed history, exploring possible etiologies.

DD$_X$ VITAMINS C
- **V**ascular: TIA, stroke, drop attack, syncope, aortic stenosis, and chronic subdural hemorrhage
- **I**nfectious: Dehydration (hypotension, orthostatic changes)
- **T**raumatic: Chronic subdural hemorrhage
- **M**etabolic: Hypoglycemia, electrolyte disturbance, and diabetic neuropathy (impaired sensation/proprioception)
- **I**diopathic/**I**atrogenic: Deconditioning, adverse effects of medications, seizure disorder, and normal-pressure hydrocephalus (ataxia)
- **N**eoplastic: CNS tumor
- **S**ubstance abuse and **P**sychiatric: Intoxication, drug withdrawal

Age-Related Factors Contributing to Instability
- Decreased proprioception
- Diminished peripheral sensation
- Orthostatic hypotension
- Deconditioning
- Osteoarthritis
- Sensory impairment: Vision, hearing
- Cognitive decline, depression
- Nocturia (e.g., congestive heart failure [CHF], diuretic therapy, prostatism) leading to bathroom trips in the dark

History
- **Ch**aracter: Describe what happened to you today. Were you alone (a witness may offer valuable collateral history)? Are "falls" a problem for you? How did you fall?
  - Trip or slip and fall?
  - Orthostatic symptoms (stood up, weak, and fell)?
  - Loss of consciousness (LOC) leading to a fall?
  - Drop attack (sudden leg weakness without LOC)?
  - Vertigo or ataxia leading to a fall?
- **L**ocation: Where did you fall?
- **O**nset: Did you have any warning of the impending fall?
- **I**ntensity: How bad was your fall? Could you get up by yourself afterward? Are you able to walk? Are you injured? Are you having pain? Delineate the character, location, and intensity of any identified pain.
- **D**uration: When did you fall? How long before you were able to call for help?
- **E**vents associated:
  - Environmental factors: Unstable furniture, poor lighting, uneven stairs, throw rugs, and loose wires or cords (e.g., home O_2)
  - Do you live alone?
  - Did you strike your head? Did you lose consciousness after you fell?
  - Was there any incontinence?
  - Any preceding chest pain, shortness of breath (SOB), or palpitations?
  - Do you use any walking aids (e.g., cane, walker)?
  - Inquire about ability to accomplish ADLs (feed yourself, cook, toileting, bathe, dress yourself)?
- **F**requency: Has this ever happened to you before? When? How often?
- **P**alliative factors: Is there anything that seems to help? If so, what (e.g., walking aids)?

- **Provocative factors:** Is there anything that seems to make it worse? If so, what (e.g., environmental factors such as poor lighting)?
- **PMH/PSH:** Diabetes, cerebrovascular disease, arrhythmia, ischemic heart disease (IHD), valvular disease, Parkinson's disease, or previous surgeries
- **MEDS:** Anticholinergic medications, diuretics, sedatives, insulin, diabetic medications (hypoglycemia), recent medication changes, or new medications
- **SH:** Smoking, EtOH, recreational drugs, and occupation and recreational activities
- **FH:** Malignancy, neurovascular disease

PEARLS
- Falls are a major cause of morbidity in elderly persons. The 1-year survival after hospitalization for a fall in this age group is approximately 50%.
- A fall may be an indication of underlying frailty, and one should take the opportunity to identify risk factors for future falls such that preventative measures can be instituted (Figure 13-1).

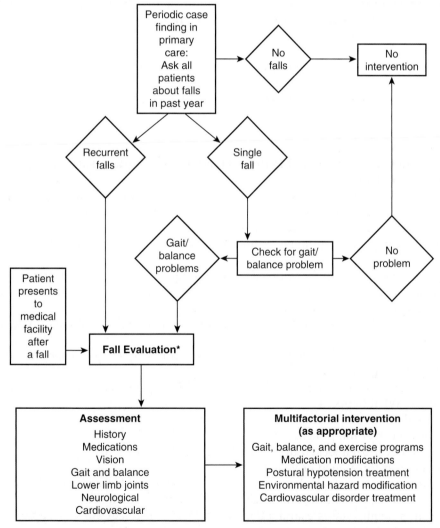

Figure 13-1 Algorithm for assessment and management of falls in elderly persons. (From American Geriatrics Society, British Geriatrics Society, and American Academy of Orthopaedic Surgeons Panel on Falls Prevention: Guideline for the prevention of falls in older persons. Physical examination and health assessment. *J Am Geriatr Soc* 49:666, 2001, Figure 1.)

INSTRUCTIONS TO CANDIDATE: A 75-year-old female is brought to your office by her daughter for a checkup. This patient has been dependent on her family for her care since having a stroke last year. Before you see the patient the nurse tells you that she noted several bruises and decubitus ulcers. Take a detailed history, focusing on risk factors for abuse and neglect.

Definition and Risk Factors

- Elder abuse represents a spectrum that encompasses physical abuse, sexual abuse, emotional/psychological abuse, neglect, abandonment, and financial or material exploitation. Neglect accounts for the majority of elder abuse.
- Abuse and neglect are more likely to take place when the elder patient is physically or functionally impaired and dependent. The presence of cognitive impairment also increases the risk. Other elder-oriented factors include female sex, advanced age, incontinence, and aggressive behavior.
- Caregiver-related factors include alcohol or drug abuse, mental illness, financial or psychosocial stress related to caring for the elder, lack of caregiving skills, and longer duration as primary caregiver. Social isolation, shared living, and lack of support (resources, family support) further increase the risk.

History

- A thorough history with emphasis on risk factors and direct screening is the most important tool to detect abuse and neglect.
- The history should be taken from the caregiver and the patient separately and alone.

Patient History

- What brings you here today? Perform an appropriate history surrounding her presenting complaints.
- Ask for a list of medications. Do you take your medications yourself, or does your caregiver give them to you? Do you take them regularly? Do you ever have trouble getting your medications when you need them?
- How are things going at home? Who do you live with? Do you feel safe where you live?
- How much can you do for yourself? How mobile are you? Can you dress yourself, feed yourself, cook, go to the bathroom, and take a bath/shower? Are you continent? Do you handle your own finances?
- Do you get outside the home? Do you spend time with friends? What do you do for recreation?
- Who helps you with the things you cannot do yourself? Do you ever have trouble getting the help you need?
- Do you ever have disagreements with your caregiver? How are disagreements handled? What happens?
- I notice that you have some bruises, how did that happen?
- Has anyone ever hit, punched, or kicked you? Who?
- Have you ever been locked up or tied down against your will?
- Are you ever threatened or yelled at?
- Note any tension or fearfulness between the patient and her caregiver. Observe the behavior of the patient in your office (e.g., reluctance to make eye contact).
- Perform a mental status examination, and note any signs of anxiety, depression, or cognitive decline.
- For patients who are unable to communicate with you because of aphasia or cognitive decline, for example, you will have to rely on the caregiver's history, collateral history, mental status examination, and physical examination.

Caregiver History

- Avoid creating a confrontational situation with the caregiver. The history should proceed in a nonjudgmental fashion. Remember that being the caregiver of a dependent adult is often difficult and challenging. Demonstrating sympathy to the caregiver may help you create an alliance with them and facilitate information gathering.
- Direct the initial history to the reasons for the visit today.
- Have you noticed any changes in your mother lately? How is she doing?
- How have things been going at home? Describe the current living arrangements?
- Any recent stressful events? Are there any financial strains with the new living arrangements?
- With what activities do you help her (e.g., feeding, cooking, dressing, bathing)?
- Ask the caregiver about routine medications and daily care. Poor knowledge of these essentials may herald neglect.
- What community resources are you currently using (e.g., respite care)?
- Are you working outside the home? What do you do for recreation? Social isolation is a risk factor for abuse and neglect.
- I noticed that your mother has some bruises and skin breakdown/ulcers. Can you tell me how this happened?
- Throughout the interview be alert to clues to depression, anxiety, substance abuse, hostility, or indifference.
- Failure of the caregiver to accompany the patient or provide essential belongings, such as glasses, hearing aid, or walking aid, is a warning sign.

Red Flags

- Evidence of tension or indifference between the patient and caregiver
- Implausible or vague explanations of mechanism of injury
- Inconsistent history of injury between the patient and caregiver
- Unexplained injuries
- Evidence of old injuries not previously documented
- Patient lacking glasses, hearing aid, or walking aid
- Caregiver not able to give details of the patient's routine medications and daily activities

PEARLS

- Like intimate partner violence elder abuse tends to increase in frequency and escalate in intensity over time. Abuse and neglect exacerbate underlying medical problems, and abused elders appear to have a greater risk of dying compared with unabused elders.
- Most states mandate reporting of elder abuse.

SAMPLE CHECKLIST

> INSTRUCTIONS TO CANDIDATE: A 76-year-old female presents to her family doctor with a history of leaking urine. This limits her activities outside of the home. Take a detailed history, exploring possible etiologies.

Key Points	Satisfactorily Carried out
Introduces self to the patient	❏
Determines how the patient wishes to be addressed	❏
Explains the purpose of the encounter	❏
Asks for a description of the problem	
• Does it occur with coughing, laughing, sneezing, or lifting?	❏
• Is there any urinary urgency?	❏
• Sense of incomplete emptying? Continued urge to void despite termination of urinary flow?	❏
Asks when the incontinence started	❏
Asks when this poses the greatest difficulty (e.g., overnight)	❏
Asks about quantity of leakage	❏
Asks about continent voids	❏
Inquires about mobility (e.g., difficulty getting to the toilet)	❏
Asks how she deals with the problem	
• Does she wear an incontinence pad or diaper?	❏
• How often does she have to change it?	❏
Asks what strategies have been tried thus far to manage the problem	❏
Asks how this affects her daily activities	
• Is she able to participate in activities outside the home such as grocery shopping?	❏
• Is there someone helping her?	❏
Asks whether it is getting better, worse, or staying the same	❏
Asks how frequently it poses a problem (e.g., everyday?)	❏
Asks whether she has any abdominal or flank pain	❏
Inquires about constipation (stool impaction can cause incontinence in the elderly)	❏
Asks about irritative symptoms	
• Dysuria	❏
• Strangury	❏
• Urgency	❏
• Frequency	❏

Key Points	Satisfactorily Carried out
Asks about obstructive symptoms	
• Hesitancy	❏
• Increased force needed for urination	❏
• Sense of incomplete emptying	❏
Asks about hematuria (blood in the urine)	❏
Asks about palliative and provocative factors	❏
Asks about normal pattern of fluid intake	❏
Asks about past medical problems and past surgeries	❏
• GU trauma: Child birth	❏
• GU/pelvic surgeries	❏
• Diabetes	❏
• CHF	❏
• Neurologic disorders, conditions that decrease mobility	❏
Asks for a complete list of medications including dosages (prescription, OTC, and herbal medicines)	
• Clarifies any recent changes to medications (e.g., addition of diuretics)	❏
Makes appropriate closing remarks	❏

PEARL

• Potentially reversible etiologies for urinary incontinence using the mnemonic **DRIP**:
  Drugs, **d**elirium
  Restricted mobility, **r**etention (overflow incontinence)
  Infection, **i**mpaction (stool)
  Polydipsia

CHAPTER 14

Ethics

OBJECTIVES

SAMPLE OSCE SCENARIOS

- A 68-year-old female is brought to the emergency department by her husband with worsening shortness of breath. She has cyanosis, is tachypneic, and is having difficulty speaking in complete sentences. She is known to have end-stage chronic obstructive pulmonary disease. In the past year she has been admitted to the hospital three times, and her functional abilities have continued to decline despite optimal medical management. She does not have an advance directive. When asked by the attending physician about intubation and resuscitation, she says, "Let me die." Talk to the patient about her wishes.
- A 47-year-old male presented to the emergency department via ambulance, intubated, ventilated, and comatose. Paramedics were called to the scene after he had a "seizure" at home. On arrival he was "decerebrate" (i.e., rigid extension). He was previously in good health. His pupils are now fixed and dilated. Computed tomography scan shows a major intracerebral hemorrhage. The consulting neurosurgeon says that the chances of meaningful recovery or even survival are negligible. His wife arrives and would like to be updated on his condition.
- A 61-year-old female presents to her family physician for the results of a recent screening mammogram. You inform her that something suspicious has shown up, and you are recommending a biopsy. She had a biopsy 3 years ago that came back negative. She was not pleased about the scar from that procedure. Discuss the proposed procedure for the purposes of "informed consent" (or refusal).
- A 56-year-old male with a complicated in-hospital course of recovery from pancreatitis is now having an upper gastrointestinal bleed. As the intensive care unit staff person on call you have been asked to see this patient. His hemoglobin is 56 g/L but he is currently refusing blood products because of religious convictions. He is now having chest pain and you note acute ischemic changes on his electrocardiogram but he continues to refuse the blood. His wife pleads with you in the hallway to "do something to help him." Discuss the situation with the patient and his wife and ascertain his wishes.
- A 14-year-old female presents to the emergency department with right lower quadrant pain and "spotting." On investigation she is found to have an ectopic pregnancy and requires surgery urgently. She understands the importance of having the surgery. She came to the hospital with a friend but would like to see her parents. She does not want them to find out what kind of operation she is having because they do not know she is sexually active. Discuss these concerns with her.
- An 18-year-old female is in the intensive care unit for 36 hours. She was intubated for acute decline in level of consciousness. Although previously healthy she is now known to have extensive thrombosis of her cavernous sinus. Her family has expressed concern to the nursing staff about the idea of organ donation and worry that we are only interested in her organs. You have confirmed that she now meets the criteria for brain death. Approach the family, and discuss her current condition.

OBJECTIVES

The successful student should have an understanding of the following core ethical principles:

- Autonomy: Principle of self-determination in setting of intact decision-making capacity, even if that decision is in contradiction to that which is recommended.
- Nonmaleficence: Based on the Hippocratic principle *primum non nocere,* first do no harm. This also includes preventing harm when possible.
- Beneficence: Do as much good as possible.
- Justice: Principle that persons with similar conditions, under similar circumstances, should be treated alike. This principle also includes the concept of fairness in resource allocation.

The successful student should have an understanding of the ethical issues involved in the following topics:

- Advance care planning
- End-of-life decision making
- Do not resuscitate (DNR) orders
- Medical futility
- Withholding or withdrawing medical care
- Substitute decision making (proxy)
- Euthanasia and physician-assisted suicide
- Informed consent
- Refusal of care and capacity to decide
- Truth telling and breaking bad news
- Confidentiality
- Dealing with mature minors
- Maternal-fetal conflicts
- Organ donation
- Resource allocation

SAMPLE OSCE SCENARIOS

> INSTRUCTIONS TO CANDIDATE: A 68-year-old female is brought to the emergency department by her husband with worsening shortness of breath. She has cyanosis, is tachypneic, and is having difficulty speaking in complete sentences. She is known to have end-stage chronic obstructive pulmonary disease. In the past year she has been admitted to the hospital three times, and her functional abilities have continued to decline despite optimal medical management. She does not have an advance directive. When asked by the attending physician about intubation and resuscitation, she says, "Let me die." Talk to the patient about her wishes.

Advance Care Planning

- Like informed consent, advance care planning is a process rather than an event. Using this process, capable patients make decisions with respect to their future health care (in the event that they should become unable to express their wishes). This may take the form of a written document called an advance care directive that outlines specific wishes, usually with respect to resuscitative measures, and/or appoints a substitute decision maker to carry out these wishes. In this process patients may identify the standard of living/quality of life that would be acceptable for them. Alternatively the patient may simply make family members and/or friends aware of his or her wishes in the expectation that they would make decisions consistent with these expressed wishes.
- An advance directive takes effect only when the patient is not able to make his or her own decision.
- Advance care planning should be reevaluated on an ongoing basis as the patient's disease changes.

End-of-Life Care

- Quality end-of-life care is often recognized as a deficiency in modern medical care.
- Singer and MacDonald identify three main elements in quality end-of-life care:
  - Control of pain and other symptoms (e.g., breathlessness, nausea, fatigue)
  - Use of life-sustaining treatment
  - Support of dying patients and their families

The Student Should

- Ask the patient about resuscitative measures (intubation, noninvasive positive pressure ventilation, defibrillation, cardiopulmonary resuscitation [CPR]).
- Provide information about the likelihood of success of resuscitation.
- Ascertain that the patient understands her disease process and the proposed treatment.
- Ascertain that the patient understands the consequences of her decision (i.e., death).
- Ask the patient's husband about their previous discussions regarding resuscitation.
- Agree to respect the patient's request (if applicable).
- Reinforce the fact that withholding resuscitative measures does not imply withdrawal/withholding of all treatments.
- Describe a plan for treatment in light of the discussion (may include admission or transfer to a quieter area of the department, symptomatic treatment).
- Offer to answer any questions or address patient concerns.
- Ask what else can be done to help (e.g., access to phone to contact other family members, access to clergy).
- State that the patient can change her mind.

INSTRUCTIONS TO CANDIDATE: A 47-year-old male presented to the emergency department via ambulance, intubated, ventilated, and comatose. Paramedics were called to the scene after he had a "seizure" at home. On arrival he was "decerebrate" (i.e., rigid extension). He was previously in good health. His pupils are now fixed and dilated. Computed tomography scan shows a major intracerebral hemorrhage. The consulting neurosurgeon says that the chances of meaningful recovery or even survival are negligible. His wife arrives and would like to be updated on his condition.

Medical Futility

- Medical futility is a controversial concept that refers to situations in which medical treatment is not likely to benefit the patient. In situations such as these, futile treatments need not be offered at all and may be refused if demanded by family members. This idea has not been universally accepted. There are two types of medical futility:
  - *Quantitative futility:* when the treatment is essentially useless
  - *Qualitative futility:* when the gain produced by an intervention (quality) is exceptionally poor (e.g., a permanent state of unconsciousness)
- In catastrophic situations whereby prognosis for recovery or survival is bleak, timely communication with family is essential. They should be apprised of the prognosis and what it means for their loved one in terms of treatments and outcomes. The attending physician should assure the family that everything will be done to ensure patient comfort, but no further life-sustaining treatment will be offered.

Withdrawal of Care

- There is no ethical or legal distinction between withholding and withdrawing treatment that has already been started.
- It is appropriate to withdraw a life-sustaining measure when it is no longer of benefit to the patient or at the request of a capable patient or substitute decision maker.

The Student Should

- Assure the wife of the certainty of her husband's diagnosis and prognosis.
- Ask whether the patient had made an advance directive or living will.
- Ascertain whether the wife is the substitute decision maker.
- Offer to facilitate a family meeting.
- Ask about discussions regarding the previously expressed wishes of the patient.
- State that life support should be stopped.
- Reinforce the fact that withholding further life-sustaining measures does not imply withdrawal/withholding of all treatments.
- Offer to answer any questions or address her concerns.
- Describe a plan for treatment in light of the discussion (discontinuation of ventilation ± extubation, transfer to a quieter area of the department, availability of clergy or other support).
- Ask what else can be done to help (e.g., access to phone to contact other family members, access to clergy).
- Mention that the patient is a candidate for tissue donation (organ donation can only be considered with the determination of brain death).
- Ask about any previous discussions with her husband about tissue/organ donation.

INSTRUCTIONS TO CANDIDATE: A 61-year-old female presents to her family physician for the results of a recent screening mammogram. You inform her that something suspicious has shown up, and you are recommending a biopsy. She had a biopsy 3 years ago that came back negative. She was not pleased about the scar from that procedure. Discuss the proposed procedure for the purposes of "informed consent" (or refusal).

Informed Consent

- The need for informed consent arises from a fundamental societal tenet that the human body be protected from violation by another and the ethical duty to involve patients in their health care decisions. Within the law medical treatment without consent can be interpreted as assault and/or battery.
- Informed consent is a *process*, not a form; completing a consent form in itself does not imply that "informed consent" was obtained. Consent is a two-part process that involves disclosure of information and the patient's subsequent decision (to consent or to refuse the procedure).
- Using understandable language the physician should disclose the nature of the procedure and its purpose, including how the outcome will alter further management plans. This discussion should also include the possible benefits and the severity and likelihood of risks (using the standard of what a reasonable person would want to know under the circumstances). The patient should be offered possible alternatives to the procedure, including the possibility of doing nothing.
- The physician should present an opportunity for the patient to ask questions or express concerns. Seek confirmation that the patient understands the procedure and its risks and benefits before making the decision.
- The patient's decision must be voluntary and not coerced. The patient may elect to take further time to consider her options or have discussions with her family or friends.
- The setting may also be of importance. For example, it would not be appropriate to seek informed consent for nonemergent surgery in the hallway outside the operating room. Arguably this setting is coercive in itself.
- **Mnemonic for essentials of informed consent: Dduv (pronounced "dove")**
  - **D**ecision-making capacity
  - **D**isclosure
  - **U**nderstanding
  - **V**oluntariness

Capacity

- Although often used interchangeably, capacity and competency are not equivalent. Competency is generally stable over time and tends to be legally determined. Capacity is applied to particular decisions and may fluctuate over time and across domains (e.g., finances, place of residence, health decisions). The treating physician and health care team determine capacity in the health care setting.
- If a patient has been deemed capable of making a particular decision, it must be respected whether it is in line with your recommendations or not. Refusal to comply with treatment recommendations is not evidence of incapacity nor is difficulty in making the decision.
- Criteria for patient capacity:
  - Ability to understand the medical problem, the proposed treatment, and possible alternatives
  - Ability to appreciate the consequences of undergoing the proposed treatment
  - Ability to appreciate the consequences of refusing the proposed treatment
  - Ability to make the decision within a stable set of values (not based on delusions or depression)

The Student Should

- Explain the nature of the procedure, its purpose, risks, and benefits.
- Offer alternatives to the procedure, including the possibility of doing nothing and the consequences.
- Ask if the patient has any concerns
- Confirm whether the patient understands the information, including the consequences of refusing the procedure.
- Ask whether the patient needs more time or information to make the decision.
- Allow the patient to make a voluntary decision.
- Explore reasons for refusing to consent (if applicable).

INSTRUCTIONS TO CANDIDATE: A 56-year-old male with a complicated in-hospital course of recovery from pancreatitis is now having an upper gastrointestinal bleed. As the intensive care unit staff person on call you have been asked to see this patient. His hemoglobin is 56 g/L, but he is currently refusing blood products because of religious convictions. He is now having chest pain and you note acute ischemic changes on his electrocardiogram but he continues to refuse the blood. His wife pleads with you in the hallway to "do something to help him." Discuss the situation with the patient and his wife and ascertain his wishes.

Substitute Decision Making

- A substitute decision maker is one who makes decisions on behalf of a patient who is not capable of doing so. These decisions should reflect what the patient would want in a particular circumstance as much as possible rather than the wishes of the decision maker for the patient.
- Ideally the substitute decision maker would be appointed by the still capable patient who has informed the decision maker about his or her wishes in particular situations.
- In the absence of an appointed decision maker, the task falls to the spouse, child, parent, sibling, or other relative. Decisions should still be based on the patient's beliefs and values. A parent's religious beliefs do not include the right to deny life-sustaining treatment, including blood transfusions, for a child. In this case the child would be made a ward of the court, and all necessary treatments would be provided in accordance with the principles of nonmaleficence and beneficence.

Informed Consent

- Consent is a two-part process that involves disclosure of information and the patient's subsequent decision (to consent or to refuse the procedure).
- Using understandable language the physician should disclose the nature of the procedure and its purpose, including how the outcome will alter further management plans. This discussion should also include the possible benefits and the severity and likelihood of risks. The patient should be offered possible alternatives to the procedure, including the possibility of doing nothing.
- The physician should present an opportunity for the patient to ask questions or express concerns. Seek confirmation that the patient understands the procedure and its risks and benefits before making the decision.
- The patient's decision must be voluntary and not coerced.

Capacity

- Criteria for patient capacity:
  - Ability to understand the medical problem, the proposed treatment, and possible alternatives
  - Ability to appreciate the consequences of undergoing the proposed treatment
  - Ability to appreciate the consequences of refusing the proposed treatment

 - Ability to make the decision within a stable set of values (not based on delusions or depression)

The Student Should

- Explain the seriousness of the patient's condition and that in light of ongoing bleeding and acute myocardial ischemia, no transfusion likely means death.
- Ask whether the patient has discussed his wishes with his wife.
- Ascertain the reason for refusing blood products (e.g., Jehovah's Witness teachings).
- Ensure that the patient is not depressed, suicidal, or delusional.
- Ascertain that the patient understands the seriousness of the consequences of refusing blood products (i.e., death).
- Allow the patient to make a voluntary decision.
- State that the patient's wishes will be respected.
- Address any additional concerns raised by the patient and his wife.
- Ask the patient whether he desires other life-sustaining treatments (intubation, defibrillation, CPR).
- State that the patient can change his mind.

INSTRUCTIONS TO CANDIDATE: A 14-year-old female presents to the emergency department with right lower quadrant pain and "spotting." On investigation she is found to have an ectopic pregnancy and requires surgery urgently. She understands the importance of having the surgery. She came to the hospital with a friend but would like to see her parents. She does not want them to find out what kind of operation she is having because they do not know she is sexually active. Discuss these concerns with her.

Confidentiality

- Confidentiality is a fundamental underlying premise of the physician-patient relationship. Trust is necessary to maintain the therapeutic relationship such that patients are secure in being forthcoming with their symptoms and concerns. Withheld information may prove detrimental.
- The autonomous patient has the right to decide when to disclose information to others (provided there is no risk of harm).
- Specific information should be disclosed in cases of:
  - Suspicion of child abuse
  - Reportable diseases (matter of public health)
  - Public safety risk such as unsafe drivers
  - Imminent serious harm to an identifiable individual

Mature Minor

- A mature minor is one who meets criteria for capacity and is able to participate in informed consent. Canadian law generally does not have an age below which one is presumed incapable.
- Criteria for patient capacity:
  - Ability to understand the medical problem, the proposed treatment, and possible alternatives
  - Ability to appreciate the consequences of undergoing the proposed treatment
  - Ability to appreciate the consequences of refusing the proposed treatment
  - Ability to make the decision within a stable set of values (not based on delusions or depression)

Informed Consent

- Consent is a two-part process that involves disclosure of information and the patient decision (to consent or to refuse the procedure).

- Using understandable language the physician should disclose the nature of the procedure and its purpose, including how the outcome will alter further management plans. This discussion should also include the possible benefits and the severity and likelihood of risks. The patient should be offered possible alternatives to the procedure, including the possibility of doing nothing.
- The physician should present an opportunity for the patient to ask questions or express concerns. Seek confirmation that the patient understands the procedure and its risks and benefits before making the decision.
- The patient's decision must be voluntary and not coerced.

The Student Should
- Explain the nature of the surgery, its purpose, risks, and benefits.
- Offer alternatives to the surgery, including the possibility of doing nothing and the consequences.
- Ask if the patient has any concerns.
- Confirm whether the patient understands the information, including the consequences of refusing the operation.
- Ask whether the patient needs more time or information to make the decision.
- Allow the patient to make a voluntary decision.
- Assure the patient that her confidentiality will be respected.
- Inform the patient that her parents' enquiries will be redirected to her (i.e., you will not lie to them about the nature of her surgery).
- Address the nature of the patient's relationship with her parents.
- Encourage her to consider being honest with her parents.
- Offer to be present for her discussion with her parents.

INSTRUCTIONS TO CANDIDATE: An 18-year-old female is in the intensive care unit for 36 hours. She was intubated for acute decline in level of consciousness. Although previously healthy she is now known to have extensive thrombosis of her cavernous sinus. Her family has expressed concern to the nursing staff about the idea of organ donation and worry that we are only interested in her organs. You have confirmed that she now meets the criteria for brain death. Approach the family, and discuss her current condition.

Brain Death
- Brain death is the complete and irreversible cessation of all brain function.
- The brain-dead patient is comatose, apneic, and does not have brainstem reflexes.
- At the time of brain-death declaration the patient is considered for all intents and purposes to be dead even though with the assistance of a ventilator and critical care vital signs may still be present.
- Brain death is an ethically challenging concept for some. Some cultural and religious groups may not be able to accept death until the cessation of all vital functions.
- Brain death can usually be determined at the bedside. Electroencephalography (EEG) is not required to determine brain death and may be unreliable. Clinical criteria for the declaration of brain death (in a patient aged >2 months):
  - Rule out reversible causes of cerebral unresponsiveness, such as hypothermia and depressant or sedative medications. This may require a period of observation.
  - Absence of brainstem reflexes, including oculovestibular (cold calorics), oculocephalic (doll's eye maneuvers), pupillary, corneal, gag, and respiratory (apnea testing) reflexes. Apnea testing includes disconnecting the ventilator for approximately 10 minutes to allow the partial pressure of arterial CO_2 to increase to 60 mm Hg (pH <7.28). Absence of respiratory effort at this point confirms apnea (absence of respiratory reflexes).
  - Absence of motor responses in the cranial nerve distribution to stimuli applied anywhere on the body. Spinal reflexes may remain intact.

Organ Donation

- Organ retrieval cannot be considered unless the patient is no longer alive.
- Brain-death declaration for the purposes of organ retrieval should be declared by two separate physicians not involved in the care of potential organ recipients. Furthermore physicians who participate in the declaration of brain death should not participate in the transplant procedures.
- Most institutions have dedicated teams of personnel for organ donation and retrieval.
- Laws about organ and tissue donation and criteria for brain death may vary from province to province and state to state. Ensure that you are aware of the laws in your region and the policies of your institution.

The Student Should

- Explain the meaning of "brain death" (e.g., complete and irreversible cessation of brain function, including the brainstem).
- Assure her parents of the certainty of the diagnosis (i.e., clinical criteria have been satisfied and verified by two separate physicians).
- Assure her parents of the certainty of the prognosis (i.e., brain damage is complete and irreversible; there is no chance of recovery).
- State clearly that their daughter is dead now (i.e., brain death is a legal definition of death).
- State that ventilatory support and other critical care measures should now be stopped.
- Ask about previous discussions with the patient about organ donation and whether she had an organ donation card.
- Explain that their daughter is now a candidate for organ donation.
- Ask the family's views regarding donation of the patient's organs.
- Address their concerns if possible (e.g., organ donation does not affect burial).
- Offer the family the option of discussing this further with the organ donor personnel at your institution.

Sample In-Depth OSCE Case

by Dr. Graham Bullock (used with permission)

> INSTRUCTIONS TO CANDIDATE: You are a clerk working in the emergency department (ED). M. Bartholomew presents to the ED with a 2-day history of "jaundice." During the next 10 minutes, take a detailed history of the onset and nature of his symptoms, exploring possible etiologies. Perform an examination of the liver. Describe to the examiner what you are doing and your findings. At the end of the examination, communicate your impressions to the patient.

PATIENT SCRIPT—MARK BARTHOLOMEW

Demographics
Age: 24 years
Sex: Male
Marital status: Single
Educational background: University student, Computer Science

Chief Complaint
"I think I have jaundice."

Patient Behavior, Affect, and Mannerisms
The patient is a young male (female could be substituted) of average build. He is wearing an examining gown and shorts. He appears a little anxious but is otherwise in no distress and is cooperative. No makeup is required.

On examination he complains of mild discomfort with deep palpation of the epigastric area and right upper quadrant (RUQ). There is no guarding or evidence of peritoneal irritation.

History of Present Illness
He has been feeling essentially well until approximately 7 days ago when he experienced onset of nonspecific symptoms, including nausea, chills, and loose stools. These symptoms continued for several days but have now largely abated and left him with a general feeling of fatigue, muscle aches, and vague abdominal discomfort. He has been sleeping much more than usual—up to 10 hours per night—and has had to skip classes. Today his roommate told him that she thought he looked yellow and told him to get to a doctor. He has not yet sought other medical help for this current illness.

Past Medical/Surgical History
Nothing of significance. Has never had hepatitis testing or vaccination that he is aware of. No previous blood transfusions. No previous hospitalizations or surgeries.

Medications
Prescription medications: None

Over-the-counter (OTC) medications: Takes caffeine tablets on a regular basis when studying. Also takes acetaminophen and ibuprofen occasionally but not recently and never to excess.

Allergies
None known.

Relevant Social History
He is a third-year university student studying computer science. He is not aware of any exposures to infectious hepatitis. No past employment or history to suggest exposure to hepatotoxic drugs.

He is currently dating and has no fixed partner. Although he has had several different sexual partners in the past year, he uses condoms "religiously." He has no children.

Nonsmoker. Drinks a "case" (24 beers) per week, mostly on the weekends.

Has dabbled with amphetamines and "wake-ups" to help him study for exams. Denies intravenous (IV) drug use but has smoked marijuana and tried cocaine nasally in the remote past.

He enjoys skiing and extreme sports. Took part in a cross-country adventure race in the southern United States (Nevada) 4 weeks ago. He drank filtered water on that trip and is not aware of any other participants who are sick. He did not have any immunizations before this trip.

Relevant Family History
Father, aged 58 years. High blood pressure, angina.
Mother, aged 52 years. Pretty healthy.
Brother, aged 28 years. Not aware of any health problems.
No known family predisposition to cancers or liver disease.

Review of Systems
* **General:** Chills last week. No documented fever. No weight change. Appetite is poor this week.
* **Head, eyes, ears, nose, and throat (HEENT):** Nil
* **Respiratory (Resp):** Nil
* **Cardiovascular system (CVS):** Nil
* **Gastrointestinal (GI):** Vague dull, constant upper abdominal pain for the last week. The pain does not radiate. No exacerbating or relieving features. Several loose, non-bloody stools last week. Now bowel movements are about normal—no color change. Had some diarrhea while in the United States for a few days that resolved spontaneously.
* **Genitourinary (GU):** No urine color change. Otherwise negative.
* **Skin:** Possible jaundice. Otherwise negative.

Physical Examination
The patient appears anxious but is otherwise in no distress.

He should not have any visible surgical scars.

He is able to cooperate with the history and physical examination.

On examination he complains of mild discomfort with deep palpation of the epigastric area and RUQ. There is no guarding or evidence of peritoneal irritation.

EXAMINER'S CHECKLIST—JAUNDICE

Please indicate which items were satisfactorily completed.

General/Introductory

❏	1. Introduces self to the patient	
❏	2. Refers to the patient by name	
❏	3. Establishes the purpose of the encounter	
❏	4. Uses open-ended questions to obtain story	
❏	5. Establishes presenting complaint in the patient's own words	

Presenting Complaint—Jaundice and Associated Symptoms

❏	6. Establishes onset	Noticed by roommate today, otherwise not sure
❏	7. Preceding symptoms	Yes, unwell for 1 week
❏	8. Fever/chills	Chills earlier this week
❏	9. Nausea/vomiting	Nausea with reduced appetite, no vomiting
❏	10. Abdominal pain	Yes
❏	11. Onset of abdominal pain	Not sure, about 1 week
❏	12. Nature of abdominal pain	Dull, ache
❏	13. Severity of pain	Mild
❏	14. Location of pain	Upper abdomen
❏	15. Aggravating or alleviating factors for pain	None
❏	16. Nature of stools—diarrhea?	Yes, last week
❏	17. Color of stools	Normal, brown

Review of Systems—Other Relevant

❏	18. Skin rash	No
❏	19. Myalgias	Yes, mild and generalized
❏	20. Urine color	No change

Relevant Social History

❏	21. Alcohol consumption	Yes
❏	22. Quantifies recent alcohol consumption	24 beers per week
❏	23. IV drug use	No
❏	24. Sexual contacts—number of partners and frequency	
❏	25. Sexual practices—barrier precautions	
❏	26. Recent travel	Yes, southern United States
❏	27. Possible exposure to contaminated water	Yes, recent trip

Past Medical History

❏	28. Previous hepatitis	No
❏	29. History of biliary/gallbladder disease	No
❏	30. Previous vaccinations against hepatitis	No
❏	31. Prescription medications	None
❏	32. OTC medications—specifically acetaminophen	Occasional

Physical Examination

❏	33. Drapes the patient appropriately	
❏	34. Inspects for rash/discoloration	Faint jaundice?
❏	35. Percusses liver span—from above	
❏	36. Percusses liver span—from below	
❏	37. Palpates for liver edge beginning in the right lower quadrant	Not enlarged
❏	38. Palpates liver for tenderness, including Murphy's sign	
❏	39. Palpates RUQ/liver edge for mass, including gallbladder	None

Closure

❏	40. Makes appropriate closing remarks	

OSCE Checklist Template

Use the template below to create your own OSCE checklists for the sample OSCE scenarios in this handbook.

- Fill in the "instructions to candidate" with the desired scenario.
- Fill in the key history and/or physical examinations to be carried out for the scenario, in addition to the points that have already been filled in for you. Think about the **ChLORIDE FPP, VITAMINS C,** and **IPPA** format to organize your thoughts.
- Be sure to fill in *all* the points you intend to carry out. Your checklist will probably be longer than the examiner's checklist because credit will not be given for everything.
- Review the sample OSCE scenario in the handbook to check your list for any omissions or errors.

INSTRUCTIONS TO CANDIDATE: (Focused history)
_____
_____
_____
_____

Key Points	Satisfactorily Carried out
Introduces self to the patient	❏
Determines how the patient wishes to be addressed	❏
Explains the purpose of the encounter	❏
Develops good patient rapport	❏
Character	❏
Location	❏
Onset	❏
Radiation	❏
Intensity	❏
Duration	❏
Events associated	❏
Frequency	❏
Palliative factors	❏
Provocative factors	❏
_____	
_____	
Past history of medical or surgical problems	❏
Medications (prescription, over the counter, and herbals)	❏
Allergies	❏
Use of alcohol and recreational drugs	❏
Family history of related medical problems	❏
Makes appropriate closing remarks	❏

INSTRUCTIONS TO CANDIDATE: (Focused physical examination)

Key Points	Satisfactorily Carried out
Introduces self to the patient	❏
Determines how the patient wishes to be addressed	❏
Explains nature of examination to the patient	❏
Examines the patient in a logical fashion	❏
Drapes the patient appropriately	❏
Inspection	❏
Palpation	❏
Percussion	❏
Auscultation	❏
Special tests/maneuvers	❏
Makes appropriate closing remarks	❏

References

INTRODUCTION

Baile WF, Buckman R, Lenzi R, Glober G, Beale EA, Kudelka AP: SPIKES—a six-step protocol for delivering bad news: application to the patient with cancer, *Oncologist* 5:302–311, 2000.

Bernstein E, Bernstein J, James T: Multiculturalism and care delivery. In Marx JA, Hockberger RS, Walls RM, editors: *Rosen's emergency medicine: concepts and clinical practice*, ed 5, St. Louis, 2002, Mosby, pp 2715–2724.

Cohen R, Reznick RK, Taylor BR, et al: Reliability and validity of the Objective Structured Clinical Examination in assessing surgical residents, *Am J Surg* 160:302–305, 1990.

Cruess SR, Johnston S, Cruess RL: "Profession": a working definition for medical educators, *Teach Learn Med* 16:74–76, 2004.

Grand'Maison P, Lescop J, Rainsberry P, Brailovsky CA: Large scale use of an Objective Structured Clinical Examination for licensing family physicians, *CMAJ* 146:1735–1740, 1992.

Harden RM, Stevenson M, Downie WW, Wilson GM: Assessment of clinical competence using Objective Structured Examination, *BMJ* 1:447–451, 1975.

Hodges B, McNaughton N, Regehr G, Tiberius R, Hanson M: The challenge of creating new OSCE measures to capture the characteristics of expertise, *Med Ed* 36:742–748, 2002.

Martin IG, Stark P, Jolly B: Benefiting from clinical experience: the influence of learning style and clinical experience on performance in an undergraduate Objective Structured Clinical Examination, *Med Ed* 34:530–534, 2000.

Matsell DG, Wolfish NM, Hsu E: Reliability and validity of the Objective Structured Clinical Examination in paediatrics, *Med Educ* 25:293–299, 1991.

Mavis B: Self-efficacy and OSCE performance among second year medical students, *Adv Health Sci Educ Theory Pract* 6:93–102, 2001.

Mavis BE: Does studying for an Objective Structured Clinical Examination make a difference? *Med Educ* 34:808–812, 2000.

Newble DI, Sawnson DB: Psychometric characteristics of the Objective Structured Clinical Examination, *Med Educ* 22:325–334, 1988.

Petrusa ER, Blackwell TA, Ainsworth MA: Reliability and validity of the Objective Structured Clinical Examination for assessing the clinical performance of residents, *Arch Intern Med* 150:573–577, 1990.

Ptacek JT, Eberhardt TL: Breaking bad news: a review of the literature, *JAMA* 276:496–502, 1996.

Reznick R, Smee S, Rothman A, et al: An Objective Structured Clinical Examination for the licentiate: Report of the Pilot Project of the Medical Council of Canada, *Acad Med* 67:487–494, 1992.

Roberts J, Norman G: Reliability and learning from the Objective Structured Clinical Examination, *Med Educ* 24:219–233, 1990.

Sloan DA, Donnelly MB, Schwartz RW, Strodel WE: The Objective Structured Clinical Examination. The new gold standard for evaluating postgraduate clinical performance, *Ann Surg* 222:735–742, 1995.

Teutsch C: Patient-doctor communication, *Med Clin N Am* 87:1115–1145, 2003.

CARDIOVASCULAR SYSTEM

Cardiovascular disorders. In Berkow R, editor: *The Merck manual*, ed 16, Rahway, NJ, 1992, Merck Research Laboratories, pp 365–594.

Chobanian AV, Bakris GL, Black HR, et al: The seventh report of the Joint National Committee on prevention, detection, evaluation, and treatment of high blood pressure: the JNC 7 report, *JAMA* 289:2560–2572, 2003.

Massie BM, Amidon TM: Heart. In Tierney LM, McPhee SJ, Papadakis MA, editors: *Current medical diagnosis & treatment 2003*, ed 42, New York, 2003, McGraw-Hill, pp 312–408.

Stein EA: Management of dyslipidemia in the high risk patient, *Am Heart J* 144:S43–50, 2002.

The cardiovascular system. In Bickley LS, Hoekelman RA, editors: *Bates' guide to physical examination and history taking,* ed 7, Philadelphia, 1999, Lippincott Williams & Wilkins, pp 277–332.

The heart. In Swartz M, editor: *Textbook of physical diagnosis: history and examination,* ed 3, Philadelphia, 1998, WB Saunders, pp 275–320.

RESPIRATORY SYSTEM

Chesnutt MS, Prendergast TJ: Lung. In Tierney LM, McPhee SJ, Papadakis MA, editors: *Current medical diagnosis & treatment 2003,* ed 42, New York, 2003, McGraw-Hill, pp 216–311.

Pulmonary disorders. In Berkow R, editor: *The Merck manual,* ed 16, Rahway, NJ, 1992, Merck Research Laboratories, pp 595–736.

The chest. In Swartz M, editor: *Textbook of physical diagnosis: history and examination,* ed 3, Philadelphia, 1998, WB Saunders, pp 248–276.

The thorax and lungs. In Bickley LS, Hoekelman RA, editors: *Bates' guide to physical examination and history taking,* ed 7, Philadelphia, 1999, Lippincott Williams & Wilkins, pp 245–276.

GASTROINTESTINAL SYSTEM

Friedman LS: Liver, biliary tract & pancreas. In Tierney LM, McPhee SJ, Papadakis MA, editors: *Current medical diagnosis & treatment 2003,* ed 42, New York, 2003, McGraw-Hill, pp 628–676.

Gastrointestinal disorders. In Berkow R, editor: *The Merck manual,* ed 16, Rahway, NJ, 1992, Merck Research Laboratories, pp 737–862.

Male genitalia and hernias. In Swartz M, editor: *Textbook of physical diagnosis: history and examination,* ed 3, Philadelphia, 1998, WB Saunders, pp 390–417.

McQuaid KR: Alimentary tract. In Tierney LM, McPhee SJ, Papadakis MA, editors: *Current medical diagnosis & treatment 2003,* ed 42, New York, 2003, McGraw-Hill, pp 522–627.

The abdomen. In Bickley LS, Hoekelman RA, editors: *Bates' guide to physical examination and history taking,* ed 7, Philadelphia, 1999, Lippincott Williams & Wilkins, pp 355–386.

The abdomen. In Swartz M, editor: *Textbook of physical diagnosis: history and examination,* ed 3, Philadelphia, 1998, WB Saunders, pp 354–389.

GENITOURINARY SYSTEM

Male genitalia and hernias. In Swartz M, editor: *Textbook of physical diagnosis: history and examination,* ed 3, Philadelphia, 1998, WB Saunders, pp 390–417.

Watnick S, Morrison G: Kidney. In Tierney LM, McPhee SJ, Papadakis MA, editors: *Current medical diagnosis & treatment 2003,* ed 42, New York, 2003, McGraw-Hill, pp 867–902.

NERVOUS SYSTEM

Blumenfeld H: *Neuroanatomy through clinical cases,* Sunderland, MA, 2002, Sinauer Associates.

Bradley WG, Daroff RB, Fenichel GM, Jankovic J: *Neurology in clinical practice: principles of diagnosis and management,* ed 4, Philadelphia, 2003, Butterworth-Heinemann Medical.

Fix JD: *High-yield neuroanatomy,* ed 2, Philadelphia, 2000, Lippincott Williams & Wilkins.

Fuller G: *Neurological examination made easy,* ed 2, New York, 1999, Churchill Livingstone.

Marshall RS, Mayer SA: *On call neurology,* ed 2, Philadelphia, 2001, WB Saunders.

Victor M, Ropper AH: *Adams and Victor's principles of neurology,* ed 7, New York, 2000, McGraw-Hill.

MUSCULOSKELETAL SYSTEM

Abernethy PJ, Hurst NP: The locomotor system. In *MacLeod's clinical examination,* ed 10, Edinburgh, 2000, Churchill Livingstone, pp 259–292.

Feske SK, Greenberg SA: Degenerative and compressive structural disorders. In Goetz CG, editor: *Textbook of clinical neurology,* ed 2, St. Louis, 2003, WB Saunders, pp 583–600.

Hellmann DB, Stone JH: Arthritis and musculoskeletal system. In Tierney LM, McPhee SJ, Papadakis MA, editors: *Current medical diagnosis & treatment 2003,* ed 42, New York, 2003, McGraw-Hill, pp 783–838.

Katz JN, Simmons BP: Clinical practice: carpal tunnel syndrome, *N Engl J Med* 346:1807–1812, 2002.

Musculoskeletal system. In Jarvis C, editor: *Physical examination and health assessment,* ed 2, Philadelphia, 1996, WB Saunders, pp 645–708.

Musculoskeletal system. In Seidel HM, Ball JW, Dains JE, Benedict GW, editors: *Mosby's guide to physical examination,* ed 5, St. Louis, 2003, Mosby, pp 694–765.

Raisz LG, Kream BE, Lorenzo JA: Metabolic bone disease. In Larsen PR, Kronenberg HM, Melmed S, Polonsky KS, editors: *Williams textbook of endocrinology,* ed 10, St. Louis, 2003, WB Saunders, pp 1373–1410.

The musculoskeletal system. In Swartz M, editor: *Textbook of physical diagnosis: history and examination,* ed 3, Philadelphia, 1998, WB Saunders, pp 446–493.

van der Linden S, van der Heijde D: Ankylosing spondylitis. In Ruddy S, Harris ED, Sledge CB, editors: *Kelley's textbook of rheumatology,* ed 6, St. Louis, 2001, WB Saunders, pp 1039–1053.

DERMATOLOGY

Freedberg I, Eisen A, Wolff K, Austen KF, Goldsmith L, Katz S: *Fitzpatrick's dermatology in general medicine,* ed 5, New York, 1999, McGraw-Hill.

Freedberg I, Eisen A, Wolff K, Austen KF, Goldsmith L, Katz S: *Fitzpatrick's dermatology in general medicine,* ed 6, New York, 2003, McGraw-Hill.

Hunter JAA, Savin JA, Dahl MV: *Clinical dermatology,* Malden, MA, 1989, Blackwell Scientific Publications.

Lookingbill D, Marks J: *Principles of dermatology,* ed 3, Philadelphia, 2000, WB Saunders.

HEMATOLOGY

Hematology and oncology. In Berkow R, editor: *The Merck manual,* ed 16, Rahway, NJ, 1992, Merck Research Laboratories, pp 1135–1292.

Linker CA: Blood. In Tierney LM, McPhee SJ, Papadakis MA, editors: *Current medical diagnosis & treatment 2003,* ed 42, New York, 2003, McGraw-Hill, pp 469–521.

ENDOCRINOLOGY

Endocrine disorders. In Berkow R, editor: *The Merck manual,* ed 16, Rahway, NJ, 1992, Merck Research Laboratories, pp 1055–1134.

Fitzgerald PA: Endocrinology. In Tierney LM, McPhee SJ, Papadakis MA, editors: *Current medical diagnosis & treatment 2003,* ed 42, New York, 2003, McGraw-Hill, pp 1067–1151.

OBSTETRICS AND GYNECOLOGY

Female genitalia. In Bickley LS, Hoekelman RA, editors: *Bates' guide to physical examination and history taking,* ed 7, Philadelphia, 1999, Lippincott Williams & Wilkins, pp 405–430.

Female genitalia. In Swartz M, editor: *Textbook of physical diagnosis: history and examination,* ed 3, Philadelphia, 1998, WB Saunders, pp 418–445.

Salber PR, Taliaferro E: Intimate partner violence and abuse. In Marx JA, Hockberger RS, Walls RM, editors: *Rosen's emergency medicine: concepts and clinical practice,* ed 5, St. Louis, 2002, Mosby, pp 863–874.

The pregnant woman. In Bickley LS, Hoekelman RA, editors: *Bates' guide to physical examination and history taking,* ed 7, Philadelphia, 1999, Lippincott Williams & Wilkins, pp 431–448.

The pregnant patient. In Swartz M, editor: *Textbook of physical diagnosis: history and examination,* ed 3, Philadelphia, 1998, WB Saunders, pp 563–582.

PSYCHIATRY

Colucciello SA: Suicide. In Marx JA, Hockberger RS, Walls RM, editors: *Rosen's emergency medicine: concepts and clinical practice,* ed 5, St. Louis, 2002, Mosby, pp 1576–1583.

Hockberger RS, Richards J: Thought disorders. In Marx JA, Hockberger RS, Walls RM, editors: *Rosen's emergency medicine: concepts and clinical practice,* ed 5, St. Louis, 2002, Mosby, pp 1541–1548.

Kercher EE: Anxiety disorders. In Marx JA, Hockberger RS, Walls RM, editors: *Rosen's emergency medicine: concepts and clinical practice,* ed 5, St. Louis, 2002, Mosby, pp 1557–1564.

Mental status. In Seidel HM, Ball JW, Dains JE, Benedict GW, editors: *Mosby's guide to physical examination,* ed 5, St. Louis, 2003, Mosby, pp 82–101.

Mental status assessment. In Jarvis C, editor: *Physical examination and health assessment,* ed 2, Philadelphia, 1996, WB Saunders, pp 99–124.

Psychiatry. In Lofchy J, Lok J, Sue M, Sikka S, editors: *MCCQE review notes and lecture series,* ed 15, Toronto, 1999, University of Toronto.

Rund DA, Vary MG: Mood disorders. In Marx JA, Hockberger RS, Walls RM, editors: *Rosen's emergency medicine: concepts and clinical practice,* ed 5, St. Louis, 2002, Mosby, pp 1549–1556.

Zimmerman M: *Interview guide for evaluating DSM-IV psychiatric disorders and the mental status examination,* East Greenwich, RI, 1994, Psych Products Press.

PEDIATRICS

Austin PE: General approach to the pediatric patient. In Marx JA, Hockberger RS, Walls RM, editors: *Rosen's emergency medicine: concepts and clinical practice*, ed 5, St. Louis, 2002, Mosby, pp 2218–2233.

Brayden RM, Headley RM: Ambulatory pediatrics. In Hay WW, Hayward AR, Levin MJ, Sondheimer JM, editors: *Current pediatric diagnosis and treatment*, ed 14, Stamford, CT, 1999, Appleton & Lange, pp 201–218.

Hostetler MA, Bracikowski A: Gastrointestinal disorders. In Marx JA, Hockberger RS, Walls RM, editors: *Rosen's emergency medicine: concepts and clinical practice*, ed 5, St. Louis, 2002, Mosby, pp 2296–2315.

Lopez JA, McMillin KJ, Tobias-Merrill EA, Chop WM: Managing fever in infants and toddlers, *Postgrad Med* 101:241–250, 1997.

Moe PG, Seay AR: Neurologic and muscular disorders. In Hay WW, Hayward AR, Levin MJ, Sondheimer JM, editors: *Current pediatric diagnosis and treatment*, ed 14, Stamford, CT, 1999, Appleton & Lange, pp 622–694.

Neurological examination. In Gill D, O'Brien N, editors: *Paediatric clinical examination made easy*, ed 4, Edinburgh, 2002, Churchill Livingstone, pp 138–156.

Sampson HA: Peanut allergy, *N Engl J Med* 346:1294–1299, 2002.

The pediatric patient. In Swartz M, editor: *Textbook of physical diagnosis: history and examination*, ed 3, Philadelphia, 1998, WB Saunders, pp 583–639.

The physical examination of infants and children. In Bickley LS, Hoekelman RA, editors: *Bates' guide to physical examination and history taking*, ed 7, Philadelphia, 1999, Lippincott Williams & Wilkins, pp 621–704.

GERIATRICS

American Geriatrics Society, British Geriatrics Society and American Academy of Orthopaedic Surgeons Panel on Falls Prevention: Guideline for the prevention of falls in older persons. Physical examination and health assessment, *J Am Geriatr Soc* 49:664–672, 2001.

Anglin D, Hutson HR: Elder abuse and neglect. In Marx JA, Hockberger RS, Walls RM, editors: *Rosen's emergency medicine: concepts and clinical practice*, ed 5, St. Louis, 2002, Mosby, pp 875–882.

Birnbaumer DM: The elder patient. In Marx JA, Hockberger RS, Walls RM, editors: *Rosen's emergency medicine: concepts and clinical practice*, ed 5, St. Louis, 2002, Mosby, pp 2485–2491.

Fick DM, Cooper JW, Wade WE, Waller JL, MacLean R, Beers MH: Updating the Beers criteria for potentially inappropriate medication use in older adults: results of a US consensus panel of experts, *Arch Intern Med* 163:2716–2724, 2003.

Hirsch CH: Mistreatment of older women. In Liebschutz JM, Frayne SM, Saxe GN, editors: *Violence against women: a physician's guide to identification and management*, Philadelphia, 2003, American College of Physicians, pp 169–189.

Insel KC, Badger TA: Deciphering the 4D's: cognitive decline, delirium, depression and dementia—a review, *J Adv Nurs* 38:360–368, 2002.

Kane RL, Ouslander JG, Abrass IB: *Essentials of clinical geriatrics*, ed 4, New York, 1999, McGraw-Hill.

Siegler EL, Levin BW: Physician-older patient communication at the end of life, *Clin Geriatr Med* 16:175–204, 2000.

Zimmerman M: *Interview guide for evaluating DSM-IV psychiatric disorders and the mental status examination*, East Greenwich, RI, 1994, Psych Products Press.

ETHICS

Confidentiality, privacy and disclosure to third parties. In Rozovsky LE, Inions NJ, editors: *Canadian health information*, ed 3, Markham, Canada, 2002, Butterworths Canada Ltd, pp 83–104.

Considine R: Informed consent & informed refusal. In Fleetwood J, Novack D, Feldman D, Farber N, editors: *MedEthEx: standardized patient exercises in medical ethics and communication skills*, Philadelphia, 1997, Allegheny University of the Health Sciences, pp 68–83.

Determining life and death. In Devettere RJ, editor: *Practical decision making in health care ethics: cases and concepts*, Washington, DC, 1995, Georgetown University Press, pp 138–165.

Documenting consent. In Rozovsky LE, Inions NJ, editors: *Canadian health information*, ed 3, Markham, Canada, 2002, Butterworths Canada Ltd, pp 145–156.

Etchells E, Sharpe G, Elliot C, Singer PA: Capacity. In Singer PA, editor: *Bioethics at the bedside: a clinician's guide*, Ottawa, Canada, 1999, Canadian Medical Association, pp 17–24.

Etchells E, Sharpe G, Walsh P, Williams JR, Singer PA: Consent. In Singer PA, editor: *Bioethics at the bedside: a clinician's guide,* Ottawa, Canada, 1999, Canadian Medical Association, pp 1–8.

Ethics in medicine, Washington, DC, 1998, University of Washington School of Medicine, Available at http://eduserv.hscer.washington.edu/bioethics/topics/index.html, Accessed January 26, 2004.

Kleinman I, Baylis F, Rodgers S, Singer PA: Confidentiality. In Singer PA, editor: *Bioethics at the bedside: a clinician's guide,* Ottawa, Canada, 1999, Canadian Medical Association, pp 55–62.

Lazar NM, Griener GG, Robertson G, Singer PA: Substitute decision-making. In Singer PA, editor: *Bioethics at the bedside: a clinician's guide,* Ottawa, Canada, 1999, Canadian Medical Association, pp 33–38.

Lazar NM, Shemie S, Webster GC, Dickens BM: Bioethics for clinicians: 24. Brain death, *CMAJ* 164:833–836, 2001.

Martinelli A: Medical futility. In Fleetwood J, Novack D, Feldman D, Farber N, editors: *MedEthEx: standardized patient exercises in medical ethics and communication skills,* Philadelphia, 1997, Allegheny University of the Health Sciences, pp 100–114.

Roush H: DNR orders & end-of-life decision making. In Fleetwood J, Novack D, Feldman D, Farber N, editors: *MedEthEx: standardized patient exercises in medical ethics and communication skills,* Philadelphia, 1997, Allegheny University of the Health Sciences, pp 35–51.

Singer PA, MacDonald N: Quality end-of-life care. In Singer PA, editor: *Bioethics at the bedside: a clinician's guide,* Ottawa, Canada, 1999, Canadian Medical Association, pp 117–124.

Singer PA, Robertson G, Roy DJ: Advance care planning. In Singer PA, editor: *Bioethics at the bedside: a clinician's guide,* Ottawa, Canada, 1999, Canadian Medical Association, pp 39–46.

The ETHICS OSCE: *Standardized patient scenarios for teaching and evaluating bioethics,* Toronto, Canada, 1999, EFPO (Educating Future Physicians for Ontario), Available at http://wings.buffalo.edu/faculty/research/bioethics/osce.html, Accessed January 26, 2004.

Transplantation. In Devettere RJ, editor: *Practical decision making in health care ethics: cases and concepts,* Washington, DC, 1995, Georgetown University Press, pp 432–468.

Weijer C, Singer PA, Dickens BM, Workman S: Dealing with demands for "inappropriate" treatment: medical futility and other approaches. In Singer PA, editor: *Bioethics at the bedside: a clinician's guide,* Ottawa, Canada, 1999, Canadian Medical Association, pp 107–116.

Wolfe M: Advance directives & family decision making. In Fleetwood J, Novack D, Feldman D, Farber N, editors: *MedEthEx: standardized patient exercises in medical ethics and communication skills,* Philadelphia, 1997, Allegheny University of the Health Sciences, pp 52–67.

INDEX

A

Abdomen. *See also* Belly
  division into quadrants, 82f
Abdomen and torso, stretch marks on, 250–251
Abdominal and back pain, pregnant female with, 276–277
Abdominal masses, structures commonly palpated as, 83f
Abdominal pain, 80–81, 81–82
  female with fever and lower, 277–278
Abnormal breathing, patterns of, 45–47, 47f
Abnormalities, pulse, 8f
Abuse
  elder, 354
  and neglect, 354
Acne
  facial, 201–204
  steroid, 203f
Acne excoriée, 202f
Acne rosacea, 201f
Acne unresponsive to treatment, 202f
Acne vulgaris, 204f
Acromegaly, male with, 257
Acromioclavicular joint, 166f
Acute myocardial infarction (AMI) defined, 33
Addison's disease, 256
Adventitious breath sounds, 54f
Age, normal ranges for vital signs by, 302t
Algorithm for falls in elderly persons, 353f
Amenorrhea defined, 279
AMI (acute myocardial infarction), 33
Amoxicillin, drug exanthem following ingestion of, 217f
Anaphylactic reaction to peanut butter, 339–340
Anatomic snuff box, 170f
Anatomy
  auscultatory, 13f
  breast, 265f
  cranial nerve, 126f
  of elbow, 168f
  esophageal, 78f
  of gastrointestinal system, 77f
  genitourinary, 111f
  of hand, 172f
  of heart, 3f–4f
  of hip and pelvis, 173f
  of knee, 175f
  of lungs, 43f
  of pelvis, 173f
  of shoulder, 165f
  of skin, 197f
  of thyroid gland, 242–243
  vascular, 129
  ventral brainstem, 126f
  of wrist, 170f

Anatomy of thyroid, surface, 242f
Anemia
  classification of, 235t
  defined, 234
  differentiating microcytic, 235t
Angle of Louis, 19, 42
Angles, carrying, 168f
Ankle
  examination of left, 189
  ulcer, 213–215
Ankylosing spondylitis, 39, 178–179
Anterior approach to examination of thyroid, 244f
Anteroposterior chest-x-ray in neonate, portable, 302f
Anteroposterior view of chest, 66f, 68f
Anteroposterior x-ray of left femur, 340f
Anxiety, 293–294
  organic etiologies of, 294b
  with organic etiology, 294b
Aoric regurgitation, auscultation to accentuate murmur of, 11f
Aortic regurgitation, 39
  defined, 15
  physical examination for, 15–16
Aortic stenosis
  defined, 14
  physical examination for, 14–15
Apical impulse, palpation of, 9f
Appendix, 77
Arcs, reflex, 126
Arm and leg weakness, left, 137–138
Arm, broken, 180–181
Arterial from venous insufficiency, differentiating, 23t
Arterial insufficiency, peripheral, 38
Arthritis, rheumatoid. *See* Rheumatoid arthritis (RA)
Ascending colon, 77
Ascites
  defined, 88–89
  physical examination for, 88–90, 108
Asthma, 62–63, 315–317
  attack, 63–64
  defined, 62
  expected findings in acute exacerbation of, 64t, 317t
Asymmetric corneal light reflex, 308f
Asymmetric gluteal folds, 309f
Ataxia, physical examination of patient with, 150
Atelectasis signs and symptoms, 48–49t
Atopic dermatitis, typical flexural location for, 208f
Atrial pressure, right, 19
Atypical pneumonia defined, 69
Auscultation
  to accentuate murmur of aortic regurgitation, 11f
  heart, 9–10
  in left lateral decubitus position, 10f
  lungs, 52–54

Note: b after a page number stands for box; f after a page number stands for figure; and t after a page number stands for table.